A New

to transcend the Great Forget
ancestral practices into contemporary living

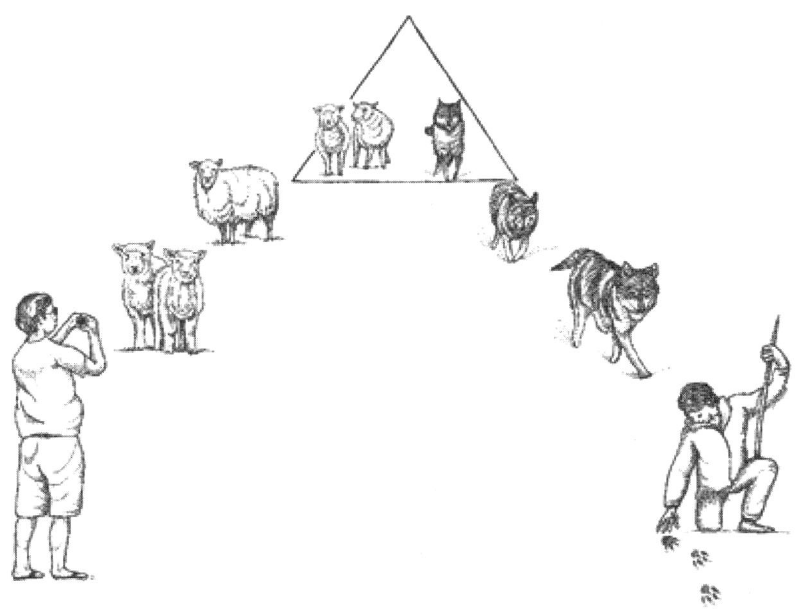

Arthur Haines

www.arthurhaines.com

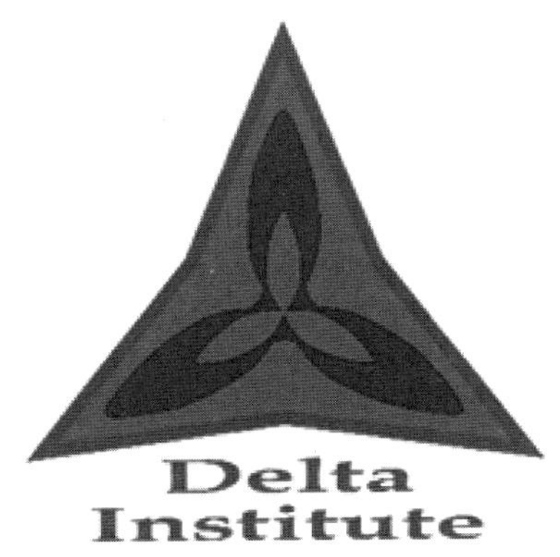

Dedication

I dedicate this book to the hunter-gatherers of the world—past, present, and future.

Acknowledgments

This book would not be possible without Daniel Vitalis. It is through countless discussions in many formats, under both the sun and moon, that has led to the refinement of the vision presented here. There are very few people that have focused as broadly and deeply on the philosophy of rewilding that could offer the development, modification, and critique of the ideas on which this book is based. Thomas Vining is thanked plentifully for the extensive assistance with the writing. He too has dedicated a lot of time to discussions of ideas and manners of expressing those ideas. Michael Douglas is also thanked here. It is his constant valuing of my person and providing assistance whenever I express the need is deeply appreciated. He supported the work behind this book. Nicole Leavitt is given here a special expression of gratitude for caring for our daughter during the long period of writing needed to allow realization of this work. And there are many others, such as Peter Bauer and Andrew Badenoch, who have engaged in discussions through cyberspace that have also freely shared their philosophy surrounding rewilding. There are also those who have specialized in particular topics of rewilding that have allowed me to present quotes from their work or have influenced my writing in these fields or both. These include Katy Bowman, Charles Eisenstein, Miles Olson, Erwan le Corre, Elizabeth Thomas, and Christopher Cantwell. Caleb Musgrave is thanked for introducing me to the Seven Fires Prophecy and sharing indigenous stories. Sara Moore, Jarrod Gutman, John Sacco, and Darren Worcester provided helpful comments on the manuscript and cover. I am also grateful for the artistic talent of Elizabeth Farnsworth, who created the cover artwork for this book.

Published by V.F. Thomas Co.

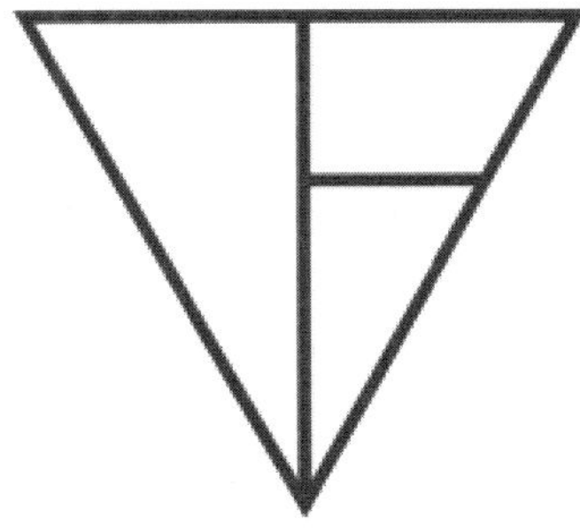

Library of Congress Control Number: 2017912760

ISBN: 978-0-9993295-0-4

Printed in Korea

Warning: You are a sovereign human (or, at least, should be striving to be one). You are responsible for your interpretation and application of the information presented in this book. The author, publisher, and printer accept no liability for any loss or injury as a result of use or misuse of ideas presented in this book.

Table of Contents

Foreword

"Do you think it's possible", I asked, as the fire crackled at our feet, illuminating the forested hollow all around us, "that modern humans are—scientifically speaking—domesticated?" Arthur and I had been discussing this idea for some time, though until now, strictly as a metaphor.

The fire our standing bodies encircled had been started with friction, in the old way, in the way of our ancestors. Our minds, now also ablaze, leaped from idea to idea, quickly linking seemingly unrelated concepts into a greater tapestry, just as the lick of the flames darted this way and that.

So many diverse elements must be brought together to birth a flame from the landscape; wood, the skeletal remnant of trees, herbs gathered at their right time, both in an ideal state of dryness and preservation, tinder, fluffed in such a way as to offer maximum surface area. The kilocalories of energy expended by the person working spindle against hearth-board, grinding out the sound heard for hundreds of thousands of years, an ancient song as characteristic of our species as our upright gate. The callouses on hands that have performed this act countless times before, revealing the mettle of one who bears the mark of a fire-starter. All these things working in tandem to bring into existence the ember that would be the nuclei at the heart of the fire—the heart of this fire.

It's the same with an idea. There is a moment when something is birthed in the mind's eye—like ignition—and there's a chance, an opportunity. If that idea is fed tinder, first small, then progressively larger, it can become the self-sustaining chain reaction that leads to a roaring fire. It burns first in the mind, but soon, like wildfire, it spreads to other minds, through a community, then out into the culture. In this case, a culture that has been locked, frozen like ice, into a way of thinking and being that has led to the extinction level event that is taking place everywhere around us, even as you read this.

For years we—just two amongst countless others—have fed this core concept, this seed crystal at the core of the lattice that would become the paradigm informing the content of this book—and the community that has rallied around this way of life.

You see, there's been an oversight in collective human thought, and its civilization-wide. Perhaps oversight is too soft a word, and taboo might be better. We see clearly, all around us, that the species we live with day to day have been domesticated. We are, in fact, quite proud of this feat, being the lords of the suite of changes science is now calling "domestication syndrome". Somehow, in our eagerness to be the masters of so many species, landscapes, and natural systems, we've failed to ask ourselves how this may have affected us, how we might have been changed by the very same influences that we've foisted upon others. This taboo is, of course, the taboo against human wildness.

Why else but taboo would we be so willing to push our wild-type—the still living, modern foraging peoples of the world—to the brink of extinction, and allow ourselves to reach a state of degeneration so profound that our very survival might be called into question? This unspoken proscription clouds our minds and keeps us from seeing the reality all around us, that we are a domesticated subspecies too, and that we are suffering from a collection of degenerative changes that are characteristic of such.

The dominant cultural meme, almost our religion, has been that we are now at the peak of our evolution and that we've achieved a lofty, god-like status elevated above all other hominins that have come before us. It appears at first glance quite simple. We, like all beasts, were struggling for survival in the wild, a savage place—"red in tooth and claw" as the popular inculcation goes. While it's certainly true that much knowledge has been gained in the estimated 10,000 years since we began the domestication experiment that would lead us to the present, there have also been unquantifiable losses, many to our own health, as will be described explicitly in the coming chapters. It's time we asked ourselves why, if domestication has been the apotheosis of our species, are we now developing degenerative diseases that were largely unheard of amongst our wild ancestors. And again, why, if this be the utopian dream fulfilled, are we less happy now—even less satisfied—than those living a still largely wild life.

Many fires have burned since that night in the forest-hollow when we began to see our modern state as one of self-imposed human domestication. Each fire we've burned together since has lent its strength to this new way of walking in the world. I can think of no one better suited to write this book than Arthur Haines. It's his unique perspective, as a scientist, an experimental archeologist, a father, a forager, a hunter, and a first-generation neoaboriginal, that lends this text such profound credibility. May this work be, in part, a torch of guiding light, illuminating the New Path before us. A path that leads us back to the balance that we—and the entire phylogeny of life—need so desperately to achieve.

May the pathway of rewilding be the path to our redemption.

I wish you health, strength, and the willingness to put the words that follow into practice.

To all our relations,

~ Daniel Vitalis

Preface

Many authors provide preceding materials to present the background story or some other crucial information that outlines the scope of their work. I would rather incorporate that story into the body of the text itself, but I find myself needing to contend with certain aspects of my writing and the topic at hand. This preface will be relatively short and merely present a few items that I request you keep in mind as you work your way through the book.

The writing you are about to embark on in the following chapters will not always leave you feeling wonderful about humanity's current situation. This book does not have each paragraph written in an uplifting tone that glosses over the harm we are doing to ourselves and the world. I'm trying to generate awareness. In doing so, I need to call egocentric acts exactly what they are—selfish. If ongoing actions can be maintained only through ignorance and lack of empathy, it is best to write exactly that. We have a tendency to use certain kinds of prose that never wholly allow an awakening because the full gravity of the situation is completely hidden behind pleasing verbiage. I ask that you allow me the freedom to describe our industrial lifeway accurately, and I'll refrain from being pejorative.

That written, this is not a book about grief. This is a book about hope and all the writing is infused with this. The intent of my words is to foster change, a transformation based on the union of information (science) and compassion (emotion) that can heal people and landscapes. I truly desire for my children's children and your children's children to experience a world where they can reach their full genetic potential and celebrate life in the unique way that humans can. However, I desire for the celebration to occur in a manner that doesn't detract from future generations also experiencing a rich and pristine world. I hope that you will be able to understand that despite writing that isn't flowery (with intention), this entire reference is about optimism and one possible path to achieving a transformation to natural health.

Many authors like to reduce complicated topics to a short sound bite that is easy to remember. Very often, such reductions lose crucial information and often don't provide the background material that allows for application of the rule to different situations. In other words, they provide a recipe and not the concepts. The problem is, life is not so easily comparable to baking a loaf of bread. Given the same ingredients and conditions (e.g., cookware, temperature, elevation, duration of cooking), one will get essentially the same product every time no matter where you are in the world. Human life is not like this. We are infinitely more complex than baking a loaf of bread and even with the same diet and environment we demonstrate variation. Each person's situation is unique and it is only through an understanding of concepts that they can build the recipe that works for their circumstances. You will notice throughout this book that I attempt to explore the complexity of situations in enough detail that will allow most people to apply the concepts—rather than providing recipes that work for the fictitious "average person".

Finally, we must also deal with the biggest misconception concerning rewilding (and likely the biggest mistaken belief about this book). Many envision the only way to remedy the tremendous nature divorcement that humans are currently experiencing is for everyone to return to a hunter-gatherer lifestyle and forgo all modern technology. If you believe that is what this book is about, please understand you are incorrect (and I intend that with politeness). It is not possible in a world with fragmented landscapes and nature-divorced humans. Therefore, this book is a collection of philosophy, information, and suggestions on how people move forward with a nature-connected lifestyle that remedies some of the dis-ease and emptiness we experience today.

It is not about all humans living in bark or thatch shelters, at least not yet (though I do recommend you experience sleeping in inclement weather protected by a well-crafted shelter you have constructed; it is a gratifying experience). Here, I advocate combining the ancestral and the modern. Specifically, this vision of rewilding is satisfying the biological, physiological, and psychological needs of *Homo sapiens* AND valuing advancements in technologies that promote life, resource conservation, and an expanded (but not one-sided) understanding of the cosmos.

As part of this vision of a nature-connected lifeway, rewilding is not seen merely as an endpoint. It is a path that is followed, with deepening awareness and greater development of proficiency in certain skillsets seen as a metaphorical continuation along this path. Where we are all heading on this course is different for everyone, in large part because each landscape is unique and requires different solutions for a truly sustainable and healthy living. Given that it has taken many generations to reach the current point of poor health and maladaptation we find ourselves experiencing, rewilding is an intergenerational path that will require multiple birth and death cycles to find our way back to a version of ecocentric living. In other words, it is likely to be our unborn descendants who will realize the ultimate goals of rewilding—humans who consider themselves part of the ecology of this planet and live with this as a guiding principle.

Everything mentioned here in this preface will be discussed in much greater detail. However, I believe it necessary to set the stage, dismiss misconceptions from the beginning, and help you understand why I have chosen a particular writing style. Keep in mind, this book could not be possible if I did not believe there existed a path forward. It is entirely based on a positive belief in the capacity of humans to transcend nature divorcement. It is based on hope. And my hope is a confidence that cannot be quenched because I have witnessed first-hand the rejuvenative ability of nature-connected living.

1. Introduction: creating awareness of the human situation

Most stories appropriately start at the beginning. This approach allows the background to be presented and the major players to be introduced. However, this is a story that is best started from near the end, where the results of a lifestyle can be plainly observed. By starting from near the end of a trajectory that humans began around 10,000–12,000 years ago, we can discuss the outcome (or rather, the consequences) of what nature divorcement has brought upon humans and the landscapes they rely on for health. Because we now have the ability to clearly observe the effects of a massive paradigm shift in humans—a shift from considering themselves part of the regional ecology to considering themselves separate from and with dominion over the globe—we can use this as a starting point to describe the effects of this change and (more importantly) how we can deviate from the current path humanity is on to restore personal, communal, and ecological health (note: they are all inextricably linked).

THE CURRENT SITUATION

Many authors who care deeply about the biosphere make a strategic mistake while trying to elicit change in the behavior of people. They begin with a description of the current predicament humans are facing by noting the harm that has been wrought on the earth through short-sighted industrial living. They launch into the statistics of the vast amount of pollutants that are emitted each year, the number of rivers that are no longer safe to swim in, and even the number of species that vanish from this planet each day (upper estimates place this at 200). There is a major drawback to starting with these figures: the statistics will be ineffective because most contemporary humans are both selfish and (as a society) unaware. This may seem very blunt, but these are necessary topics to understand (it helps explain the lack of change in the face of overwhelming evidence). The selfishness can be demonstrated by examining the many hundreds of things people do that indicate they have no concern for humans in other lands or the other-than-human persons they share their landscapes with. We could discuss pollution, resource exploitation, shipment of toxic materials to other lands, widespread radioactive contamination from nuclear weapons testing, refusal to consider other beings in our decision making (even our own children), and so on. Based on current rates of global resource use, we need 2 ½ earths to keep pace, a clear indication that our unsustainable use of resources is leaving less and less for future generations.

Perhaps a good example to illustrate the selfishness of modern humanity is the mining of coal and its burning to generate power. Miles (literally) of forested mountain tops in the southern Appalachians of the eastern United States have been torn apart with explosives and heavy equipment to acquire coal. Over 470 mountains have been sheared off, leaving a desolate ruin that can be aptly described as a polluted wasteland. The companies responsible for these acts formerly left the sites as they were until regulation forced them to replant the mined areas. People in portions of the United States power their homes through energy produced from coal-fired power plants. This practice rains arsenic, lead, mercury, and cadmium down on the northeastern landscapes, acidifying lakes, accumulating in the soil, water, and food, and contributing to fetal defects (among many other health issues). Coal-fired power plants are the number one human-produced source of some of these metals. Worse yet is that part of this energy generation is used for very non-essential activities (e.g., televisions left on when no one is viewing them, hours spent playing video games). One has to be selfish to condone a method of power generation that contributes to physical and metabolic abnormalities in infants living in other places.

Likewise, the lack of awareness demonstrated by contemporary humans indicates that even if they were to care about the excessive harm caused by the current manifestation of industrial living, they are not likely to be cognizant of it (and even if they were, most wouldn't know what meaningful steps to take to change this—which we will discuss later in the book). Again, many hundreds of examples could be listed here detailing the lack of conscious awareness; in fact, many prefer to remain uninformed of the impact our society has to the health and well-being of the world's biota ("ignorance is bliss"). Think about it: we just keep throwing disposable items "away", not realizing there is no away when live on a planet, there is really just "over there". So, we throw things "over there" expecting that they will stay put, which isn't the case. Plastic microparticles are now found in many marine regions, are consumed by the wildlife, and then ingested again when we consume the wildlife as food. Another example of muted awareness: some health conscious people are sure to seek out the "BPA-free" label on various plastic goods. Bisphenol A (BPA) is a component of some plastics that exhibits hormone-like activity in our body (i.e., it disrupts our endocrine function, which means the functioning of our hormonal system becomes interrupted to some degree). Of interest to this story is that no one asked what plastic manufacturers exchanged for the BPA. It served a function and can't just be removed without finding a replacement chemical. Using an analogy, you can't remove the yeast from dough and expect the bread to rise when it is baked. You have to replace the yeast with another leavening agent. Likewise, when you remove BPA from a plastic, it must be replaced with a chemical that serves the same function. Manufacturers did just that. They switched to using Bisphenol S and Bisphenol AF, two other compounds that disrupt hormone function and contribute to chronic disease. But most did not even ask.

These two important features of modern humans (selfishness and lack of awareness), combined with the fact that approximately 80% of the United States population lives in urban areas where the continued destruction of nature is not apparent to them, create a situation where such statistics are meaningless abstractions. Modern humans cannot see the connections they have to nature and do not understand that what they do to their landscapes they do to themselves. This means that the only statistics that have any chance of making an impact are those that affect the people themselves. So let us get started there.

But wait, this approach often proves ineffective as well. Chronic disease is now so prevalent, that people assume it to be a normal part of life. They simply expect to suffer from cancer and watch those around them die of the same (or cardiovascular disease, stroke, diabetes, etc.). Given that the lifetime odds of contracting cancer are 2 in 5 (1 in 2 if you are male), almost everyone has been touched by this disease in some way as they or family members and friends succumb to this needless ailment. Likewise, cardiovascular disease is the leading cause of death in the United States, and more than half of the people over the age of 45 will develop this disease. It is imperative to understand that our society is made up of such a high proportion of physically sick individuals, that no one considers it unusual that nearly 7 in 10 people living in the United States have used a prescription drug in the past year and that more than half of them are using two or more prescription drugs (keep in mind there is evidence that some prescription drugs cause cognitive impairment). Mentioning these health statistics simply has little effect because people don't realize that life can be different (in fact, it was very different at one time).

Sometimes, describing the health problems experienced by infants and children (and their frequency) has a little more effect. Most people do care about the health of their children. So, let us begin the discussion there (all of the following information is freely available by searching online, including on the Center for Disease Control's website). While fewer than 10% of living Americans have diabetes (of any form), that will be changing dramatically in the coming years. For those children born in the new millennium, 1 in 3 will develop some form of diabetes in their lifetime. Diabetes reduces life expectancy by 10–20 years. Given that the preponderance of diabetes is type 2 (noninsulin-dependent diabetes mellitus), it is entirely preventable (we will explain later how many "genetic diseases" are in fact the inheritance of diet and lifestyle, and are not actual genetic diseases). Continuing with the state of children's health today, approximately 1 in 9 children have asthma (a 27% increase between 2001 and 2012). One in 13 children has food allergies (a 50% increase between 1997 and 2011). Developmental disabilities now afflict 1 in 6 children (a 17% increase between 1997 and 2008). A diagnosis of attention deficit hyperactivity disorder occurs in nearly 1 in 9 children (a 28% increase over a ten-year period ending in 2009). Children with autism spectrum disorder occur at a frequency of 1 in 50 (though we are told by "experts" that there is nothing to be concerned about because this is largely attributable to increased reporting of the disease). Cancer is the second leading cause of death in children (though a recent study suggests it may now be the leading cause). And all of this is only the beginning of the numbers we could list. It should be apparent to anyone that our children are experiencing poor health—it isn't just the elderly who now have a plastic container with seven compartments filled with prescription pharmaceuticals. It should also be obvious that without change, unhealthy children grow into unhealthy adolescents. (If you need further convincing, read "A Compromised Generation: The Epidemic of Chronic Illness in America's Children by Lambert, this book consolidates a lot of research, making it easy for the reader to come up to speed on a diversity of young person's health topics.)

American adolescents suffer from a high degree of mental health and emotional disorders. Approximately 1 in 5 teenagers have symptoms or will develop symptoms severe enough to impact daily life. These are primarily anxiety, behavioral, mood, and substance abuse issues. Mood swings and identity crises are common facets of life with high school-age adolescents. While there are many causes for these issues, it is certain that unhealthy adults create or exacerbate these issues in adolescents. In other words, disease and poor health begets disease and poor health. Keep in mind that current estimates are that 1 in 6 high school students have suicidal thoughts—and nearly 1 in 12 makes an attempt on their life. Suicide is the third leading cause of death in teenagers. These numbers should be alarming. They should raise questions. How can we continue with the status quo knowing this is the outcome? How is it we can push forward with our current mode of living given the harm it is causing? (Remember selfishness and unawareness?)

Experts will speculate on the causes of poor emotional and physical health in children, adolescents, and adults. They will endlessly debate the various factors that contribute to disease, and then make recommendations they believe will correct the health issues. We will try this drug or that drug, or make alterations to the diet that amount to simply switching to different combinations of nutrient-poor food, or we will use the assistance of trained behavioral specialists who have no idea what real health is (because they live in an unhealthy society and have not actually observed it). Most of the methods have little or no lasting effects and continue the intergenerational march toward declining health. Experts never use the obvious method of dealing with health issues: find people (read "communities") who do not experience said health issues, observe what they do, and incorporate their diet and lifestyle into a treatment regimen.

What we see is the exact opposite being done in this country. An ailment is identified, a treatment plan is formulated, often one that has never been used before, and then the people undergoing the treatment become Guinea pigs as the health professionals sit back to wait and see if the treatment plan works. This is done with diet as well. We see the creation of diets new to humans, touted as life-extending regimes, but in reality there is no evidence that these diets work. Worse, there is no understanding of what the diets do many generations down the road because the diets are novel—they are an experiment.

Let me use an example to describe the process that should be used to identify root causes of ailments and how those ailments can be healed and prevented. One of the best examples involved an Ohio dentist named Weston Price. He observed high rates of poor dental health in his practice, with frequent dental caries (i.e., cavities), extensive crowding of teeth and, in particular, widespread occurrence of impacted wisdom teeth. Rather than formulating a new treatment plan (such as a diet) to try to correct these issues, Dr. Price travelled around the world to identify people who did not suffer from these dental issues. He was able to find such people on each continent that had extremely low rates of dental caries, straight and uncrowded teeth, and palates (in actuality, faces) that were wide enough to fit all of the teeth (including the wisdom teeth). Though these people enjoyed very different diets, there were commonalities amongst all these different groups that he was able to summarize. These stand as some of the best dietary suggestions that can be employed for dental and periodontal health because they are real world observations (not a hypothetical treatment approach).

This is one of the real issues today with approaches to treating illness and disease—the approaches are not grounded in the historical observation of people who lived a particular way (or employed a particular diet) for many generations. Without this information, we cannot ascertain the full impact of a treatment (or diet or lifestyle) on the people. Without this kind of anchor, we are free to drift away into a multitude of esoteric approaches, many of which are biased by the researcher's own beliefs (beliefs that may ultimately not be based on credible facts). Any suggested approach that doesn't take into account the observations of healthy people and what they did or did not do, is potentially (or actually) making recommendations that stand in contradiction to real world observations. Such approaches should not be taken as the final word. I will be discussing many unsuccessful health practices throughout this book and how the researchers failed to take into account what we know about humans. The real question that should be asked by everyone: are there healthy people to use as a benchmark for well-being in humans? The answer is yes (to qualify that, there are a few remaining, most of them no longer exist). But before we get to this group of humans, we need to discuss another topic: domestication.

DOMESTICATION

Domestication is a process of modifying a group of organisms to attenuate undesirable traits and accentuate desirable ones. It is a process that humans used to change some wild animals into livestock, or work animals, or pets. Wild animals have traits that do not make them favorable for raising in large numbers in close proximity to people. Some of them are too dangerous and would maim or kill humans that approached them. Other animals are too lean and would not produce enough food to make them worthwhile for raising. And still others would not cooperate, refusing to pull heavy loads or whatever else was asked of them. Therefore, human breeders, through many generations of selective breeding, changed the wild animals to make them more tame and, in some cases, produce more food for humans (such as larger breasts in chickens, greater milk production in some breeds of cows, etc.). The reasons we domesticate animals varies for each animal, but there are certain traits that define domesticated animals. These are: altered temperament, altered social hierarchy, altered diet, and an ability to breed in captivity (there are other traits we could discuss, but these will suffice).

Altered temperament simply means the animals have been tamed. Through taming, the animals are safe for their human captors to be around. Imagine the wild progenitor of modern-day cows (*Bos taurus taurus*), called the auroch (*Bos taurus primigenius*). These were wild bovids with large horns and a fierce temperament (the males and females engaged in aggressive behavior to establish position within the herd). Any human approaching an auroch to tend this animal would be gored and trampled (the Spanish fighting bull is a domesticated form of the auroch that has not been tamed to the extent of most cattle—envision this animal's reaction to one's approach). Of note is that the auroch is extinct today, having been wiped out due to intensive hunting pressure, extensive habitat loss (conversion to cultivated fields), and diseases transmitted by domesticated cattle.

Altered social hierarchy refers to the ability of domesticated animals to recognize leadership in a different form than would be experienced in the wild. This is an important trait of domesticated animals because they must recognize humans as their leaders. For example, the domesticated dog (*Canis lupus familiaris*) is derived from an ancestor of the gray wolf (*Canis lupus lupus*). Whereas gray wolves do not recognize humans as their leader, and if placed in a closed room with a human would not act subordinate to that individual (quite the opposite would occur), the domesticated dog accepts humans in the leadership position. It was formerly thought that gray wolf packs were led by a dominant male and female (called the alpha male and alpha female). However, these were observations of animals living in captivity, a living condition that had altered their social behavior. Recent research shows gray wolves to be more egalitarian (more sharing of food resources) than was once believed. But domesticated dogs do have a strict social hierarchy with an alpha, and that alpha is generally the human owner (i.e., captor). Without modifying the social hierarchy, domesticated animals would not perform tasks asked by humans.

Domesticated animals must be able to **tolerate an altered diet**. When they are brought into captivity and moved to different regions of the world from where their wild progenitor lived, including moving to different continents, they must be able to eat the foods supplied by their human tenders. Consider the red junglefowl (*Gallus gallus*), a medium-sized bird native to Asia that is the wild progenitor of the domesticated chicken (*Gallus gallus domesticus*). This wild bird is omnivorous, consuming plants (and their seeds) and a diversity of insects and other invertebrates, including winged ants and termites. This is its natural diet. What does the domesticated chicken eat? A variety of diets, but in industrial farming, it primarily consumes large amounts of grain (note: no green plants and no invertebrates). This is an unnatural diet for this species, but the domesticated form survives (note I did not state it thrives) on this artificial diet rich in grains.

The **ability to breed in captivity** is also a requirement for domesticated animals. If they did not reproduce, humans would not be able to replenish the herd after they consumed some of the animals (or after animals died). The only option would be to domesticate additional wild animals (which is usually a long, multi-generational process). Therefore, the ability to breed in captivity is a necessary attribute of any domesticated animal. Some species that many would think are domesticated are actually only tamed. The elephant (*Elephas maximus*), for example, does not breed well in captivity for a number of reasons, including difficulty of managing bulls in breeding condition and a limited understanding of the estrous cycle of the female. By taming them, humans calm their wild temperament and train them to perform commands. But this means that people wishing to use these animals for work usually tame young individuals from the wild, which is far more complicated than simply breeding more individuals in captivity. Other animals, such as the domesticated pig (*Sus scrofa domesticus*), originally domesticated from the Eurasian wild boar (*Sus scrofa*), have no trouble breeding in captivity. Pigs will reproduce in relative confinement, making it easy to raise additional animals and limiting the expense and difficulty of providing large, open spaces that mimic wild environments. Animals that will accept small spaces (including for breeding) are easier to manage, feed, and slaughter.

After examining these four criteria that define (in part) domesticated animals, the question that needs to be asked is: are contemporary humans domesticated? Let us go back to those four criteria and examine them objectively. First is altered temperament. Do modern humans lack a feral temperament? Another way we can ask this question is: do they accept conditions or actions that a wild human would refuse to endure (if they had a choice)? Consider that contemporary humans will live in crowded cities with poor sanitation, high crime rates, and terrible air quality, completely cut off from natural scenes. And while most have a choice as to whether they live there or not, they accept those settings, despite the fact they know them to be unhealthy and (in many cases) dangerous. They will live in close proximity to industrial mills and agricultural fields that employ conventional (i.e., chemical) methods, where the rates of physical abnormalities and autism in their young children are substantially elevated. Most of the people living near those factories and fields will do nothing about those conditions. They will accept them as part of their life story (even believe there is no other way). They will pay taxes that fund their elected leaders, leaders who are supposed to serve them—though they actually serve those lobbies that contribute significant campaign contributions. People wonder why carcinogenic compounds are still added to health and beauty products, why mills can freely discharge toxic waste into the rivers that run through countless communities, and are baffled by the fact that foods utilizing genetically modified organisms (GMOs) are still not labeled as such. They expect their elected leaders to protect them from such things. And when they don't, they grumble, but ultimately accept those conditions as well. They spend their lives as wage slaves, working jobs they don't enjoy, to buy things society tells them they must have. It is clear that contemporary humans have an altered temperament. No human would accept the modern living that many endure unless their soul's fire had been extinguished.

Humans today live in a social system that is in stark contrast to that experienced by most humans prior to the agricultural revolution. Most human communities that hunted and gathered their food were egalitarian, they shared of the resources and no member received disproportionate amounts of material wealth. These cultures valued their community and their members, as well as the local landscapes they relied on for their health and well-being. Agricultural societies (aside from some exemplary small-scale versions) are completely different. There is a social hierarchy in place where some individuals receive more wealth (in all its forms) than do most members of that society, and various privileged individuals enjoy substantial freedoms that most individuals do not. Those who have wealth remain in this position through use of a warrior class (the military) who defends the upper class and prevents the lower class from redistributing the wealth. Often with agricultural and, later, industrial societies, there is also a class of religious elites who play an important (even if unknown) role in maintaining social stratification. Yes, contemporary people have a highly altered (and very imbalanced) social system that is relatively new to human existence.

Humans currently eat a highly altered version of their ancestral (i.e., wild) diet. The human diet for 95% of our existence on this earth has involved a mix of wild plant and animal foods (primarily), some eaten raw, some eaten cooked (yes, we have always cooked some of our food—the advent of cooking predates the appearance of *Homo sapiens sapiens*). None of the food consumed would be considered highly processed. There were no artificial ingredients, no synthetic food coloring, no anticaking agents, no preservatives, and no GMO foods created by using laboratory methods to transfer genes from one organism into the genome of a completely unrelated organism. For that matter, humans did not consume cultivated plants, species that are also genetically modified (through breeding) to be less bitter, more sweet, and lacking seeds. This means the plant foods have less medicine, less fiber, and less nutrition, respectively. And it isn't just the kinds of foods people eat, but even the ratios of foods and macronutrients are drastically different today than in the past. Contemporary humans certainly eat an altered diet.

Finally, can humans breed in captivity like other domesticated animals? Not only can they, one can go so far as to say that most are now no longer willing to give birth on their own in a relatively natural setting. With infertility rates skyrocketing, many couples are dependent on drugs and other procedures just to conceive. Very few births occur outside of an institutional setting today. Whereas most deliveries prior to 1900 occurred outside of a hospital, today less than 1% of births do. Many people are terrified of birthing, considering it more of an ailment than a natural event. Forceps, vacuum extractions, episiotomies (i.e., intentional cutting of the perineum to guide tearing), synthetic hormones, various forms of anesthesia, and cesarean-section births are commonplace today—many used unnecessarily. The concept of a human infant entering the world into loving hands and taking their first breath with skin-to-skin contact of their mother in their home (where they will grow up) has been replaced with a drug-induced alteration of natural hormones, the steely grip of forceps, and the not-so-home-like setting of a hospital room. This establishes a pattern of nature divorcement that the infant will grow into during their life. Humans breed quite well in captivity, and the scariest part of it all, most are convinced that this is the only way to give birth.

Considering that modern humans fulfill these four criteria for domestication (altered temperament, altered social hierarchy, tolerate an altered diet, ability to breed in captivity), it appears that most of the people alive today are a domesticated version of *Homo sapiens*, a concept that I hope both intrigues and frightens you at the same time. Think about it: we are not wolves, we are basset hounds. We are the domesticated version of something stronger, more aware, supremely more capable, and intimately more connected to this earth. We used to belong to vital, self-reliant, and sharing communities. We now reside in towns and cities populated by people that are utterly dependent on growers and manufacturers. As a result, we must endure (i.e., submit to) anything they do to the world because we cannot live without their products. Domestication, one facet of nature divorcement, has rendered most humans incapable of healthy living and (for many) a fulfilling life. Of course, there are still questions that require answers. If we are domesticated humans, who are our wild progenitors? And who domesticated us? These questions will be answered in chapter 2.

WHAT NATURE DIVORCEMENT HAS WROUGHT

Many people realize that city builders (i.e., modern people) are not as connected to nature as they once were. For many reasons, people now see relatively natural landscapes as an unfamiliar array of shapes, colors, and textures. They are unable to identify the individual (though inextricably linked) parts. In much of the United States, where forests are common in areas that have not been cleared for homes and agricultural fields, nature is simply a wall of green (and an intimidating one at that). Such landscapes are called "undeveloped", a term that connotes these areas haven't yet expressed their true worth. Not until they have been cleared and homes or businesses have been built upon those lands are they christened "developed", even though they are often, at that point, substantially expunged of life, polluted, and geometrically simplified (i.e., lacking the amazing complexity found in natural systems). These developed landscapes do not support the diversity and vigor of life that existed prior to the land alteration. Keep in mind, humans have always altered the landscapes they lived upon, but those alterations mimicked natural processes and were often not even seen by the agricultural people who first explored lands inhabited by indigenous peoples (i.e., the explorers thought the lands were completely uninhabited).

Nature divorcement is not simply about people spending less time in forests (or prairies or mountain ranges), it is a practice of abandoning a way of thinking about ourselves. We no longer consider ourselves part of the local ecology where we live. There are the wild plants, fungi, animals, and other forms of life that interact with each other and the nonliving components on the landscape (e.g., rocks, soil, water)—and then there are the humans who live near (but outside of) those things. And while this belief is utterly false, it is the prevailing mindset. Humans consider themselves separate from and above other forms of life. Though we are unique, beautiful, and capable of amazing things, is this not true for other-than-human persons as well?

Perhaps most harmful to our health is the attitude that we are no longer wild animals. We see ourselves as civilized, risen up out of the savagery that was life prior to the advent of society. In fact, we are domesticated, not civilized (there is a big difference). Our steady march away from natural living has cost us dearly. However, we cannot truly see this disconnection from nature for what it is because a bias against nature has been designed into society for countless generations. We use the word "savage" to describe native peoples who practiced gratitude in daily life. European imperialists used an early form of the Discovery Doctrine to take land from native peoples and inflict on them cultural loss, forced-march relocations, starvation, massacres, and outright genocide (who is actually savage?). We justified this, in part, because they were wild animals and we were civilized. Consider the synonyms suggested for the word "wild" by the word processing software I am using to write this manuscript include: rough, desolate, barren, remote, and harsh. Contrast this with those suggested for the word "civilized": cultured, educated, refined, and enlightened. So, not only are we disconnected from nature, we are biased against it, and our very education system (formal and informal) seeks to amplify the degree to which we view nature as unnecessary, inferior, and a backward step for humanity.

Today, we sit in our homes or apartments, quite thrilled with what modern living has given to us (aside from the health issues we have discussed earlier in this chapter), not realizing that nature divorcement pervades many aspects of our life. Here are some examples (listed in no particular order, most of which will be discussed in greater detail later in the book):

• We eat genetically modified and cloned foods for almost every meal. Cultivated plants have had their genomes altered, sometimes substantially, through breeding (and sometimes also laboratory methods), resulting in foods with reduced nutrition, diminished levels of beneficial phytochemicals, and less fiber. Further, some produce found in supermarkets is sterile (notice the lack of seeds), and in some cases these kinds of plants were grown from clones to produce the fruit we eat.

• We have little or no understanding of natural medicine and holistic methods of healing. In fact, we even distrust herbal medicine, considering it ineffective or even dangerous, while we instead willingly ingest synthetic drugs that have a litany of side effects, one of which is death. The drugs do not cure the root issue, rather they merely treat symptoms of the underlying problem. The fact that a portion of these drugs pass un-metabolized through our bodies and into public water supplies is unknown to most—anti-depressant, antibiotic, and antifertility drugs are not treated in public water systems, meaning everyone drinking that water is subjected to small doses of these drugs.

• We raise our children in a way that does not recognize the long evolutionary history that is hard-wired into our infant's wild consciousness. In other words, our indigenous ancestors practiced certain forms of child rearing that have now created "expectations" in the infant. For example, when a new infant cries, she or he expects to be responded to. However, we consider this response detrimental to the infant, believing (erroneously) it creates a spoiled child. Refusing to respond to a new infant's only method of communication creates a stressful situation for the infant, resulting in chronically elevated levels of stress hormones that disrupt healthy brain development.

• We love plastic because this cheap material can be discarded (without reusing), which means we don't have to go through the hassle of washing it (like glasses, metal utensils, and ceramic bowls). But abandoning more natural materials comes with costs. We use approximately 260 million tons of plastic each year, accounting for 8% of the world's oil production. We never stop to think what the consequences may be from the use, recycling, or disposal of plastic. For example, polyvinyl chloride (PVC) recycling and incineration discharges chlorine, dioxins, phthalates, lead, cadmium, and BPA, all of which pose health hazards for humans (and other-than-human persons). For example, the dioxins are known carcinogens and negatively affect the thyroid gland, central nervous system, and immune system. Lead is documented to leach into drinking water from PVC pipes. Perhaps it should also be mentioned that PVC flooring is associated with higher rates of autism.

• We spend most of our time within the confines of a building, shielded from the elements. Within these geometrically simple structures, our brains become dulled and behavioral issues become exacerbated. Time spent in nature has been documented to increase creativity and cognitive ability. It has been shown also to reduce symptoms of attention deficit hyperactivity disorder (ADHD). Considering that people in hospitals recover faster if they have a view of a natural area, it is clear that humans are wired to live in nature (not indoors). But we disregard all of this, finding it easier to spend excessive time indoors, relaxed, and watching other people live their lives on reality television shows.

• We are convinced that we have bettered our lives through all of our technological advancements. Our entire day (and night) is bathed in electrical and chemical technologies. We frequently microwave our food, a process that creates novel and carcinogenic compounds in the food we eat. We cover our walls with paints that off gas volatile organic compounds, which contribute to asthma, allergies, and cancer. We drink fluoridated water, even though fluoride is a cumulative central nervous system toxin. We bathe the food we grow in various chemicals, so much so that the Gulf of Mexico has a dead zone for a portion of the year due, in part, to the agricultural runoff into the Mississippi River. In fact, people's well water in sections of this great river's watershed becomes polluted with nitrogen to the extent that warnings need to be issued to protect infants against methemoglobinemia, a condition where nitrogen compounds alter the hemoglobin in the blood resulting in impaired oxygen delivery to the tissues (coma and death are possible outcomes here).

• We have lost the ability to perform vital tasks that would allow us to survive outside of civilization. We cannot identify and gather wild plants for food and medicine. We can't make clothing from plant fibers and animal hides that one could harvest from their ecoregion. We can't make functional shelters that would protect us from the elements. We can't fabricate tools from natural items occurring on our landscapes. Without supermarkets, pharmacies, and shopping malls, we are utterly hopeless. While we are rich beyond comparison in possessions, we have lost our original affluence—the ability to craft and survive anywhere we travel. Our lives are now governed by our jobs, the economy, and the political regime. We have no other options because we are the result of The Great Forgetting, when ancestral knowledge was lost in favor of social stratification and wage slavery.

• We disregard the impacts of our living on the next generation, contrary to the cultures that came before us. Numerous statistics show that the health of our children is decreasing with each generation as inflammatory diseases, emotional problems, and developmental issues become more frequent and more severe. Wild and traditional cultures invested in the next generation, but modern society is afflicted with nature divorcement, and it has muted our awareness, impairing our ability to see the intergenerational effects of our current lifeway.

• We have abandoned true community for virtual communities. We are connected to people around the globe, sending fragments of thoughts to our faux friends at light speed. But where is the soothing voice, the caressing touch, and the supportive embrace of a real community member? Where are the other aspects of true communities, such as rites-of-passage that mark important events in people's lives, sharing enthusiasm for their accomplishments, and providing expectations for the next phase of their life? Where is the ceremony, the offering of gratitude for the people and the landscape? Where is the union experienced by people who share similar beliefs and practices? Social media are simply not acceptable replacements for actual community.

These are all examples of nature divorcement in modern humans. Notice that it isn't solely about time spent outdoors, it is also about abandoning beneficial practices of indigenous people, humans who were immersed in nature and lived as an interdependent part of their landscape (rather than believing they should gain dominion over it). Nature divorcement means we are not living as people who understand that we are part of this earth, that we are supposed to be members of forward-thinking human communities who are interwoven with the greater wild community. As such, we need to keep part of our awareness focused on the future to understand how our living sustains or degrades the health of the ecosystem. We desperately need to regain healthful practices, and not just with diet, but throughout the different aspects of our lifeways. Remember, humans didn't just appear on the planet; anatomically modern humans have been here for 200,000[1] years. And before that were the archaic humans. Prior to them were hominids who represented some of the most intelligent life on the planet. Our evolutionary line goes back

[1] Recent evidence from Hublin and colleagues, published in Nature, suggests our species may be significantly older than previously believed. A 2017 article pushes the date of *Homo sapiens sapiens* back to approximately 315,000 years before present.

seven million years as a lineage separate from our common primate ancestors. Disregarding all this is a perfect recipe for disease and discontent.

Nature divorcement is the core issue that must be addressed. This separation from the natural world can be seen to inspire many of the difficulties modern humans face. Nature divorcement creates an attitude of separation from the natural world. Once this outlook has permeated a culture, they will be willing to do terrible things to other-than-human beings for the simple reason "they are not us". This attitude eventually becomes "they are not worthy of the status we afford us" and, sooner or later, it is applied to other humans who practice different lifeways. Therefore, nature divorcement drives not only the health issues our society faces but can be seen to be a root cause of political and religious fanaticism. The only way to correct this is to participate. Participation implies integration, rather than separation, control, and manipulation—ideologies that are common in modern humans. We need to visualize (once again) the world as a complex mega-organism that we are part of. Such a worldview makes the poor treatment of its parts (whether that be other humans, other living beings, or even abiotic components like rivers and mountain chains) impossible. This would amount to a person treating their left arm worse than their right one, damaging it beyond function, and still considering themselves to be a healthy individual. Participation in local ecology enables a reunion of domesticated humans with their intrinsic wildness (more on this in later chapters).

AWARENESS CREATES GRIEF

After reading all of this, you might consider me to be a very depressed person. I have just spent pages and pages discussing facets of modern existence that rob people of their health, their happiness, and their ability to share their unique gifts with the world. I've presented only the tip of the iceberg—entire volumes could be organized around the chemicals we put in our food, the toxins we discharge into the air, the community traditions no longer practiced, the replacement of real nourishment pregnant mothers should receive with synthetic vitamins, and so on. And while I do not despair (now), that was not always the case. Learning about the harm that industrial living has caused, how it has further removed us from the sacred connection that ties us to the earth, was very saddening to me. It seemed as though each direction I turned was another piece of evidence suggesting humans could no longer live up to their full genetic potential. And as people became more and more physically, physiologically, and spiritually sick, it was clear they also became more apathetic about the environment (on which we rely).

I certainly lost a lot of sleep thinking about things. It truly hurt me to see yet another big box store being built where a forest once stood, an event that meant a tiny increment of our ability to be self-reliant was taken away from us in the name of progress (progress for what?). And while that forest provided real food and goods, the big box store sold mainly highly processed foods rich in artificial ingredients and merchandise that would soon enter some landfill. If you research enough aspects of industrial living with an open mind, you'll likely hit the wall of grief as I did. Being a biologist only magnified the sorrow. I could see how much our landscapes have been altered by invasions of non-native species, how the age structure of the trees was skewed toward younger individuals that do not produce fruit, and how many important components of the forest were now missing. Despite all this awareness, succumbing to despair wasn't (and still isn't) an option. Too much is riding on our finding real solutions. We need to regain our health so that we can help others do the same. We can't expect miracles with a world filled with sick people (in some cases these are people who aren't even aware they are experiencing an illness). Healthy people do amazing things. That is where we need to begin. So that is where I started, with my own health.

I was experiencing numerous health issues in my mid-thirties. I made huge advances by changing my diet. But I came to realize that human health is not solely about food we eat (though this is one of the most fundamental issues facing humans today). Humans are nourished by so much more. We need exposure to the elements, movement, a caring community, a lover's embrace, to feel that others appreciate our gifts, to find places that make us feel alive, to experience spirituality that is not weighed down by dogma and bureaucracy, to feel connected to a familiar landscape, and to believe we have real purpose. Most humans today, on the contrary, eat poorly, remain indoors, are sedentary and bereft of community, have loveless relationships, never find their gifts or place that calls to them, are without spirit, feel disconnected, and do not feel satisfied with their professions. We can't address everything here in this book, but we will get to much of it. Together, we will help lift the weight you may be experiencing. We will examine many aspects of life through the lens of ancestral living, bringing forward those pertinent lessons so that we can enjoy health in this time of living.

WHERE IS THE PROOF?

At this point you may be wondering where are the citations? Where is the list of studies and reports that back up the statements I am making? To be clear, most of what I write is based on scientific study, including the historical observations of *Homo sapiens*. And that which is speculation on my part can be shown to be primarily grounded in scientific thought (but see below). The reason for not providing extensive literature sources is evident: it won't do any good if you are already convinced this writing is bogus. Today, we all have our sets of information that support our world view. I'm not talking about different ways of interpreting the same data, I'm writing about different data. For example, if you consider a strict vegetarian diet to be the most healthful diet on the planet, there are studies to support your contention. There are also studies that show it can have unintended consequences, especially for young (i.e., developing) people. Do you believe in human-influenced global warming? Whether you do or not, there are studies that lend validity to your stance. We now live in an age where studies can be designed (intentionally or not) to demonstrate our own position regarding a topic or set of beliefs. We simply select those "facts" that best fit with the way we choose to live. If you come to this book staunchly opposed to its content, no amount of literature will convince you otherwise because you can cite your own studies to refute many of the statements I will make. Therefore, I urge readers to employ common sense (and keep in mind, common sense is based on reason and gut feeling, the latter is a form of emotion).

That said, throughout this work, I will often list researcher's names and/or the title of a book or study to help people find a particular reference. The vast majority of those sources I have studied are available for anyone to read. In this way, I can (at least) shorten someone's search time and help them locate supporting evidence more quickly. I will do this here and there throughout the book to reinforce to the reader that this work is based on science. To be more accurate, this work is the result of decades of personal experience made through the lens of evidence-based research that is grounded in historical observations of wild humans. The frequent mention of "science" here is important for two reasons. One, this (the scientific method) is a valuable tool for interpreting our world and creates useful lines of evidence, and while it should not (and cannot) be ignored, remember that there exist many contradictory studies. Further, you should not deceive yourself with the belief that all valuable science is repeatable, because it isn't for a number of reasons (e.g., test subjects may be substantially changed from a previous time and have a different health status, test subjects may be actually or effectively extinct, as in the case of some indigenous groups). Two, referencing scientific study is especially important in a society where the majority feels emotion is all but useless in decision making (even though it is often used without realization). It is important that everyone understand our society's over-reliance on science has led us to the predicament we are now in. Technology is not going to solve any problem if there is no will (no spirit) to do so. Will a new invention stop racism or religious fanaticism or the belief our environment is there to be exploited? An infusion of human emotion and heart-based cognition (two vital aspects of our being) are being forgotten in a society populated by automatons. Emotion provides a powerful manner of waking people up from their slumber of non-awareness. Consider that science has helped people to understand the danger of a given industrial chemical, but it is emotion that inspires people to write their representatives, hold information sessions, and work to change consumer habits and/or laws.

Our country has a large number of people that are unhealthy (to varying degrees) as a result of modern living, and many are also unhappy with aspects of their life, but determining exactly what issues should be addressed is often a major obstacle. Anyone who believes that pharmaceutical drugs (for example) will create real health and true happiness is, unfortunately, exploring an ineffectual path. But, if you come to this book with an open mind, which is a requirement of both good science and polite discourse, I am convinced you will find the statements to resonate with both of your cognitive centers (mind and heart). In other words, my writing is based on reason that is influenced by feeling. I would contend that we must use both, or our world views become too skewed toward science or toward emotion. Both of these manners of arriving at answers have strengths and weaknesses, but together they act synergistically and form a system of checks and balances on our decision making and actions (or inactions).

REWILDING

It might be useful now to describe what this book is and is not about. This book is about rewilding. More accurately, it is about starting the rewilding of humanity to undo the domestication we have experienced. Rewilding is about returning to a wild state, at first in philosophy (and eventually in practice). It is a way for us to reconnect with what is truly important and shed those things in life that only serve to distract us from real living. By rising above domestication, people can work toward restoring awareness, health, and self-reliance, while at the same time walking more softly on the planet. Rewilding, at least at this point, is not about returning to a life in bark shelters (though for some it can mean that). It is a path that everyone, regardless of where they live and what they do for work, can embark on. Rewilding will look different for each person based on their knowledge and abilities. It is not about going backwards in time, but rather moving forward in an intelligent and sustainable manner that takes into account what has worked and what has not worked on this planet. Given that it took humanity many generations to lose their wild health and proficiency, it will take generations to restore it (i.e., it is unrealistic to think people can return to self-sufficient living in the span of a few years). Because rewilding can take different forms, for some it will be about building hunter-gatherer and herder-gatherer communities who practice horticulture and (possibly) limited agriculture. For others, it will be about merging the material knowledge of modern people with the nature skills and philosophy of the indigenous people. Evidence clearly indicates that a new path forward is urgently needed, and moving beyond domestication (i.e., rewilding) is unmistakably a healthy alternative for all involved.

Rewilding is considered, by some who do understand what this lifeway is about, to be a backward step for humanity, reverting to some point in history when humans lived as hunter-gatherers and abandoning all forms of technology. Let us be clear about several items. First, we cannot go back to living as hunter-gatherers (not most of us) because agriculturalists have populated the world with too many people and fragmented the land with cities, industries, and fields. Hunting and gathering requires more land per individual than does agriculture because it does not intensely manage the land (and while hunter-gatherers did manage lands, they did so in less extreme ways than utilized today). There is simply not enough space in the world for everyone to live as hunter-gatherers, even if everyone wanted to. There is no going back to this mode of living for billions of people, except for some individuals and small communities who have enough space to utilize this life history strategy (and that would be a good thing because hunting and gathering is proven to be sustainable, something that cannot be said about industrial living). Second, humans have always utilized technology and have been on a mission to create novel ways of securing the things they need. One of the hallmark traits of humans is their ability to innovate. There was a time when the bow (hunting weapon) was a novel piece of technology that allowed humans to hunt with great efficacy because it permitted them to launch a projectile with unparalleled accuracy at substantial distances (relative to what was possible prior to this invention). Earlier still, the controlled use of fire represented an amazing technological innovation that literally changed the anatomy of hominids and made possible the appearance of *Homo sapiens* (more on this in chapter 3). Finally, any suggested path forward that requires the abandonment of all modern technology will be ignored by most humans. Such a suggestion, regardless of its potential value, will fall on deaf ears. As has been presented thus far, ignoring the past is what generated the conditions we are experiencing today. Therefore, the only path forward must initially marry the new with the old (a form of transition culture). This is one vision of rewilding, a strategy that can be called the neoaboriginal path.

I want to reiterate that because different people will be in different stages of rewilding and have different abilities to rewild based on their past experiences and living situations, this book is meant to provide a range of solutions to all categories of people. Whether you live in Brooklyn, NY (highly urbanized), or in Grafton, ME (very rural), there will be information in this book that can make major inroads towards the recovery of personal health, the generation of native awareness, development of a road to self-reliance, and the deepening of one's connection to nature. Recommendations provided here will be based on modern science, but only those that do not contradict what we have observed in living people. Most "health movements" center on diet, or possibly including movement as well (e.g., Paleo Diet). What is being described here is a holistic approach to an entire lifeway. This reference will describe ways to reconnect with more of the requirements for human health. Through diet, medicine, movement, community, ancestral skills, and nature philosophy, we can exist as humans were meant to exist: healthy, relatively long-lived, at peace, and fully conscious.

THINK ABOUT IT

Agricultural humans have long been working toward an idea of a perfect world where we have abundant food and leisure time, no chronic disease, and meaningful lives. The sad fact is, we had all this and gave it up (see chapter 2). Now that we have saturated our lives with industrial technology, most people are unable to achieve all of these features simultaneously, but must, instead, choose which one they will pursue (most choosing abundant food and leisure time, but simultaneously experiencing chronic disease and lives without meaning). Even extreme wealth does not guarantee health today (there are examples of company CEOs and similar wealthy people passing at relatively young ages). Each new technological innovation is supposed to set humanity free and move us one step closer to complete dominion over the natural world, where hunger, fatigue, and illness are just distant memories. But if you carefully study "the ascent of humanity", you will see this path has led to a multitude of unforeseen consequences, which have impacted our lives in dramatic (and often not so beneficial) ways. Now, we are dependent on technologies we can't replicate ourselves (i.e., we can't make the things we use in daily life). This has forced us into wage slavery where leisure time is a priceless commodity and chronic illness is a common side effect of our modern lifeway. Each day, we need to create new fixes for the problems the last technology created. As Charles Eisenstein[2] writes:

> "The myth of technological utopia is uncannily congruent to the religious doctrine of heaven, with technology as our savior".

But, we march forward on the same path. If we can just cure this or invent that, then (finally) everything will be better. Every step forward on this industrial, nature-disconnected path brings a whole new suite of problems. Maybe a path where we recognize we are meant to be wild beings (and not technological automatons) has some promise—a path where human creativity is guided by a deep nature philosophy. Such a path—a neoaboriginal path—is completely within our ability to create. We simply must take off the blinders of domestication and truly see the current state of the world.

---

[2] Charles Eisenstain. 2013. The Ascent of Humanity. Evolver Editions, Berkeley, CA.

2. Ancestral lessons: the relevance of indigenous lifeways

"Nasty, brutish, and short"—this is one often repeated description that has been provided of hunter-gatherer (i.e., indigenous people) lives. And while wrong on every account, it is what most people consider to be an accurate description of the people who came before us (i.e., the people who are our ancestors). The truth of the matter is much different, and many people will not want to hear an accurate recounting of indigenous life because they want so much to believe we are living during the best conditions humans have ever experienced. Belief in this helps us to consciously overlook all of the things we know to be wrong with modern living (such as the shockingly high rates of cancer, the increasing frequency of depression and suicide, and the blatant ecocide occurring in every corner of the world). While it is certainly true that not every aspect of indigenous life was idyllic, there are features of that mode of existence that need to be understood in order to fully appreciate what we are missing out on today. Unfortunately, many are content thinking that indigenous people had it truly terribly, allowing them to tolerate everything they instinctively know to be unhealthy, unfair, and even oppressive aspects of contemporary life. They simply say to themselves: "at least it isn't like it used to be". But what if how it used to be was better than we have been told?

OUR BIASED VIEWS

Before we embark on an examination of indigenous life, we need to overcome the usual bias that occurs in discussions of indigenous people—bias that extends in both directions. Many people are fond of romanticizing indigenous lifeways and believe life in that time was a veritable utopia. Likewise, anyone who notes that hunter-gatherers have valuable aspects of their life are quickly targeted by other people who point out that indigenous life wasn't perfect. The naysayers note that starvation, homicide, inclement weather, risks associated with travelling in rugged terrain, dangerous animals, and various other hardships did occur in indigenous people's lives. It is even frequently stated that rape existed in hunter-gatherer villages. I do not disagree with these statements. Further, I'm not implying that life was perfect for hunter-gatherers (because it wasn't). What I am stating is that there were aspects of their life that were much better than today, and we need to bring forward those aspects into the present. While I do appreciate many facets of human culture that the indigenous practiced, I'm not without an understanding of the difficulties that wild living requires. And for the record, while rape was known in some hunter-gatherer cultures, there are plenty of well-studied indigenous groups where rape was not observed.

We have tremendous societal bias when it comes to indigenous people. There are so many examples of this it is difficult to know where to begin. Consider English explorers who believed that the Aborigine of Australia must have been on the verge of starvation due to the foods they were observed consuming with frequency—insects and lizards. These foods were considered starvation foods by the English; therefore, the wild people of this continent must be starving. The reality of course is that the Aborigine did not abhor these foods and can be said to have experienced greater overall health than the people who were judging them. (I encourage you to read "Hunter–gatherers have less famine than agriculturalists", written by Berbesque et al. in 2014 for further information on this topic.) Even in arenas that do not pertain to health, we see great issue taken by European colonists to traditional ceremonies that were offering gratitude, mourning those that had passed, or were seeking answers through the use of entheogens (i.e., plants, fungi, and animals that can produce an altered state of conscientiousness). These practices were halted by the European colonizers because they were believed to be an affront to Christianity. The historical literature is replete with examples of people of European descent considering indigenous people to be subhuman and in need of saving (while in actuality, the health of many indigenous groups was severely impacted by the loss of their ancestral lifeways).

Bias is especially true today where most people have never seen a hunter-gatherer (they are, in fact, a globally imperiled "species"). What they have seen are Native Americans, or other First Nations People, who are no longer living their ancestral lifeway (i.e., they are no longer hunter-gatherers). These people are often succumbing to various chronic diseases at even higher rates than the general population, likely due to a combination of factors. These include low income (resulting in poor diets and poor healthcare), alcoholism, and fewer generations spent on a modern diet (their physiologies have had less time to adapt to a menu based largely on cultivated grains and highly processed foods). In some cases, people have seen on-line images of hunter-gatherers, but most of these images are of people that have been displaced by agriculturalists or have been extensively contacted. These people, with altered lifeways, are now consuming a large proportion of modern foods. Throughout this chapter, we are going to be discussing the health, longevity, and relative absence of chronic disease found in hunter-gatherers who were still living on their traditional diet and practicing their traditional lifeways (i.e., prior to disruptive contact). Any observations taken from people who practice extensive agriculture, consume modern foods, drink heavily or utilize modern addictive drugs, live in marginal land, or are otherwise prohibited from practicing their ancestral lifeways are potentially unrepresentative or even misleading. This means that many ancient cultures, such as the Aztecs, Mayans, and Mississippians, are not representative because they practiced extensive agriculture to feed their populations. Keep in mind also we are discussing those hunter-gatherers (or sometimes herder-gatherers and forager-horticulturalists) who have lived relatively recently (over the last several hundred years), where direct observations could be made prior to the destruction of their lifeways. We are not discussing Paleolithic people who lived prior to the advent of agriculture for one very significant reason—many important manners of processing foods to reduce antinutrients and maximize nutrition had not yet been invented (these will be discussed in detail in chapter 3).

LONGEVITY

Perhaps one of the most persistent (and grossly inaccurate) myths is the idea that indigenous people lived very short lives. Considered to be common knowledge is that hunter-gatherers passed away from old age after 35–40 years of life (these figures are what I commonly hear reported to me from members of the audience when I am lecturing). The short life myth is one of the most important legends we need to address because it allows people to entertain the notion that cardiovascular disease and cancer (for example) were rare among hunter-gatherers because they didn't live long enough to acquire these diseases. And while many hunter-gatherers did enjoy long lives, the short life myth would not explain the prevalence of childhood cancer, asthma, autism, allergies, and the like. So, where do these low numbers (35–40 years) come from?

First, we need to understand how life expectancy has been misunderstood. Let us assume that the life expectancy of a particular group of hunter-gatherers is 35 years (which is close to the actual figure for many groups). That means that each individual, starting from birth, is likely to live to be 35 years old. If this is the average life expectancy, it means many people needed to live longer (much longer) to offset any infant and childhood mortality. The figure 35 is an average—but it has been interpreted in discussions occurring in recent years to be the general upper limit of life in foraging communities (i.e., the life span). This misinterpretation of "average life expectancy" for "life span" has been a major obstacle for understanding that hunter-gatherers had many individuals who lived long lives (longevity that rivals some affluent countries).

For example, Stephen Guyenet collected mortality data from a Russian mission in Alaska where the age of death was recorded for the Inuit in the early half of the 1800s. Examining the data that had been collected, he found that a significant number of individuals in the Inuit culture lived past the age of 80, and some exceeded 90 years of age. In fact, excluding infant mortality, 25% of the population lived past the age of 60. The work of Hill et al., who examined the Hiwi of South America, also documented a significant number of individuals living past the age of 60, with 79 as the oldest recorded individuals in their study. These results (and others that could be listed) don't support the typical narrative of death at 35 years for wild humans.

Ryan and Jetha, in their book "Sex at Dawn", describe another interesting misinterpretation of age of death data. Archeologists use dental eruption measurements to estimate the age of human remains. Researchers examine the distance that the third molars have grown out of the jaw bone to arrive at an approximate age of death for the human being examined. At around 35 years of age, the molars are no longer growing further out of the jawbone, which means individuals older than 35 years old cannot be distinguished from one another as to their actual age. Therefore, these individuals are noted as "35+". If you examine papers that utilize dental eruption, you will note that the researchers are examining primarily teenagers and young adults because of this limitation. But somewhere along the line, the notation of 35+ became simply 35 (note the loss of the plus sign). It then became entrenched in minds of some who read about archeological remains of hunter-gatherers that the general upper limit of their lifespan was 35. This is, of course, incorrect.

Consider also the age that women undergo menopause. This life stage has important ramifications for family life, as this loss of fertility in women helps to ensure that children are not borne to women experiencing declines in reproductive health and it frees up older women from the responsibility of bearing children so that they can provide their child-rearing experience to their grandchildren (who have less experienced mothers). In the United States, menopause usually occurs between the ages of 40 and 61 (with most women beginning menopause in their 52nd year). If indigenous women died as young as most believe, it would mean that menopause is a new phenomenon. Such an important aspect of female life would have evolved much earlier, given the value it would have to the next generations. In fact, we know that indigenous women did experience menopause, and that the average age of menopause was not much different than women in the United States (mid-40s to early 50s).

One of the best papers written on the topic of hunter-gatherer longevity is the one prepared by Gurven and Kaplan that examined several hunter-gatherer groups (along with foragers who practiced horticulture and hunter-gatherers with significant outside contact). Their work showed that hunter-gatherers experience relatively high mortality in the first fifteen years of life, which brings down the average life expectancy. Once passing this milestone, the frequency of individuals that live until 45 is significantly higher. Those living to the age of 45 can expect an additional 21 years of life (on average). Gurven and Kaplan's work showed the mode of highest adult mortality (averaged across five groups) was at 72—in other words, the highest frequency of adult death occurred at age 72 (though in some groups this figure was as high as 76 and there were individuals within some hunter-gatherer groups who lived more than a decade longer).

As can be determined from the previous paragraphs, indigenous people did have members of their cultures living into elderhood, long enough to experience the chronic disease that is so frequent in American society. It is clear that the short life myth is just that—a myth. While hunter-gatherers did experience greater mortality during the younger years, there were a significant proportion of the individuals that lived into their 60s and 70s, and even later in some groups. Seeing an unbiased picture of indigenous longevity will be important to framing much of the information that will be presented later in this chapter.

Before we get to the remaining discussion, it must be stated that Americans have no business setting longevity standards for world. Further, longevity is not the ultimate criterion by which we should judge the success of anyone's diet and lifeway. The United States is an incredibly wealthy nation and it uses its wealth to take a disproportionate amount of global resources. While Americans represent only 4% of the world's population, they use 25% of the world's resources. This means they are able to have much of the hard labor and repetitive tasks performed by migrant laborers and fossil-fuel-powered machines. Americans make up for health in old age with prescription drugs and hip replacements and other invasive surgeries. But more important than all of this is the fact that longevity is a very selfish goal for a particular diet and lifestyle. It focuses on the individual—which is one of the contributing issues that have brought us to the place we are at today. We should be focusing on the health of the next generation. As I stated earlier, modern people are selfish (some knowingly, some not), and so they focus on long life even though intergenerational health can be seen to be declining. I would consider a diet that produces healthy, well-formed children a better diet than one that adds a decade of life but produces health consequences in the next generation.

CHRONIC DISEASE

The term cancer is used to describe a suite of diseases that are characterized by abnormal cell growth that frequently (but not always) results in one or more neoplasms (i.e., tumors). This abnormal cell growth is capable of spreading to other regions of the body. Cancer is problematic to the body since the cells have nearly limitless replication ability because the usual safeguards (such as apoptosis, or programmed cell death) have been eluded. Apoptosis is process by which old and defective cells are killed in a controlled manner by the body so that they cannot cause harm to surrounding tissues or (ultimately) the entire organism. Cancerous cells are different from normal cells in that apoptosis has been thwarted, so that the cells continue to proliferate, damaging the function of one or more organs. Cancer has become a common affliction in the United States. It has also become big business (more on that in chapter 5). Its frequency today—lifetime odds are 1 in 3 women and 1 in 2 men—means cancer has become a routine part of life. Almost no families go long without being touched by this illness. But surely the reason it is so common today is because we live much longer (right?). In other words, cancer is a trade-off we have experienced with longer life. Many authors would have you believe it isn't something we should be concerned about preventing because our new-found longevity is the actual root cause of cancer. Fortunately, we have a method of verifying such assertions. As has been outlined previously, indigenous cultures had many members living into elderly years. If cancer is part of growing old, then it would have been seen in wild people as well.

Of course, it is difficult to know the real frequency of cancer in wild cultures because the diagnostic tools we have access to in hospitals and similar facilities allow more detailed screening of this illness. Further, we no longer have the ability to examine large groups of people living as hunter-gatherers in different regions of the world because either they do not exist in most locations or they have been acculturated (which is a euphemistic way of writing that their lifeways have been forced aside by colonizers). With those limitations in mind, it is worth noting that there have been extensive searches for cancer in indigenous groups by trained medical professionals during the 1800s and 1900s. Some of these surveys occurred as late as the latter half of the 1900s, at a time when doctors would have certainly observed cancer in some individuals if it occurred (and using those same methods they could find cancer in people living within modern societies). So, what were the results of those surveys?

Stanislas Tanchou was a French physician who performed surgeries in the 1800s. In an 1843 address to the Academy of Sciences in Paris, he told the audience of several medical professionals who had reported on the frequency of cancer they encountered in frontier locations away from modern civilization. For example, he spoke of Dr. Bac, a surgeon-in-chief who had spent six years working in Senegal and had not observed a single case of cancer. He described the work of Dr. Baudens, a surgeon-in-chief working in Algiers for eight years, who encountered only two cases of cancer. He also spoke of Dr. Puzin, who had seen 10,000 people and found only a single case of breast cancer. Many of the people observed by these physicians were indigenous people with varying degrees of contact with civilization, but none were living highly modern lifestyles from which the doctors had come (where cancer was much more frequent).

Albert Schweitzer was a physician, medical missionary, and Nobel laureate who visited Gabon (west central Africa) in 1913. He and his wife (an anesthesiologist) established a small hospital 200 miles upstream from the mouth of the Ogooué River. Schweitzer noted that he did not discover a single case of cancer in the aboriginal population. He observed 2000 patients in the first nine months of establishing the hospital at Lambaréné on the Ogooué River. While he stated he could not positively state there was no cancer at all, he elaborated that it must be quite rare if no cases could be found.

Francois Fouché was a surgeon who spent over six years in southern Africa among the Sotho people. He reported in 1923 having observed 14,000 native people during that time—not one person amongst the natives living a relatively traditional lifestyle was found to have cancer. However, he notes that cancer was frequent in the Caucasian population and he did find cancer amongst modernized indigenous. What is interesting about the article authored by Fouché is that he realized that lifeway was a predictor of the frequency of cancer. He also realized that his observations (and others he was aware of at the time) demonstrated research should focus on the specific factors of civilization that are promoting cancer in people.

"These facts are well known to all medical men in South Africa who have practised [sic] amongst the native races. In view of the present stimulus given to research in the causation of cancer, I think the article and facts quoted above ought to receive serious consideration."

Unfortunately, the medical industry in the United States has not put much effort into the prevention of cancer (and some oncologists actively dismiss the huge role that diet and lifestyle play). Rather, all the focus is located where income can be earned: pharmaceutical drugs and other therapies to treat cancer once it has occurred (more on this in chapter 5).

Lyman Buckley, who was an associate editor of the journal Cancer, contributed an article in 1927 on his observations of cancer frequency among Alaska natives. Doctor Buckley had spent 12 years among several different indigenous groups, during which time he never observed a single case of malignancy. From this he became aware that it was civilization itself that contributed to cancer, including the increasing frequency of this illness in contacted tribes no longer living their traditional lifeways.

Weston Price, a US dentist, spent years travelling to different regions of the world to observe people living in isolation from modern foods. As part of this research, published in 1939 (titled "Nutrition and Physical Degeneration"), he interviewed different physicians who lived amongst relatively isolated indigenous people (i.e., people who still enjoyed their traditional diet and practiced many aspects of their ancestral lifeways). One physician he interviewed, Joseph Romig, had 36 years of contact with Alaska natives. In all that time, he did not observe a single person afflicted with cancer, except for the natives who had become "modernized", where it was described as frequent. Doctor Price also interviewed Dr. Nimmo, a government physician who worked on the Torres Straight Islands. In his work with 4000 natives, Dr. Nimmo saw only one case he suspected to represent cancer. During that same time period, Dr. Nimmo had performed several dozen surgeries to treat cancer on the Caucasian population, who numbered around 300 (and did not consume the traditional foods of the natives).

Alexander Berglas authored "Cancer, its Nature, Cause and Cure" in 1957, where he described the work of Dr. Eugene Payne. Spending over 25 years in portions of Brazil and Ecuador, Dr. Payne examined approximately 60,000 people native to this region. He reported finding no evidence of cancer among the natives.

Vilhjalmur Stefansson was an explorer and ethnologist who spent time in the early 1900s in northwestern North America among indigenous people. In 1960 he published "Cancer: Disease of Civilization?: An Anthropological and Historical Study" that discussed the prevalence of cancer among relatively isolated groups. Stefansson published in this work a letter written to him in 1958 from Dr. White, a physician who worked amongst Aleutian Islands natives from 1934 until 1948. During that time he observed only a single confirmed case of cancer. Stefansson noted in his 1960 work that among missionaries working around the world, cancer was extremely rare among the indigenous people, though it was found among the modernized groups.

These reports (and others not presented here) indicate indigenous people who had not been acculturated were highly resistant to malignancies. Frederick Hoffman, who authored a large report on cancer for Prudential Insurance in 1915 titled "The Mortality from Cancer Throughout the World", described the situation well: "cancer is exceptionally rare among the primitive people". And while you may be thinking that there must have existed cancer that was missed (which is likely true to some extent), keep in mind that cancer was being found in Europeans, Americans, and other people with highly modernized lives using the same techniques and resources available to the physicians examining the indigenous groups. Today, the same indigenous people who were once so resistant to cancer are now succumbing in large numbers to this illness. It is very clear that there are detrimental aspects of contemporary living that produce sickness in humans (of any race). The loss of traditional lifeways is correlated with an increase in cancer (and other chronic disease, as we will discuss shortly). Work with Inuit populations (and published by Fellows in 1934 in a work called "Mortality in the Native Races of the Territory of Alaska, With Special Reference to Tuberculosis") demonstrated that the more modernized indigenous people became, the higher the rates of cancer they experienced. This is also true of contacted and acculturated indigenous of the Amazon Basin. While they do not experience the rates of malignancy of those who live in urban areas, the incorporation of various aspects of modern living have degraded much of their native resilience to this collection of illnesses. I do hope the full weight of these paragraphs is hitting you (with force)—cancer is not part of the human condition. It is not something we need to experience, not even in age. We don't need to seek a cure for cancer because prevention is plainly possible (and will be detailed in this book). Alexander Berglas demonstrated his understanding of the situation when he wrote:

"Civilization is, in terms of cancer, a juggernaut that cannot be stopped... It is the nature and essence of industrial civilization to be toxic in every sense... We are faced with the grim prospect that the advance of cancer and of civilization parallel each other."

What about cardiovascular disease and diabetes? Did indigenous groups experience similar rates of these illnesses as do modern people? There have been many papers in recent decades that have attempted to demonstrate that hunter-gatherers experience similar high rates of cardiovascular disease (and other chronic ailments, such as neurovascular disease) as contemporary Americans do. All these papers suffer an important shortcoming in that they have observed populations long after contact with civilization, in times when traditional diet and lifestyle practices were significantly altered and modern foods had become common place. Only studies that examine populations prior to displacement of traditional foods (i.e., prior to disruptive contact) provide a real look at the situation.

To frame the historical indigenous experience of these chronic ailments, we need to re-state the occurrence of these ailments observed in the United States today. Cardiovascular disease is the leading cause of death in the United States, with over half of the people over 45 in this country experiencing this disease. As for the prevalence of diabetes, the current Center for Disease Control (CDC) estimate is 9% of Americans, or 1 in 11 people (a figure which represents a doubling over the period of 1990 to 2008), experience some form of this illness. Further, the CDC estimates that the younger generation will experience much higher rates of diabetes. Given the prevalence of these two diseases, we would expect them to be present, to some degree, in all populations, past and present, if these are natural conditions experienced by humans (especially if one wishes to consider that Americans are a healthy people). Let us examine the medical anthropology literature and find out.

The first reported case of diabetes in Australian Aborigine was recorded in 1923 in Adelaide (see Basedow's publication in 1932 titled "Diseases of the Australian Aborigines"). What is remarkable about this is that medical missionaries were present in Australia since at least 1838. Prior to acculturation, there was no evidence of diabetes among this indigenous group.

Doctor L. White, who we discussed earlier regarding cancer, in his 1958 letter to Vilhjalmur Stefansson, noted that among the Aleutian Islands natives that arteriosclerotic diseases were practically non-existent and diabetes was extremely rare. He stated that he saw no coronary heart disease amongst the indigenous of this region after 17 years of practice. What is noteworthy about this is the fact far northern populations consume a higher proportion of animal foods and a higher proportion of fat than many other cultures in the world (and were still free of illness and lived relatively long lives). This clearly indicates that the abundant literature "demonstrating" that animal foods (in general) cause cancer and that fat always leads to heart disease are erroneous—these generalizations that are made in the contemporary medical literature are contradicted by examinations of people consuming such foods. It clearly points to the need for a revision of these statements. We will see that this research does suggest that the kinds and proportions of animal foods and the kinds of fats consumed by industrialized people are the problem (not animal foods and fats in general; see chapter 3).

Over a period of 1967 to 1969, Truswell and Hansen made three medical trips to assess the !Kung of the Kalahari (southern Africa). During their visits, they noted that obesity, high blood pressure, coronary heart disease, and neurological disease were not seen. While the !Kung did experience some health issues (e.g., infection, traumatic injury), they did not experience the usual suite of chronic ailments that afflict people in financially affluent countries.

Taylor and colleagues in 1971 published an editorial on medical research performed on the Masai of east Africa, which cited several earlier papers looking specifically at cardiovascular disease among members of this herder-gatherer group. Fervent interest in this group was being generated by their peculiar diet because it consisted of a high proportion of animal fat and protein, especially from milk, meat, and blood of the animals they tended. Other studies have suggested approximately 66% of their diet is fat. Atherosclerosis and heart disease were unknown (note that multiple independent researchers have found similar results).

Staffan Lindenberg and colleagues in 1989 examined 2300 residents of the island of Kitava, one of the Trobriand Islands in Papua New Guinea's archipelago. These people were forager-horticulturalists who also consumed some wild animals (e.g., fish). It was estimated that only 0.2% of the calories came from western foods. They did not find any cardiovascular disease in the inhabitants, even though 6% of the population was from 60 to 95 years old. Diabetes was also noted to be absent. In this case, the majority of calories were obtained from carbohydrates found in root vegetables (which indicates that carbohydrates, in and of themselves, do not cause disease, as asserted by advocates of a very low carbohydrate diet).

There are abundant reports of a general lack of chronic disease (of all kinds) found in hunter-gatherer populations. These reports, though varied in source and detail, all present a surprisingly similar story: cancer, heart disease, diabetes, and other chronic ailments are not a compulsory part of the human story, rather, they can be tied to a lifeway that contributes to poor health. We are living in a period of evolutionary mismatch, where our bodies have certain requirements that are not being met by modern living. As we continue our examination of indigenous people living on their traditional diet and practicing their traditional lifestyle, it will become clear that evading chronic disease is not the only benefit provided by an approach to living that incorporates human history.

SKELETAL STRUCTURE AND PHYSICAL FITNESS

Indigenous people possessed an active lifestyle that, along with dietary elements, contributed to excellent physical fitness. Their muscular development, strength of bones, and beauty of their bodies (especially their faces) were best developed prior to extensive contact with European colonizers and conquerors. This statement is defensible through several lines of evidence (which we will briefly explore). Details concerning specific movement patterns (daily and seasonally) will be presented in chapter 8.

Human skeletons contain a record of how people lived. Bones are not inanimate, rather they are dynamic structures that respond to the stresses placed upon them in ways that can be observed (even long after death). Differences in diet and lifestyle—including differences in nutrition, movement, and overall health—can be detected in the skeletal remains between groups of people who practiced different manners of subsistence. Multiple studies from different locations in the world have shown that the skeletons of hunter-gatherers show denser (i.e., stronger) bones, no signs of iron deficiency, little or no signs of infection, very low incidence of dental caries (i.e., cavities), and fewer signs of arthritis compared with the remains of agricultural people. These studies make clear that our transition to a more sedentary way of life left its mark on our frames, such that those skilled in bioarcheology can observe differences between our bones and those from hunter-gatherers.

One such researcher (Claire Cassidy) presented a very compelling story of the effects of different lifestyles on our skeletons. This study was important because it compared a large number of remains of two groups of people living in the same region and experiencing the same climate but differing in their diet (and the subsequent activity required to secure their dietary elements). Both groups lived in what is now the state of Kentucky. One group utilized hunting and gathering to acquire their nutrition, the other relied primarily on agriculture (growing corn, squash, and beans), with some wild animal and plant foods supplementing the cultivated crops. There were significant differences between these two groups. Certain infections, in this case ones that cause periosteal inflammation, while occurring in both groups, were thirteen times more prevalent in the agriculturalists. Iron deficiency resulting in poor bone health was present in the agriculturalists, but absent in the hunter-gatherers. Tooth decay was rampant in the agricultural group, with nearly seven teeth per mouth showing signs of decay (vs. an average of less than one in the hunter-gatherers). No hunter-gatherer children had caries, while the agricultural children developed caries in the second year of life. Overall, Cassidy's work showed the hunter-gatherers were healthier, had lower infant mortality, suffered fewer infections, and lived longer than the early agriculturalists.

Movement and physical loading of the skeletal system is critical for strong bones. Two different groups of researchers have examined the skeletons of a suite of primates with particular emphasis on the trabecular bone, which is the spongy tissue at the ends of the bones that is part of the joints. These two research teams studied remains from other-than-human primates, early hominids, pre-agricultural foragers, and humans from agricultural societies. They found that trabecular bone tissue was less dense in agricultural groups than in previous primates. Wild humans (i.e., pre-agricultural people) had, on average, 20% more bone mass than those practicing agriculture. While this might not seem like a significant difference, this is approximately the amount of bone mass that would be lost after three months of weightlessness in space. This change in bone density indicated a more sedentary lifestyle, one that involved less overall movement (i.e., less stress on the skeletal system). Ultimately, agriculturalists have more gracile and more fragile bones than in hunter-gatherers. Given that industrial technology has allowed modern humans unprecedented levels of inactivity, this trend has continued today with industrialists (i.e., modern humans) showing even weaker bones than early agriculturalists.

Bones require stress from movement and load bearing to make them strong. Observations of hunter-gatherers demonstrated they are generally much more mobile than modern humans, covering larger distances in their search for food and other resources. For example, living groups such as the !Kung (Kalahari Desert, Africa) and Aché (Paraná River watershed of Paraguay) have been documented covering average distances of 8 to 16 km (5 to 10 miles) a day. Both genders of adults were active. We could also examine the yearly movements of hunter-gatherers (i.e., their home ranges) as a way of assessing the amount of activity they experienced. Estimates vary widely for different groups, in part, due to the availability of resources (especially food) in their ecosystems. The Aka of west-central Africa were estimated to have travelled an area that covered 400 km^2 (98,842 acres) over the course of a year. The Hadza of present-day Tanzania were estimated to cover an area of 2520 km^2 (622,705 acres). The Mi'kmaq of northeastern North America travelled an area that was upwards of 5200 km^2 (1,284,947 acres). The Inuit of Baffin Island covered an area that was 25,000 km2 (6,177,634 acres). These figures indicate a level of activity that is not experienced by many contemporary people.

The active lifestyles of the indigenous are well demonstrated in the fact that a typical foraging mother is estimated to have carried her infant a total of 4800 km (3000 miles) during its first four years of life. But it wasn't all work, as indigenous activity also included play and celebration. Dance was an important aspect of social life, and communal dancing could occur several nights a week and last for hours. Hunter-gatherer physical movement would best be described as light to moderate throughout much of the day with occasional need for high-intensity activity. The volume of activity experienced by hunter-gatherers contributed to excellent physical (musculature) and physiological (cardiovascular) health. It is important to keep in mind that exercise also benefits many other aspects of personal health, including insulin sensitivity, brain health, mood, life span, energy levels, and libido. Further, it is one of the key aspects of lifestyle that protect the body from chronic disease.

There are many ways one could demonstrate a superior physical conditioning of the average hunter-gatherer to the average contemporary human. An important hunting weapon among many indigenous is the bow, a technology that dates back over 65,000 years. This shaped piece of wood is flexed by pulling a string attached at each end, this stored energy transferred to the projectile (the arrow) once the string is loosed. The stiffer the bow, the harder it is to flex, and the more strength it requires to draw it back. If we were to examine the most frequently purchased draw weight of traditional (i.e., non-compound) bows today, they fall in the range of 22–25 kg (50–55 pounds) of force needed to bend the bow to its full draw. A study done on the Hadza by Marlowe found the average draw weight on their bows was 31.5 kg (69.4 pounds), with the highest pull (in that study) at 43.1 kg (95 pounds). Some Hadza bows have been recorded (in other studies) to require 60 kg (132 pounds) of force to draw them. If one were to shop for traditional bows today, they would find that such draw weights would not be widely available because few, if any, people could hunt with such bows (most traditional bows today are made in a range of draw weights that peak at 27 kg, significantly below the average draw weight of a Hadza hunter-gatherer).

Not only did native people around the globe have significant differences in skeletal development, but there were substantial differences in facial structure compared with modern people. These differences were primarily the result of features of their diet—features that can still be enjoyed today (but aren't). The facial structure possessed by many people today can actually be described as a deformity. What is most troubling with this is not merely that the differences occur but, rather, the fact that some of these changes are not even recognized today (i.e., many people possess distinctive facial deformities that we believe to be the norm for *Homo sapiens*). Therefore, the first step to learning how to correct these skeletal deficiencies is to learn they exist.

Weston Price (the Ohio dentist) travelled to all six continents where people isolated from modern foods could still be found during his research in the 1930s. What he thoroughly documented through careful notes and thousands of photographs were striking skeletal differences between indigenous (and some traditional) people and those who consumed the foods of civilization (e.g., white flour, highly processed sugar, vegetable oil). Throughout his journeys, people who consumed their traditional wild (and in some cases, cultivated and pastured) foods had broader faces, wider noses, and mouths with room to fit all their teeth. What this meant is that their teeth emerged straight and uncrowded—and this includes their third molars (i.e., wisdom teeth). Relatively isolated indigenous people did not display impacted wisdom teeth, a feature that is quite common in the mouths of modern people. While many today believe that humans have an inherent flaw in the design of their mouths because their teeth often don't all fit (without crowding and impacting), the fact is, they all used to fit. Regardless of the continent, and regardless of the specifics of the diet, indigenous people had broader faces and maxillae (i.e., upper jaw and palate), and correspondingly had straighter teeth and proper growth of their wisdom teeth.

How do we know these differences in facial and dental form were diet related? Because Weston Price inquired as to the diet of the people that displayed differences in dental structure. When the parents consumed their traditional foods, the children grew into adults with broad faces and beautiful dentition. If the parents consumed the foods of civilization, then the children demonstrated narrow faces and various dental issues, especially as adults. Two items are important here—diet mattered, but it wasn't just the diet of the person, it was also the diet of person's parents (i.e., poor nutrition in the parents results in deficiencies in the next generation). These observations were consistent from group to group, which included indigenous people on the North American, African, and South American continents, groups in Polynesia, and isolated people in Switzerland and islands off the northwestern coast of Scotland. All of this was photographically documented in his work "Nutrition and Physical Degeneration". Modern food produced the altered dentition so commonly observed today. Therefore, crowded teeth are a skeletal deformity based, in part, on poor nutrition (as well as food texture, not discussed by Price, which affects the stresses, or lack thereof, experienced by the mandible and maxillae and are also important to proper facial form).

Weston Price's work not only catalogued the dental form and occlusion of people he visited, but also the prevalence of dental caries. In every case, significant differences occurred between relatively isolated people and those engaging in a modern diet. For example, he examined Native Americans living near the mouth of the Kuskokwim River (Alaska) who consumed almost exclusively wild food and found the incidence of cavities to be 0.1% (specifically, 1 tooth in 820 observed had a cavity). In the same region were people of similar or mixed ancestry that were consuming almost entirely modern foods. In this group, 252 of 1094 teeth observed (21.1%) were found to be carious. Another example, visiting the Lockhart River on the island-continent of Australia, Price found in those isolated Aborigine that of the 1784 teeth observed, 4.3% were carious. These results stand in stark contrast to those living on a reservation at LeParouse (near Sydney) where 47.5% of the teeth demonstrated cavities. These results were relatively consistent regardless of the continent he visited. Dental caries, while not limited to modern people, is profoundly more common in those consuming modern foods. Again, the diet and lifestyle of the indigenous provided them with supportive factors that protected them from various issues we commonly face today.

COMMUNITY EXPERIENCES AND HAPPINESS

Perhaps one of the most compelling reasons to consider the lessons in indigenous lifeways is to understand that they possessed happiness. It was a happiness that did not require the latest version of the smartphone of choice, or a particular brand name of clothing, or a certain make of vehicle with higher social status. Therefore, their happiness did not involve the mining of rare earth metals. It did not promote the cultivation of a fiber crop that is extremely harmful to grow (using the methods of most cotton farmers) and condone horrific work conditions in overseas clothing factories. And their happiness did not generate pollution as one drives around in class. While Americans are not the happiest people on the planet, they do rank within the top twenty (a respectable showing). But I would politely argue for most that their happiness requires financial wealth, one that produces industrial pollution, creates wage disparities, and maintains social stratification (which is a euphemistic way of writing "some people have more privilege than others"). If achieving personal happiness causes harm to the world, how long can such happiness be achieved before the world is unable to support it? I would go further and state that most Americans who experience happiness are actually experiencing something different—momentary pacification of a desire to own more and more material goods (I will expand on this concept in chapter 12). This is very different in indigenous groups with intact lifeways, where visitors and researchers universally reported the same thing: these people were happy and content. Further, features of depression, such as suicide, were virtually non-existent.

There is little doubt that the happiness experienced by hunter-gatherers is due, in part, to a strong connection to family and other tribal members (i.e., to the community). Hunter-gatherers do not live in broken societies where on-line social media stand in for actual human relationships. They experience true community that is supportive and sharing. Their happiness is also based on their social dynamics. They do not experience high levels of within-group competition for resources, as our society practices today. Unlike agricultural and industrial societies, there are no repressive forms of socialization. This means that there are not classes of people that experience less happiness than others. They practice a more consensual decision making, with everyone having a real (rather than illusionary) part in the choices they are confronted with. They implement equality and uphold personal autonomy. Happiness also comes from their attitude toward life. They approach work (at least more of it than we do) with a playful attitude; therefore, their life is not consumed by hours of complaining about life chores. And they celebrate with their community (often).

Most of us, at some point, have engaged the erroneous belief that indigenous people were constantly on the verge of starvation and had little to be thankful for. The reality is quite different. While certainly the late winter period for north-temperate Native Americans (for example) was a difficult time of year, there were also multiple periods of substantial food abundance. Keep in mind that, on average, hunter-gatherers spent three to six hours a day acquiring food, and much of the rest of the day was spent in leisure, repairing clothing and other light tasks, visiting, storytelling, singing, dancing, engaging in ceremony, and intimacy. There is little wonder these people were happy—they could locate or craft everything they needed for living and had more spare time to enjoy life.

OUR WILD PROGENITORS

In chapter 1, we discussed four features that (in part) define a domesticated animal. These are altered temperament, altered social hierarchy, tolerating an altered diet, and ability to breed in captivity. Remember that modern humans possess all four of these criteria. There are also morphological changes that occur with domesticated animals (i.e., they look different from their wild progenitors). For example, the domestic dog shows many traits different from the animal it was derived from (the wolf). These traits include different coat patterns, floppy ears, shortened muzzles, smaller teeth, smaller brains, and curly tails (among many others). This means that a biologist can view a living domesticated dog and identify that it is not a wolf. Similarly, an archeologist can examine the skeletal remains of a domesticated dog and determine they do not belong to a wolf. Even when domesticated dogs approximate the size and shape of a wolf, they display various skeletal features that allow identification, such as shorter muzzles and more crowded teeth. In other words, domestication produces visible changes in the morphology of the organism.

Likewise, noticeable skeletal changes have occurred in modern agricultural and industrial people, as discussed earlier in this chapter. These include lighter bones and narrower maxillae, the latter of which often resulting in crowded, crooked, and impacted teeth. Therefore, an archeologist could examine the bones of a human and determine if they belonged to a hunter-gatherer (wild human) or a contemporary person (domesticated human). To be perfectly clear: through diet and movement, or more accurately, poor diet and lack of movement, we modern humans have changed our physical form to the point we no longer resemble our recent hunter-gatherer ancestors. These aren't cosmetic or cultural differences in dress, make-up, and hair styles, rather, we are discussing fundamental alterations to our being—none of which can be described as beneficial. Weaker bones cannot handle heavy stresses and crowded and crooked teeth are more difficult to clean, leading to periodontal disease (half of Americans over 30 years of age have this disease). Not to mention, we have, on average, smaller brains than hunter-gatherers. If we also include our propensity to develop chronic disease (e.g., cancer, cardiovascular disease, diabetes), it can be seen that modern people are changing what it means to be human.

Given that a name is provided to the domesticated form of various animals to indicate their distinctiveness from their wild progenitors, one could argue the same should occur here. Choosing an appropriate scientific name that portrays the changes that have occurred in modern people would be useful to help describe the current situation. Considering the fact that contemporary humans spend a great deal of time in the home—the average American spends 90% of their time indoors—use of the Latin *domesticus* would seem appropriate, a word that means "belonging to the house". Another set of related traits for modern humans is that they are, on average, physically weaker with more slender bones, and less adept at dealing with extremes in temperature (because most people need a thermostatically controlled environment to be comfortable). These traits suggest another word from the Latin language: *fragilis*, meaning "fragile" (while this may seem derogatory, it is meant to present a powerful statement of what many humans have become, especially in financially affluent countries where sedentary lives lead to weak musculoskeletal systems and almost complete avoidance of uncomfortable weather). Combining these two Latin words into a single epithet, we get *domesticofragilis*. Modern humans and hunter-gatherers are clearly the same species, the morphological and anatomical changes are not extensive and they have the ability to interbreed. Therefore, this new name would be used to designate a novel subspecies of human as *Homo sapiens domesticofragilis*[3]. This would translate as the "domesticated, fragile, wise man", a suitable name for contemporary humans (note: the use of man here is intended as a gender neutral term). The anatomically modern hunter-gatherer would still be referred to as *Homo sapiens sapiens*.

---

[3] This is meant to be an informal, but educational, use of scientific names and not an official publication of a new taxon. Following the rules of zoological nomenclature, the name *Homo sapiens sapiens* is actually tied to the domesticated species as Carl Linnaeus is considered to be the type specimen of anatomically modern humans.

Of course, there are many differences that could be highlighted between hunter-gatherers and modern humans to support the distinction that has been made here. The method of acquiring nutrition is profoundly different between these two kinds of people. Hunter-gatherers participated on their landscapes as predators of plants and animals; modern people modify their landscapes to make them conducive to (in most cases) non-native plant cultivation and animal husbandry. Most hunter-gatherers lived in relatively egalitarian cultures without social classes; modern people live in highly stratified societies where a small proportion of the people experience wealth and privilege that most of the members do not. Most hunter-gatherers demonstrated well-rounded skill sets, with division of labor occurring primarily between the genders; modern people are highly specialized with extreme division of labor occurring along educational and professional lines, and most alive can only perform a tiny fraction of the skills needed for living (therefore, they must purchase the things they need for survival). Hunter-gatherers procured raw materials from (primarily) their local landscapes and crafted these with great skill into the items they needed for daily living; modern people, especially those in financially affluent countries, acquire little or nothing from their local environments. Instead, they have raw materials in distant lands crafted into goods they need or want by laborers and machines, and have these goods shipped to their home or to stores where they can secure them with financial resources (rather than using physical and artistic skill). We could go on and on. The differences between hunter-gatherers and modern people are substantial. While many would express marvel for the immense accomplishments of modern humans and their technological progress, these achievements (while amazing) have created an epidemic of weakness, disease, blunted awareness, and separation from that which sustains life. This doesn't suggest we should abandon modern science and technology (as some would declare), but that these developments should be grounded in an understanding of humans' long immersion in nature (i.e., our material knowledge should be infused with a nature philosophy).

AGRICULTURE: HUMANITY'S BIGGEST MISTAKE?

The advent of agriculture is sometimes described as humanity's biggest mistake. Many authors believe that agriculture is ultimately to be blamed for much of what has befallen humans. However, the fact that small-scale egalitarian farming communities who did not destroy their land bases have existed suggests that agriculture alone is not entirely responsible for dramatic shifts in social organization and world view. Perhaps most forms of agriculture utilized today are merely symptoms of the core issue (nature divorcement). While agriculture revolutionized the ability of humans to provide themselves with food (through concentrating food production), early forms of this mode of subsistence were not reliable and people experienced crop failures leading to starvation on a scale rarely experienced in hunter-gatherer cultures. While aboriginal people had a large diversity of different foods they utilized, agriculturalists relied on relatively few—and when these failed, the consequences were devastating. The switch to utilizing a smaller number of plant foods to provide a larger proportion of calories, even in the absence of crop failure, was harmful to human health. The shrinking bodies (and shrinking brains) of early agriculturalists, along with other aspects of health (e.g., dental caries, infections) demonstrate that these fewer foods (i.e., lower dietary diversity) could not sustain the physical form and certain aspects of health possessed by the indigenous that came before them.

Important to this discussion is that ancient people did not immediately transition to agriculture as a method of acquiring nutrition. It took people time to develop complete crop packages, whereby they could abandon hunting and gathering because their form of agriculture could supply most or all of their nutrition. Many eastern North American natives, for example, never developed complete crop packages and relied extensively on wild foods until colonization by Europeans interrupted their living. It should also be noted that indigenous people did practice the tending of certain plant populations, which would involve selective harvesting, weeding, coppicing, burning, and intentional planting of seeds and other propagules. However, these methods were generally targeting perennial species that could grow within intact natural communities (i.e., their methods did not require the felling of forests and tilling of the soil). What indigenous people practiced is better described as horticulture.

Understanding the difference between agriculture and horticulture requires an understanding of natural succession. Ecosystems are subjected to disturbances on a periodic basis. Such disturbances can include fire, flooding, landslides and avalanches, insect hordes, and intense wind storms. Disturbances that are severe enough to remove the existing plant life restart the vegetation sequence that occurs at a given site. For example, a catastrophic disturbance can kill a forest and eradicate the trees. In some cases, these catastrophes can remove the top layers of soil needed to support tree growth (e.g., high-intensity fire). After the disturbance, this open area is colonized by various lichens and/or herbaceous plants that ultimately contribute to soil by breaking down parent material and building organic matter through the death and decomposition of their bodies. Over time, a soil capable of supporting a diverse array of plants is formed. Ultimately, woody vegetation will return to the site and a forest canopy will again be formed. This process, of short-lived plants adapted to colonizing a disturbed site that are eventually replaced by (on average) longer-living, shade-tolerant species is called natural succession. It begins with a catastrophe and continues along through time until reset by another catastrophe.

Agriculture, as is commonly practiced in the world, requires the forest to be removed to create abundant light and eliminate competition for soil moisture and nutrition (i.e., it requires substantial manipulation of the landscape). Humans enter the site and, in most cases, fell the trees or burn the forest down, opening up the site. Then, to some degree, the soil is disturbed (through plowing and tilling) to allow planting of seeds or propagules and further removes competing vegetation (unfortunately, this process also causes losses in soil moisture and kills beneficial, symbiotic fungi). This process is, in effect, a catastrophe (from an ecological perspective). Agriculture continues the removal of unwanted plants, prevents tree growth, and breaks the soil again each year. This is necessary because the plants utilized in agriculture are primarily annual species that require open areas (i.e., they cannot grow in the shade of a forest). Therefore, it is completely appropriate to refer to agriculture as an endless cycle of catastrophes the land must endure. Such a process of producing food has, in most cases, led to the loss of topsoil, the pollution of waterbodies, and the inability of an area to support the array of life it did prior to commencement of agriculture. This stands in stark contrast to horticulture, which can utilize perennial species that can grow in intact plant communities (including the interior of forests). Many hunter-gatherer groups have practiced some form of horticulture. Its effect on the landscape was often so minimal that European colonizers did not even recognize that wild people were living (or had recently lived) in the area.

As marvelous as agriculture may seem, it did not come without costs (some of which we have already described). In addition to the physical changes that humans experienced when they began to consume a large proportion of their calories from a less diverse diet based and the human-induced catastrophe the landscape experienced, deep changes in human culture began to manifest in the different regions that took up extensive agriculture. Agriculture required a change in lifestyle from nomadic to sedentary (or largely sedentary) as crops were tended through the growing season. This delayed return system of providing nourishment also allowed the first form of storable wealth in the form of dried grain—a wealth that could be used to pay others to accomplish work and other tasks. It was not until agriculture appeared that substantive and widespread social stratification emerged, and with it different classes of people emerged, such as political or religious elite, warriors, and bureaucrats. An abundance of storable food, as sedentism and farming allow, created the first groups of people who were freed from the rigor of food procurement—the upper class. Entire ranks of people came into being who were fed by the toils of others. Prior to this time, all people (except those physically unable) took part in hunting and gathering (including the children).

Equally important, agriculture forced people to endure subservience. As a mobile hunter-gatherer, whenever someone came along and demanded something of them (such as labor or possessions), they simply refused and moved to a new location out of range of the demanding party. But as a sedentary agriculturalist that practices delayed-return food systems, you have too much invested in a plot of land. If the crops are still a month away from being harvested, and you were to leave to flee the demands of a ruling group, you would lose your investment and all of your potential food resources. Instead of fleeing, agriculturalists learned to submit and pay some of their wealth to avoid losing everything. Agriculture required that people yield to ruling parties and pay taxes (in some form) to people who were not part of an intimate community that shared resources for the benefit of all. This was a monumental change in human social dynamics that continues (in some form) today.

Finally, agriculture changed one of the fundamental goals of humanity. Species are required to adapt to their landscapes in order that they survive. Humans have a long history of technological advancements that have helped them to thrive everywhere they lived, including some of the world's most extreme climates. Better clothing came with the invention of the awl and needle, providing protection from inclement weather. The atlatl and bow allowed for greater food acquisition (especially for larger animals) at safer distances than previous methods. Humans learned to detoxify plants, allowing greater utilization of species and maximizing food resources from their landscape. Agriculture changed all of this. The goal was no longer to learn to adapt to the landscape. Rather, we endeavored to change the landscape. With adaptation no longer the goal, our bodies have suffered as we have attempted to control our world (a process that continues today). We now experience physical and physiological degeneration, processes that continue (progressively) as we move into the industrial age (a period of time where we are making larger and larger scale changes to our environment). Our bodies are now, in many ways, maladapted to the very land we occupy and the experiences we live. Agriculture was not humanity's first or biggest mistake, but, as commonly practiced, it has furthered us along a path leading to human weakness, illness, and advanced nature divorcement.

SUSTAINABILITY

The word "sustainable" is a too often used word in the world today. One cannot discuss sustainable practices without also discussing what it is that one is sustaining. For example, if one practices something that sustains the current level of habitat alteration (read "ecocide") or pollution being produced today, then such a practice cannot be deemed beneficial (even if it is sustainable). In other words, we need to take a new stance on the word sustainable, and request to know from growers and manufacturers what it is in fact they are sustaining. While the world actually needs rejuvenative practices (i.e., activities that heal people and landscapes), rather than just sustainable practices, that is another discussion for later in the book.

Let's step back and examine contemporary human's track record for sustainability. It is important to start with the region where agriculture on a large scale was invented: the Fertile Crescent. This region, which includes modern-day Iran, Iraq, Jordan, and Syria, was once an area so productive that it gave rise to civilization. It wasn't just farming and the domestication of plant and animals that this region produced, but also metal tools, writing, labor specialization, and full-time professionals. But, the agriculture they practiced, which had originally fed the growing population, also destroyed the land base and resulted in the conquering of this region by other people. Deforestation removed the trees that were, in part, responsible for holding the soils in place. Grazing domesticated animals (sheep and goats) prevented the forest from returning. Irrigation also caused an increase in salinity of the soil, resulting in a loss of soil productivity. All of the facets of the agricultural lifeway, including burgeoning human population, turned the forests of the Fertile Crescent into deserts in the span of approximately 8000 years.

The examples of civilizations falling due, at least in part, to human-induced ecological degradation or human population issues (or both) are not uncommon. They are historically attested and/or in the process of occurring in present day on all continents humans have lived. Specific features of ecological degradation include habitat destruction, soil fertility losses, water issues, overhunting, overfishing, introduction of invasive species, and increasing levels of toxins (the last one primarily a modern-day phenomenon). Overpopulation and increasing impact (to the landscape) of individual people are human population issues. These features have been written about extensively by Jared Diamond (such as in his book "Collapse: How Societies Choose to Fail or Succeed"). It should be noted that most of these human-induced ecological or human population issues are not (or rarely) observed in hunter-gatherers cultures.

But wait, didn't Paleoindian hunters wipe out the megafauna on the North American continent (i.e., isn't that an example of overhunting)? Actually, no. This idea, that humans caused the extinction of the large mammals found on this continent, such as the mammoth and mastodon, is called the overkill hypothesis. However, these mammals actually experienced substantial population declines prior to the arrival of humans on this continent. It has been estimated that between 75 and 90 percent of the original populations were gone when early hunter-gathers arrived here. There was a brief period of partial population recovery and a time spanning approximately 1000 years when humans and the megafauna coexisted. And while Paleoindians in some regions of the continent did hunt these animals, there also exist regions (e.g., northeastern North America) where the animals occurred in large numbers but their modified remains, as would occur during butchering, have not been found in early hunter-gatherer camps (as presented in research by Boulanger and Lyman). This does indicate that humans are not the sole cause of the extinction of these animals (evidence actually points to climate and environmental change). Certainly, this is not to say that hunter-gatherers have not caused any extinctions because they have, including the large flightless birds of New Zealand called moas (genus *Dinornis*) and several large animals on the Australian island-continent. But if we want to compare statistics, it is estimated that between 35 and 200 species now go extinct every day, largely as a result of human activity on the planet, a rate that is over 1000 times the background rate of extinction. And while there are real issues with attempting to calculate extinction rates (and that these figures may be exaggerated), it is also considered by most biologists that we have entered the earth's six mass extinction period (again, as a result of human activity).

I believe a brief discussion of a single food species will help to better illustrate the issue of sustainability and the differences between indigenous and contemporary resource management. Rick and colleagues (published in 2016 in the Proceedings of the National Academy of Sciences of the United States) examined the collection history of the eastern oyster (*Crassostrea virginica*) in the Chesapeake Bay of Maryland. This wild species of shellfish has been harvested for food for at least 3500 years by Native Americans. In that time, despite frequent harvesting, climate change, and rising sea levels, the indigenous people did not cause declines in the oyster populations. This sustainable use can be evidenced by studying the shell middens, which are piles of discarded shells from the oysters after the organism was removed from their protective valves. Within these prehistoric middens, the abundance of shells and size distribution of gathered mollusks were examined closely by the researchers. Studies on shellfish from around the world demonstrate that as collecting intensity becomes too high, the size of the shells decreases because the mollusks do not have sufficient time to grow to a large size prior to being collected. In this case, the continual presence of large shells in the Chesapeake Bay demonstrates that the oysters were being collected in a sustainable fashion. Today, the eastern oyster has been depleted to 1% of the former populations. Reasons for the depletion include over-harvest, polluted waters, destruction of estuarine habitat, and diseases (brought on by water quality declines). It took domesticated humans a few centuries to destroy an abundance of life that indigenous people utilized for a few millennia. It is important to note that the modern-day declines of important wild food species, like the eastern oyster, are rarely based exclusively on over-collection—it is often the concurrent habitat degradation that results in greater losses of life.

Using North America as an example, humans have occurred on this continent for approximately 19,000 years (give or take, research concerning this date is ongoing, see Bourgeon and colleagues study published in 2017). In that time, they spread to all corners of the continent and lived as hunter-gatherers for most of that time. Agriculture first appeared in the eastern half of the continent 3800 years ago; however, the agriculture did not represent a complete crop package, so some hunting and gathering was still practiced. In most parts of the country, agriculture did not arrive until significantly later (or not at all prior to contact). In that time, the natural resources of this continent were used and tended. When the Europeans began to arrive in large numbers (primarily after 1620), they believed that in some parts of the country they were entering an uninhabited wilderness. Early explorers commented on the pristine nature of the forests, not realizing that these lands had been recently occupied and, in some cases, modified by indigenous people (using techniques that resembled natural processes). This speaks volumes as to the kind of land management that was primarily utilized. But once Europeans arrived, things began to change rapidly and dramatically. In less than 400 years, contemporary humans have taken a landmass with vast wilderness and converted much of it to an agricultural and industrial region. At present, 99% of the tall-grass prairie has been lost. Tilling of the soil and loss of native, deep-rooted grasses resulted in the loss of ten feet of topsoil in some locations during the Dust Bowl of the 1930s. We have lost over half of our original wetlands in the United States, these converted to other uses through landscape alteration. Over ⅔ of United States estuaries and bays are degraded due to agricultural runoff. Twenty-five percent of US beaches are closed every year due to pollution, this owed (in part) to over 10 trillion gallons of untreated sewage, waste water, and industrial waste entering American water ways every year. Even our own drinking water is not safe—73 different pesticides have been found in US groundwater (which forms part of our drinking water supply). Apex predators (such as the grizzly bear and gray wolf) have been extirpated from most of the regions they formerly occurred. Even in my home state, Maine, where we pride ourselves on natural resources, there is a sizable list of species that no longer occur here after Europeans arrived, including the woodland caribou, wolverine, eastern wolf, timber rattle snake, mountain lion, and Atlantic walrus (this list does not include species that are now extinct, such as the great auk, sea mink, and passenger pigeon). These facts (and many pages more of them that could be listed) indicate that the agricultural/industrial mode of existence, at least as currently practiced, is anything but sustainable.

As a final line of evidence for the lack of sustainability of civilizations that practice nature divorcement, we can examine the track record of longevity of agricultural societies. The longest continually existing civilization was the Roman Empire, which lasted 1480 years. While some would contend China's current civilization to be the oldest (stating an age of 3600 years), it has been overthrown many times and was conquered by the Mongol Empire in the late 1200s. Even the National Aeronautics and Space Administration (NASA) recently funded (in part) a study that demonstrates the near inevitable collapse of complex, socially stratified societies (this study was based on the "Human And Nature DYnamical" (HANDY) model). If we compare hunter-gatherers, it is easy to find continually existing cultures that have survived much longer. For example, the Hadza of Tanzania have existed for approximately 10,000 years. Even longer are the Australian aborigines, who have persevered for approximately 50,000 years as hunter-gatherers. These timespans strongly suggest that worldview and the consequent manner of interacting with the world are strongly correlated with a culture's longevity. Said another way, cultures that practice nature connection (i.e., ecocentric living) have demonstrated sustainability on a scale not matched by those who exercise nature divorcement (i.e., egocentric living).

THE UNANSWERED QUESTION

Recognizing that contemporary humans share many features in common with domesticated animals relative to their wild progenitors, and that our wild ancestors were hunter-gatherers, we still have an unanswered question. And that is: who or what is responsible for the domestication of humans? Asked another way: who or what changed the selective pressures to produce the plainly visible traits of domestication found in modern humans? If we were to examine other domesticated animals, such as cows, pigs, or sheep, it can be seen that humans domesticated these animals through altering aspects of the animals' physical and social environment, producing something different from the wild forms of these species. One interesting hypothesis declares that species of wheat, including emmer (*Triticum dicoccum*) and einkorn (*Triticum monococcum*) (and other cultivated plants) were responsible for our morphological, anatomical, and ecological changes. Essentially, wheat's value to humans led us to change the very nature of our species in order to reap the benefits of its cultivation. However, the forms of wheat that ultimately came to exist did not occur in nature—humans created them through a selective breeding process. Therefore, the real task is to determine what allowed humans to remain in one place and focus on tending fields and breeding plants to produce desired qualities.

Agriculture is a process of food intensification, it generates more food per unit area than that observed in other food production systems (e.g., foraging, perennial horticulture). To manage this delayed-return system, humans had to transition away from nomadism to sedentism, a strategy that allowed them to remain in place and focus on growing annual grasses for nourishment. And what allowed this sedentary behavior was none other than the constructed environment, including significant landscape alterations that did not mimic natural processes (e.g., tilling, irrigation canals) and the house, a structure that provided substantial protection from the elements but also accelerated the process of separation from nature. This constructed environment was responsible for a decline in nutrition and dietary diversity because early agriculturalists consumed fewer hunted and gathered foods and ate more cultivated plants. This setting meant that humans received enough calories (though not necessarily enough nourishment) to spend less time roaming the landscape, leading to a measurable reduction in the robustness of musculoskeletal system. The protection afforded by the home led to real changes in what we could endure in environmental extremes and began a process of psychological dependence on the indoor setting.

The constructed environment, with its greater food production, fostered an increase in local human populations. This led to the perceived necessity of leaders (hereditary, elected, or otherwise) who would represent a larger group of people, which was the beginning of social hierarchy. Without a need to carry all of one's belongings to new encampments, the home became a location where material wealth could be stored and accumulated, which would eventually contribute to the appearance of wealth inequality. It changed the way we viewed our landscape and facilitated nature divorcement as we spent more time behind the walls of our domiciles and more effort modifying the landscape to grow desirable crops. This environment, epitomized by the house, can be seen to have created new selection pressures that changed the physical body and human social organization. It is the very place you are likely sitting now, while you read this book, that facilitated the taming of humans. Who created the constructed environment? Clearly, it was humans themselves. They were responsible for their own domestication—they self-domesticated through interacting with the constructed environment.

REGAINING ANCESTRAL HEALTH: THE NEOABORIGINAL PATH

We have been discussing in this chapter many positive features of indigenous living. While focusing on physical health, we have touched on other aspects of living, such as happiness, philosophical outlook, and effects of different world views on the surrounding landscapes. To be very clear, there is no attempt being made here to suggest that all aspects of hunter-gatherer life were superior to today's living. Further, there is no suggestion being offered that we should (or even can) return to this lifeway. Our landscapes have become too fragmented for most people to return to a hunter-gatherer style of living, and in places where this is possible, most people are either unskilled or too weak (or both) to live in this manner. Therefore, what is being posited is that we should incorporate those practices that produced better health outcomes. In some cases, we can practice hunter-gatherer lifestyle elements without modification. In other cases, the various elements of their lifeway would require modification into something we can perform today. The indigenous people of the world (prior to extensive and disruptive contact) demonstrated that humans are capable of living long, happy lives free of chronic disease (including cancer) in a way that was not destructive to the world. Moreover, it produced health through the generations (rather than escalating illness) while demonstrating actual sustainability. Where possible, it would be desirable to emulate aspects of their living to achieve similar results.

The examination of indigenous cultures was necessary for two important reasons: (1) this is our ancestry and (2) we must examine entire groups of people to identify health outcomes. The hunter-gatherers (past and present) are our wild ancestors. Aspects of the environment that they experienced and became adapted to are now built into our genetic framework. It is clear that our genes and their genes are very similar. We are essentially (from a genetic standpoint) hunter-gatherers who experience a tremendous incongruity in what our bodies require and are adapted to and what our bodies currently receive and experience. Humans have practiced a hunter-gatherer lifeway for most of their existence (archaic humans appeared approximately 500,000 years ago, agriculture around 10,000 years ago, though later for many parts of the world). Given this, our bodies (and our genes) are designed for a style of life that we do not experience and it is illogical not to consider these facts when designing a strategy for health. In other words, diets and lifestyles that do not consider human evolutionary history are unlikely to succeed through the generations. Equally important, one needs to examine entire communities living a similar lifeway to fully understand the effects of their diet and lifestyle on their health. This is perhaps best demonstrated by observing the Standard American Diet, which is documented to have deplorable health outcomes for many people. Yet, many of us know someone who has lived a long and relatively healthy life despite this diet. These resilient individuals are not proof that this diet is healthy (abundant research states otherwise), only that some mitigating factors (such as healthy prior generations) have allowed them to survive despite a diet bereft of nutrition and filled with synthetic additives. Making a dietary gamble based on a few individuals that demonstrate a measure of health in an otherwise unhealthy population is not good practice. We must look at what a diet and lifestyle usually produces in an entire population to assess its actual impact.

Now, if it has been possible, through the writing thus far, to convince you that something is amiss, that contemporary humans have taken a horrible turn by leaving a nature-connected mode of living, the next most difficult task may be to convince you that you have control of your health. You are much more than merely your genes and your family history. It is very clear today that many diseases considered to have a strong genetic influence are, in fact, not genetic diseases at all. People don't simply inherit genes from their parents, they also inherit lifestyles (that produce similar results). In other words, if the diet and lifestyle of your parents produced type 2 diabetes in one or both of them, it is likely to do the same to you. However, that does not imply you were fated to experience diabetes—beneficial alterations to your diet and exercise patterns can prevent diabetes from occurring (and a host of other ailments). Additionally, it is now realized that genetic expression (i.e., how our genes function) can be influenced by nutrition, exercise, positive experiences, and other beneficial features of life (likewise, poor diet, lack of exercise, and chronic stress can negatively affect genetic expression). This concept, that we are not merely our genetic code, but how our genetic code is influenced by our environment, is referred to as epigenetics. It is a key that frees us from the lock made by previous generations. It is such an important concept that we will dedicate space in chapter 3 to its understanding. In summary, you can alter your path, and with the right tools, experience health and fulfillment.

Earlier in this work (chapters 1 and 2), I presented evidence that contemporary humans are a domesticated subspecies of our wild progenitor. In those discussions, hunter-gatherers (the wild progenitors) were referred to as *Homo sapiens sapiens*, and modern people (the domesticates) were named *Homo sapiens domesticofragilis*. Present-day humans became domesticated by following a path that led to various changes in their physical form, social structure, food procurement methods, world view, etc. This path can be shown to have weakened humans physically, creating tamed versions of our wild ancestors. But this is not a path we need walk. We can forge a new path that reclaims our wild health, strength, and awareness. Most importantly, we can walk a path that generates deep nature connection, so that once again we can travel through forests (or prairies, or deserts) as part of those landscapes, familiar with the life that exists there. We can walk of a path of forward-thinking people who reclaim biological equality and seek to participate in our local ecology. Imagine a life with the following attributes:

- knowledge of what to eat that creates healthy adults and healthy children who do not succumb to chronic disease, whereby nutritional dogma and dietary fads can be recognized and avoided;

- grasp of the fact that human nourishment includes much more than just food, and without these elements, true health is not possible;

• comprehension of how the modern water supply (in its many forms) is harmful to a long life free of cancer, and how to go about acquiring wild water;

• an understanding of what true medicine and holistic healing are, allowing many people to break free from failed therapeutic approaches promulgated by rigid practitioners of western medicine;

• a deep desire to move on a daily basis, this yearning created by an accurate understanding of what happens to our bodies when we sit motionless day after day, building a strong body that is adapted to the place it resides;

• similarly, building a body that is infused with nature strength, allowing a body to cope with the elements and better experience the regional landscapes as a wild animal;

• movement through life fully aware, with an ability to see the real and potential connections that exist around us, enabling every person to build their own relations for well-being;

• having a set of factual criteria that help us minimize harm as we navigate the market place, criteria that are free of green-washing and other false claims;

• truly feel like an integral member of the biosphere, to feel that your place is a special one, and that your gifts can be realized and shared for the benefit of all life.

All of this is possible by rectifying our past with our present and setting our sights on a possible future. If one manner of living can create health problems, blunted awareness, and loss of connection to nature, then another manner of living can heal these ailments. Rather than continuing on the path of domestication, we can choose a feral road, one that leads to the recovery of wildness. This is not a call for anarchy, rather a call for the special attributes found in wild humans. Because we cannot go back to being hunter-gatherers (at least not all of us), we must find a new path forward that allows anyone living in any location to progress down a wild path, with each generation further transcending the current domesticated condition. In essence, we need a new indigenous person, one that knows how to walk intelligently and softly on this planet. To provide a name to this person, we can combine the Latin *neo* (meaning new) with *aborigine* (meaning original, indigenous, from the beginning) to create a new epithet: *Homo sapiens neoaboriginalis*, the new aboriginal wise man.

This book is about the rewilding path, one named "the new aboriginal". Contained within this work are successful strategies for reversing and ultimately rising above human domestication. It is not simply a book about diet, or medicine, or movement, or community, because all of those things (and more) are needed for health in humans. Taking a more holistic examination of *Homo sapiens*, and grounding modern study with historical observations, we can generate individual awareness that will build, with time, into communal awareness. Most importantly, we can treat the actual root issue of the ailments we experience today: the belief we are separate from the earth. To do this, we must stop living in a short-sighted fashion and understand everything we do to the world today to appease our need for material wealth, instant gratification, and perpetual comfort is preventing future generations from experiencing a vital life. As Wendell Berry stated in his 1971 article in the magazine Audubon:

"We can learn about it from exceptional people of our own culture, and from other cultures less destructive than ours. I am speaking of the life of a man who knows that the world is not given by his fathers, but borrowed from his children; who has undertaken to cherish it and do it no damage, not because he is duty-bound, but because he loves the world and loves his children."

I will expand on Berry's statement to advance that if you truly love your children, then you will desire to give them health (at birth) and a world capable of supporting their health (throughout life). This is cannot be accomplished by adhering to the Standard American Lifeway (and that practiced in other affluent countries). However, a life that creates healthy individuals and healthy ecosystems can be had by embracing a new path. This path is one where humans consider themselves part of the earth, and, therefore, understand that what we do to the world we do to ourselves. Which path will you choose, that of *Homo sapiens domesticofragilis* or *Homo sapiens neoaborigalis*?

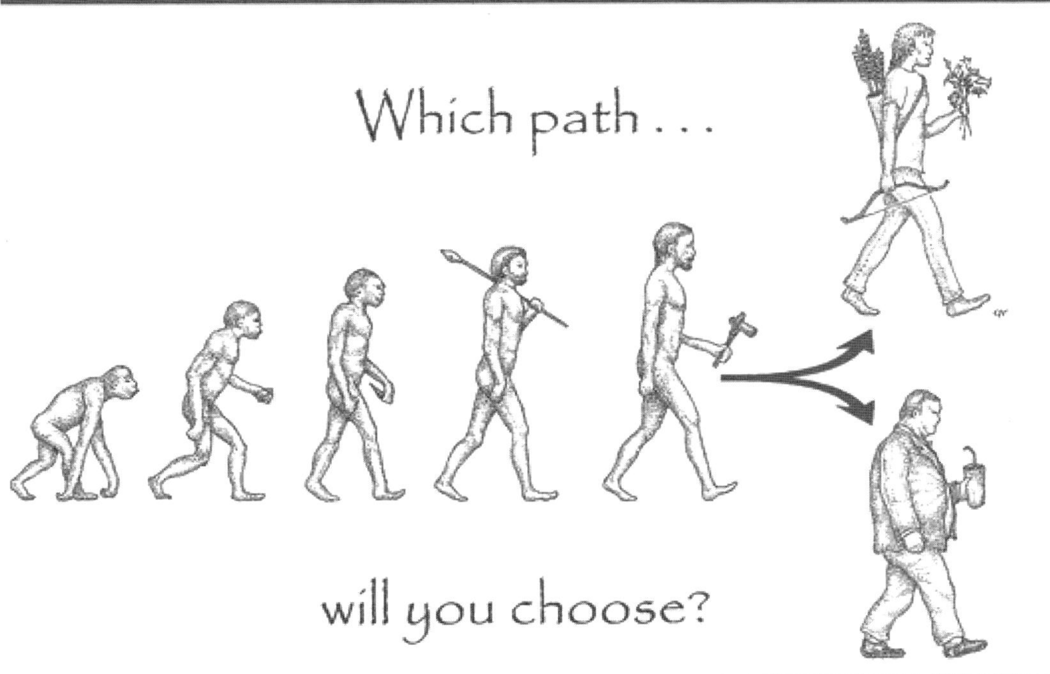

Illustration by Elizabeth Farnsworth.

3. Deep nutrition: the real human diet

There was a time when there were no questions about what you were to eat. Dietary wisdom was part of your cultural heritage. You (or members of your community if you were very young) knew exactly what organisms would be gathered as nourishment, where and when they could be found, and how they would be prepared. This latter step (preparation) was elaborate for some species to maximize nutrition and reduce or eliminate antinutrients and toxins. This information was handed down from very early on and became part of the individual's understanding of their landscape. It was a component of human ecology. There were no debates, no arguments, and no factions based on foods that were to be avoided. Scientific study was not needed because the foods were not highly processed, did not contain synthetic ingredients, were not sprayed with chemicals, and were not genetically modified in a laboratory (though some were genetically modified; more on this later in the chapter). Today, this is all different. Individuals, organizations, and governmental agencies all have different information and assert that different foods (or ratios of foods) should be eaten. They all have studies that support their stances, though some of these studies can be shown to have major shortcomings (primarily because many begin with *a priori* assumptions about a particular food or study the food out of context). Any individual who is actually open to new information will be completely confused because of confounding and contradictory published research. As importantly, diet has become a major defining characteristic of some people; therefore, anything that impacts their belief system is to be blocked, ridiculed, and/or systematically attacked, often with substantial amounts of pejorative language. The interesting part of this entire debate—almost all of these diets (even those with ardent supporters) fail to include a necessary characteristic for any diet.

INTERGENERATIONAL HEALTH

Diets are not simply supposed to nourish adults in a manner that protects them from chronic disease. This is low hanging fruit—many diets can accomplish this objective. Diets are supposed to create healthy and well-formed children. This is a much more difficult to achieve objective and many diets fail to deliver it. It is, in fact, the highest measure of the success of a diet—transferring health through the generations. Isn't it an obvious question: what value is a diet that can sustain adults but fail to provide the necessary nourishment for a developing human? It is surprising how infrequently this question is asked. If you examine the list of accomplishments of any fad diet, they include such things as losing weight, looking younger, boosting energy levels, and helping build muscle. These are all valuable goals but they are also selfish goals as they focus on the individual and not the next generation. Extending life is also an often-touted goal of certain diets, which (to put it bluntly) plays to the individual ego and fails to take into consideration what shortcomings a diet may have for fetuses, children, and young adults.

The clear goal of any diet should be to nourish a developing human to reach adulthood in a manner that is free of any ailment or deformity (i.e., the child should become a healthy and well-formed adult). If we were to hypothetically examine a young child with rickets, which could present as severely bowed femurs, it would be clear (in most cases) that the child's diet was inadequate because rickets is usually caused by insufficient vitamin D in the diet (though other causes are known). Assuming normal vitamin and mineral metabolism, everyone would agree that the diet (and, potentially in this case, the lifestyle) did not supply the child with adequate nutrition. Now, continuing with this idea, if a child grows into an adult with crowded, crooked, and/or impacted teeth with malocclusion (i.e., poor bite pattern), very few people will consider this a deformity, and fewer still will examine the actual cause—which is diet, one lacking deep nutrition and enough substantive texture to properly stress the bones of the jaw and maxillae. The primary reason for this is because this deformity, to lesser or greater extents, is so prevalent in Americans that we do not want to consider the common situation to be a defect based, in large part, on insufficient nourishment. Surveys of malocclusion rates in US adults place this as high as 70% (that is, 7 out of 10 adults have a deformity of the skull). Just over 65% of Americans have one or more impacted third molars (i.e., wisdom teeth), indicating there is not enough room in the mouth to fit all the teeth. The work of Weston Price has documented the role of diet in malocclusion and impacted teeth. Further, archeological work demonstrates shape changes in the skull, especially the mandible (i.e., jawbone), when humans began farming, which represented a major shift in diet (one that did not supply adequate nutrition). Based on this, any diet that does not provide for healthy skull formation with a broad palate and room in the mouth for well-aligned teeth is deficient in one or more elements. Hunter-gatherer diets almost universally produced proper alignment and spacing of teeth (i.e., good occlusion, no impacted teeth). It should be disturbing to anyone that today we infrequently produce skulls with our ancestral form (i.e., we rarely express what our genes sequences are capable of producing).

This book will discuss diets that have been practiced for, in some cases, many thousands of years. These are diets that have a track record of producing health, vitality, and proper physical form generation after generation. Many diets that are promulgated today have no such evidence of benefit. Even though they may have existed for decades or centuries, few if any people have relied exclusively on those diets from birth to death for multiple generations—which is the only way a diet can actually be examined for its long-term effects on human health and build. We are facing the dietary predicament that we experience today because people have forgotten that diets need long-term proof of value (which can be attained through historical observation and archeological study). Many people convert to a specific diet as adults, experience relative improvement in their health (which would occur for many on almost any diet that avoided chemically grown, highly processed foods) and become convinced this diet should be practiced by everyone. Think about what they have done: they have experienced a level of healing from a new diet (which is valuable), and then gone on to assume this diet will be appropriate for all ages of all races living in all places with absolutely no evidence of how this diet will transfer through the generations. Looking at it from a scientific perspective, all they have actually determined is that the diet they are trying out (i.e., experimenting with) has increased **their** health in this time and place (the emphasis on the word "their" is to highlight the diet may not benefit their children or, for that matter, other-than-human persons). Another stage in their life or another environment with different demands on their body and said diet may not offer the same advantage or provide enough of certain nutritional elements. Given that many people do not practice a diet that has been used continuously for many generations, any statements they provide about its value are merely anecdotal. This is not to say they are without value, but, again, the long-term effects of novel diets are largely unknown, meaning that people who practice these diets are acting as Guinea pigs in a nutritional experiment. This is certainly not a gamble I want to take with myself or my child.

THE DIET OF *HOMO SAPIENS*

People today are highly confused about diet. They simply cannot determine any longer what the actual human diet is (and there is one, with many variations). Having lost their connection to nature and living without realization of their own domestication creates a situation where they are unable to see how arbitrary (for lack of a better word) many diets actually are. Confounding the situation further is the overwhelming amount of literature stating one thing or another about nutrition. Many statements that can be found in print and online are directly contradicted by observations of people who practiced various diets (details to be provided later in this chapter). In order for us to determine what a healthy diet that can provide intergeneration health is, we must realize that seeking answers from data gathered exclusively on domesticated humans will have major shortcomings. Said another way, do you want to be a wolf or poodle?

Let us use a hypothetical example. In this example we have a zoo that has just acquired a chimpanzee (*Pan troglodytes*). This particular zoo has never housed a primate before, so they are unsure about its diet. Fortunately, this zoo is wealthy, and they have the funding to follow several different avenues for determining what they will feed the chimpanzee. The zoo keepers have essentially three options they could follow:

(1) research what wild chimpanzees eat in their native range and acquire those foods;

(2) build a diet using domesticated foods that most closely mimics the ancestral diet of the chimpanzee;

(3) make up a diet based various factors (some of which may not relate to nutrition at all) and wait and see how the chimpanzee responds to the diet.

Each one of these potential diets has advantages and disadvantages, though from a nutritional standpoint, it is likely that number 1 would be best, and number 3 would be worst. The chimpanzee hails from western and central Africa, where it has a long evolutionary history of living in this region. Chimpanzees split from their closest extant relative (bonobos, *Pan paniscus*) about 1 million years ago. Therefore, their nutritional needs would be closely tied to the foods they have experienced over that time. Studying wild chimpanzees to identify the kinds and ratios of foods they consume would best provide the same nutrition to the captive chimpanzee (even better, if the zoo keepers could provide a habitat that allowed for similar movement as in the wild, the captive individual would experience even better health while in the zoo setting). However, a fully wild diet for this captive chimpanzee might be impossible from a practical sense. Gathering wild foods requires time and expertise. Such foods would also require transport and storage to the zoo location (which could be a continent away).

The second option might be a best practical solution. Research into the macro- and micronutrient profiles of wild chimpanzee food could then allow a replicated diet using cultivated foods. While the replication would not be perfect (there are differences, sometimes manifest, between wild and cultivated plant foods), such foods would be widely available and much easier for the zoo keepers to acquire. Keep in mind, human study has shown that a diet based primarily on cultivated plants does not support human health and form in the way a wild one does (as discussed in chapter 2). Also note that in this diet, the practical ability to acquire wild foods is a driving factor in what the captive chimpanzee is fed (i.e., the nutritional requirements are no longer the sole criteria for what to feed the animal). Therefore, while perhaps the best practical solution, this is unlikely to be the best nutritional solution.

Diet number 3 would likely be the worst diet of all for the captive chimpanzee. Such a diet would have no track record of producing health in this species of primate and might offer highly distorted nutrient profiles compared with what the chimpanzee physiology requires (even in captivity). This "made up" diet would likely use several criteria that have nothing to do with nutrition, including use of foods that are available in abundance (but not necessarily the most nutrient dense), avoiding foods that are deemed off limits by a certain religions, relying on human cultural bias to drive food choices, or prohibiting foods based on personal beliefs that do not relate to nutrition. While these might seem like odd criteria to use, they are commonly utilized to fabricate contemporary human diets (often with poor consequences). Of course, with this diet, there would also be an ethical issue for consideration—feeding a captive chimpanzee a diet that is new to chimpanzee existence is using the individual as a test subject (and likely against the test subject's wishes).

So what is the diet of *Homo sapiens*? We can use the chimpanzee example above almost without modification to identify the best possible human diet. For now, we will be discussing nutritional considerations only (other important factors will come into the discussion later in this chapter). If you were tasked with finding out what a chimpanzee eats, would you visit a zoo or research wild populations (assuming you had the means to accomplish either approach)? Given that the zoo would be feeding the chimpanzee a diet based, in part, on considerations other than nutritional, clearly these animals would not be experiencing a diet that best matches what they acquired from their landscape (and what their bodies are adapted to consuming). Visiting a zoo to acquire information on the dietary habits of a chimpanzee would only provide information about what they are fed in captivity. Would you visit a jail to identify the best possible diet for humans? Wild chimpanzees would hold the key to understanding their species' nutritional requirements and intake.

We could use any number of similar examples to frame this dietary question. If one wanted to determine the actual diet of the dog, would it be more useful (and accurate) to study the diet of the wolf (wild) or a poodle (domesticated)? The poodle would likely be eating a dried kibble, a food that would include a proportion of grain (the fruit of a grass—something not consumed by wolves) and other filler ingredients (like cultivated legumes and potatoes) that would not be part of the ancestral diet of the dog. Further, many brands of dog food provide an altered macronutrient profile (e.g., kibble is richer in carbohydrates than the ancestral dog diet), contains foods new to canines (as noted above), contains foods less nutrient-dense than the wild foods they evolved to consume, includes synthetic preservatives (in less expensive brands), and sometimes has artificial coloring. And, as it turns out, domesticated dogs suffer a suite of health problems due to the food provided to them, including allergies, anemia, organ failure due to toxic exposure, dental caries, periodontal disease, gastrointestinal issues, inflammation, obesity, heart disease, and cancer. This occurs because dog food kibble is a poor match to their wild-type diet. It is important that you note the similarities here between some of the health issues faced by domesticated dogs and those faced by domesticated humans (i.e., us). Given that most people today eat the human equivalent of dog food, let us agree that the diet of *Homo sapiens* should not be determined by people who are unable to live without chronic disease and altered physical form (again, us). Therefore, to identify what the human diet is, we should examine wild humans (i.e., indigenous people practicing their traditional lifestyle) and study what they eat.

TRAITS OF HUNTER-GATHERER DIETS

Since long before anatomically modern humans appeared on this planet, human ancestors have been hunting and gathering wild food from their landscapes. Early on in hominid history, most foods were selected that could be gathered with relative ease (i.e., no specialized tools were required). As time passed, specialized tools began to appear, such as a sharpened digging stick to unearth carbohydrate-rich storage organs of plants (e.g., tubers, bulbs, taproots, rhizomes) and simple stone blades that could cut flesh from the bones of scavenged animals. A progression of increasingly sophisticated tools occurred, culminating in items like fishing nets and lures, various traps and weirs, the harpoon, and the hunting bow. Each landscape required its own set of tools and techniques to secure nourishment (including energy) because each landscape had its own set of plants and animals that interacted with a unique setting and climate. Therefore, each group of people around the world could be identified, in part, by the foods they ate and the tools they used to acquire, transport, store, and prepare the wild foods that formed their diet. Further, these tools did not include just hunting weapons, but also the skillfully woven baskets and other containers that foods were gathered in, the ceramic vessels they were cooked in, and the bark vessels they were stored in. And while each hunter-gatherer group was distinct in its assemblage of tools and foods items, there were commonalities among all of them that define the human diet prior to domestication (i.e., as long as humans have occurred, they have practiced the following dietary traits). The twelve traits of hunter-gatherer diets follow.

1. Omnivory. All hunter-gatherer cultures consumed plant and animal foods (as well as fungi and bacteria). In other words, there were no strict vegetarian groups. In fact, this would not have been possible in most places on earth due to seasonality of plant foods. Only with the advent of long-distance transportation did it become possible for people in affluent countries to practice such a diet. The proportion of different kinds of foods eaten by hunter-gatherers was dependent on location and season. Those living in the far north consumed diets that were very rich in animal foods (up to 99% of the diet); though they did not eat exclusively animal foods and prized many plant foods while available. Some hunter-gatherer groups ate a higher proportion of plant foods (only 26% of the diet coming from animal foods), and even consumed plant foods only for weeks at a time during certain periods of the year. Ominivory assured that the people received not only a diversity of nutritional elements, but also received the most active forms of certain vitamins and essential fats (e.g., vitamin A, vitamin D, omega-3 fatty acids), resulting in much higher actual vitamin levels than contemporary people receive (more on this later in the chapter). Omnivory has been practiced by hominids long before anatomically modern humans appeared (cut marks on bones demonstrate that early hominids were consuming animal foods ca. 3.4 million years ago; anatomically modern humans are much younger than this at approximately a few hundred-thousand years old).

2. Uncooked and Cooked. Hunter-gatherers ate a mixture of uncooked and cooked foods. Even in tropical locations, where fires were not required for heat, fires were maintained for cooking (and other purposes). Some plants were consumed without being heated, others required cooking to detoxify them or help reduce antinutrient concentrations. Likewise, animal foods were sometimes cooked, and other times, some portions (or the entirety) of animals were eaten raw. This dietary trait ensured that heat-sensitive nutrients were acquired in the diet. However, contrary to popular belief, many nutritional elements are not destroyed with heat, and cooking makes some dietary features more bioavailable to the body. Cooking serves not only to kill pathogens, but also pre-digests food through denaturing proteins and gelatinizing starches, which allows more energy to be acquired from certain food items. Cooking food dates back over 1 million years (i.e., it predates the appearance of *Homo sapiens*); therefore, humans did not start cooking at some point in their history, they inherited cooking from their hominid ancestors. Note that the term "raw" is not being used here to denote uncooked foods. While raw (in some dietary circles) simply means uncooked, some uncooked foods, including those that are dried, soaked, leached, and sprouted, are chemically altered (sometimes significantly) from the foods actual raw state (i.e., fresh from the landscape). These methods of preservation and/or preparation are not here treated as raw (though they are uncooked).

3. Full Utilization. Indigenous people consumed a larger portion of the animal than contemporary people, eating marrow, organs, fat, roe, skin, and other parts of the animal (when possible). Such utilization of the animal meant they did not consume the relative amount of lean muscle meat that contemporary people do (which has important ramifications for cancer, as described later in this chapter). Modern practices in urbanized regions focus on consumption of what is essentially the least nutritious part of the animal, in contrast with hunter-gatherers who prized organ meats (the most nutrient-dense part of the animal), which is further indication our loss of dietary wisdom. Some organ meats, like the liver and heart, supply massive amounts of nutrition and are true super foods. Further, organs often accumulate specific nutritional elements that they require lots of for vital functioning; therefore, consumption of organ meats benefits that organ in the people who consumed them. The full utilization of the animal by hunter-gatherers also means they received a higher proportion of certain lipids in the diet than many contemporary people do and wasted less of the animals they killed.

4. Food Diversity. Wild people ate a large number of plant and animal species, incorporating a great diversity of kinds in their diet. The exact species were dependent on location, and were influenced by many variables, including latitude, elevation, rainfall, climate, proximity to large water bodies, etc. Diversity in the diet protects against nutritional deficiencies as different foods contain different amounts and, equally important, ratios of vitamins, minerals, essential fatty acids, and kinds of fiber. Food diversity also protects against food scarcity (i.e., the more choices one has, the more likely one can secure adequate nutrition). Many hunter-gatherer groups in temperate regions and those closer to equator easily exceeded 100 species of plant in the diet, and this number does not include medicinal plants that were also ingested and contributed to the phytochemical diversity experienced by humans. People in affluent countries actually eat far fewer plant species than they realize because many kinds of plants found in supermarkets actually belong to the same species (more on this later in the chapter). Part of the nutrient deficiency experienced by modern humans relates to a diet consisting of too few foods.

5. Food Processing. Hunter-gatherers often employed specific processing techniques to reduce toxins, remove or deactivate antinutrients, and initiate breakdown of the foods (promoting improved digestibility). Food processing was a very important detail of the diet and resulted in chemical alterations to the food. Examples exist where toxic plant species were used as staples (i.e., the plants were toxic raw). Food processing techniques included cooking, drying, soaking, leaching, and diluting. None of these processing methods relied on industrial machines or chemicals, nor did they result in significant losses in food nutrition (as commonly occurs today). While modern methods of food processing are considered detrimental to the organisms eating the food (because they create highly processed foods), indigenous methods actually promoted health.

6. Seasonality. They ate seasonally (except for stored foods) and many foods were not consumed year-round (e.g., bird eggs, sweet fruits, migratory animals, greens and shoots) because they were not available. This limited the potentially harmful effects of any food that can be consumed in excess today. Some people had access to a variety of plant foods year-round, while others were extremely limited and relied extensively on animal foods. There were certainly many examples of foods that were stored, such as dried eel (*Anguilla rostrata*) among the Penobscot of central Maine, annual wild rice (*Zizania palustris*) among the Ojibwa of the Great Lakes region, and cloudberry (*Rubus chamaemorus*) among the Iñupiat of far northwestern

North America. However, hunter-gatherers did not store many kinds of foods and did not store the majority of the calories they would take in during the winter season (for temperate and more northern groups). The indigenous, in many ways, practiced a true seasonality of food that was not dependent on long-distance transportation from warmer regions.

7. Food Refinement. They utilized relatively simple means of refining the foods, including (but not limited to) grinding, drying, cooking, and soaking. They did not produce highly refined foods that had certain microscopic components removed. For example, though they did grind nuts and grains to produce flour, they did not remove the bran prior to grinding (a method that produces white flour). As such (and along with other details of their diets), there was no need for artificial ingredients or nutritional supplements. With few exceptions, seed oils were not consumed separate of the seed. Likewise, fructose was not consumed separate from the fruit. Therefore, isolated food components that can be harmful in quantity were almost always consumed within the context of whole food (i.e., with associated fiber and/or lipids).

8. Lipids. Hunter-gatherers had no social fear of certain kinds of fats. Saturated fats were consumed and were important components of their diets. The ratio of the essential fatty acids ω6 and ω-3 were consumed at approximately 1:1 to 3:1 ratios (the Greek letter ω is read as "omega"). However, most contemporary humans in urbanized countries consume a ratio between 8:1 and 24:1 (with notable exceptions, such as the Japanese). Hunter-gatherers consumed far less polyunsaturated fats than contemporary people, not utilizing the tremendous volume of plant seed oils (e.g., corn, soy, cotton, safflower) that contemporary people ingest. Further, the plant seed lipids were ingested with the food intact (i.e., not extracted), so the polyunsaturated fatty acids were protected from exposure to oxygen and sunlight, features that create oxidized fats that are damaging to cardiovascular health. The relative amount of lipids in the diet varied by location, but was generally within the range of 28–58% of the dietary calories (exceptions exist). It should be noted that no group consumed enough fat to remain in chronic ketosis (more on this in the section FATS FOR HEALTH later in this chapter).

9. Simple Sugars. Sweet, mono- and disaccharide sugars were part of indigenous diets (aside from fructose in fruit). Foods such as sugar and syrups (made from tree sap) and honey were highly sought after and specialized techniques and tools were employed to collect such foods. For example, in North America, several species of maple (genus *Acer*) and birch (genus *Betula*), among other trees, were tapped to collect their sap for creating syrup and sugar by evaporating the water. Honey was gathered on several continents, including Africa (Hadza), South America (Guarani), Asia (Onge), and the island-continent Australia (Aborigine). Reports exist of certain groups consuming large amounts of such foods during periods of the year and (in some cases) these foods were stored for later use. Sweet fruits were gathered by virtually all hunter-gatherers, including far northern peoples, and often dried or otherwise preserved for later use. Of course, such foods were not separated from their nutrition (i.e., refined) and contained vitamins, minerals, and antioxidants.

10. Natural Ingredients. The entire diet of hunter-gatherers was formed of natural ingredients that could be foraged, gathered, hunted, or collected from the landscapes they lived in. There were no synthetic ingredients, artificial preservatives, or chemical coloring agents in the diet. Further, there were no residual solvents, deodorizers, bleaches, herbicides, pesticides, fungicides, and other chemicals that were inadvertently consumed (as there are in industrial food systems). That said, not all dietary components were organic. For example, salt was used by some indigenous groups, this being sourced from mineral deposits, brine springs, or the ocean. In some cases, even plant ashes were used to flavor foods because of their salty taste. Geophagy (i.e., consumption of certain kinds of soil) has also been practiced by some hunter-gatherer groups to detoxify bitter foods (especially those soils rich in charged clay particles that can bind to certain plant toxins). While naturalness does not necessarily mean safe, hunter-gatherer diets are not barraged with novel ingredients that are new to humans (and the ultimate safety of such ingredients in concert with other new additives is poorly known).

11. Nutrient Dense. Wild foods are, on average, more nutrient dense than cultivated foods. The discussion here of nutrition is not limited to vitamins and minerals, but also plant compounds (i.e., phytochemicals), essential fatty acids, fiber, conjugated linoleic acid, and other important dietary components. The nutrient differences are most profound in plant foods because of the genetic changes from breeding in favor of sweeter taste, fewer seeds, larger size, less bitter taste, uniform ripening, ability to survive long-distance transport, etc. These genetic changes (due to breeding) have most affected the phytochemistry found in food plants such that modern foods provide less "medicine" (it has been, to various extents, bred out of cultivated plants). This lack of overall nutrition means that modern food supplies less protection from cancer, inflammation, and pathogens. With regard to animal foods, much of the differences in nutrition between domesticated and wild animals results from the diets they are fed (i.e., grain-fed animals have lower amounts of key nutritional elements). Due to a number of factors, hunter-gatherers were estimated to receive ten times the fat-soluble vitamins and four times the water-soluble vitamins and minerals that many contemporary people receive in their diets.

12. Wild. Hunter-gatherers consumed wild foods. While they did tend and even actively managed some plant populations (through burning, weeding, etc.), they were not consuming highly modified organisms (until they became agriculturalists). While many people today have an aversion for what are labeled as GMO (genetically modified organisms), those same people fail to realize that virtually all cultivated produce has been changed (often significantly) from the wild progenitor (i.e., modern produce is also genetically modified). These forms found in the supermarkets did not exist until humans created them. Wild foods are what humans have consumed for almost all of their existence, and it protected them from chronic diseases while preventing massive alterations to the landscape (which are required for cultivated produce and feed for domesticated animals).

These twelve traits are found in every hunter-gatherer group that has ever been observed. Given their health and longevity, and the fact this diet is what humans have evolved to consume (in its many variations), modern diets should attempt to emulate (as closely as possible) these traits. Trait 12 (wild) will be the most difficult to follow (but there are ways to approximate this; see Wild and Minimally Modified Plant Foods later in this chapter). Kinds of foods consumed and macronutrient profiles can vary significantly and still stay true to these twelve traits (allowing for tremendous flexibility). For example, plant foods in the diets of hunter-gatherers ranged from 1% of the total calories (Nunamiut of far northwestern North America) to 74% (Gwi of Kalahari region of Africa). Further, every region has its original wild foods (sacred foods, if you will) that each person today can still find and acquire (to some extent). Certainly not every aspect of hunter-gatherer diets was perfect. Starvation did occur at some frequency; however, that is no different from today, especially outside of affluent countries where hunger and starvation are not infrequent. Again, this is a call to bring forward those beneficial aspects of hunter-gatherer diets to provide nutrient-dense diets for contemporary people. Any diet that deviates significantly from these twelve traits is a novel diet that has no proven track record of intergenerational health (or, worse, has a well-documented consequence of chronic disease; e.g., Standard American Diet).

HOW FIRE HAS SHAPED US

One of the things that is critical for understanding the form of any organism is to realize how it derives its energy and nutrition from the landscape in which in lives. Consequently, a downy woodpecker is shaped very differently from a broad-winged hawk, in large part as result of differences (and resulting consequences to the body form) in how these two animals gather (i.e., capture) their food. Likewise, and more dramatic, the moose and gray wolf are tremendously dissimilar because they utilize manifestly different food sources—the moose utilizes plant foods that cannot flee from it and the wolf, primarily, utilizes animal foods that must be captured. All the animals discussed here are well suited to derive nutrition from their landscape. It can be viewed not only in their gross physical form, but also in their teeth, their digestive tracts, their brains, and their limbs.

If we were to examine anatomically modern humans, we would note what appears to be a disparity between their physical form and what they consume. As previously noted, all humans (until some recent domesticated humans) have consumed an omnivorous diet (which includes animals). We do not have the sharp claws and the prominent teeth of other mammalian predators. We also have digestive systems that do not act like a carnivore's digestive system. Briefly, most carnivores like canids (dogs) and felids (cats) hold food in the stomach much longer than humans and have intense muscular contractions to break down the lumps of food into small pieces. But anatomically modern humans also do not have the grinding dentition and large digestive tracts of herbivores. We are little like many plant predators. Even our close relatives, such as the chimpanzee (*Pan troglodytes*) and gorilla (*Gorilla gorilla*), who consume a large proportion of their food as plants, have powerful jaws, strong teeth, and larger digestive systems (to allow more time for fermentation of plant material by symbiotic bacteria). In fact, the human digestive system is only about 60% of the size it would be expected to be based on measurements of other primates. Further, we have much larger brains than would be expected compared with other primates. So what does all this say about the human species?

One of the interesting features that has changed over our evolutionary history is the size of our digestive system. It has gotten smaller over time as assessed through examination of the rib cage and pelvis. As discussed by Richard Wrangham in his book "Catching Fire: How Cooking Made Us Human", a more flaring rib cage and a wider pelvis are needed to house a larger gastrointestinal tract. Looking at the skeletons of extinct hominids, we can see that older forms have more flared rib cages and wider pelvises (such as *Homo habilis*, who lived approximately 2.1 to 1.5 million years ago) compared with younger forms like *Homo erectus* (who lived approximately 1.9 million to 70,000 years ago). Likewise, the rib cage was even less flared and pelvis proportionally narrower still in *Homo neanderthalensis* (who lived approximately 250,000 to 40,000 years ago). And while this was happening, there was a concurrent increase in the size of the brains. Why these two features of humans would be inversely correlated is not a mystery. The digestive system requires vast amounts of both energy and neural cells to coordinate the functioning of moving food along from the mouth to the anus and digesting that food. Over 100 million neurons make up the neural system that regulates digestion, approximately equal to the number found in the spinal cord. The body can only commit so many resources to this neural center without compromising resources to other neural centers, such as the brain. Therefore, a large enteric nervous system (that associated with the digestive tract) limits a large central nervous system (that associated with the brain and spinal cord). Therefore, any behavioral feature that would reduce the size of the digestion system could allow a larger size of the brain.

Studying the remains of extinct hominids also demonstrates other significant and progressive changes. These include decreasing size of dentition, decreasing mass of muscles associated with chewing, and weaker jaw bones. These traits indicate that there was an increasing proportion of softer food entering the diet. Softer food could include a higher proportion of animal foods, but as already noted, our teeth and stomachs are unlike carnivores. Further, we know from archeological sites and analysis of starch grains found on the teeth of ancient hominids that these species consumed a diversity plant foods. Raw plant foods of many kinds require extended chewing and digestion times (i.e., fermentation by bacteria), as can be seen in many animals, including primates, that are primarily herbivorous. Plant foods require strong teeth and jaw muscles for grinding the material in small pieces. This fact does not align with our anatomy and physiology (i.e., we are not adapted to eating large amounts of raw plant foods).

All of these changes that have occurred in hominid form can be explained by the cooking of food. The heat of cooking softens food, requiring less robust dentition and the associated skeletomuscular features to support and power those teeth. Further, the heat of cooking acts to predigest food through the gelatinization of starches and denaturing of proteins. This, in turn, means the gastrointestinal tract is no longer constrained by the digestive needs of raw foods (especially plant foods that require extended fermentation) and more energy can be derived from the food. Raw food requires more energy to digest and, therefore, supplies the body with less energy to power various systems (including portions of the nervous system). The next logical question becomes: does the archeological record support the controlled use of fire far back into our evolutionary history. The answer is: sort of.

Finding evidence of cooking is very difficult to do because of the impermanence of that kind of evidence. Tools for starting fire or carrying fires from another location (such as a lightning strike) are most likely made of plant material. Further, both ash and cooked food remains are biodegradable and simply don’t last forever. While some authors suggest that controlled use of fire (for cooking food) is only 300 to 400 thousand years old (which is older than most estimates of the age of anatomically modern humans), there is evidence of this practice going further back. A site in Israel called Gesher Benot Ya'aqov pushed the evidence of controlled fire use back to about 790,000 years ago. Another site, recently described in a paper by Francesco Berna and colleagues in 2012, called Wonderwerk in South Africa, showed evidence of controlled use of fire dating back 1 million years. While Wonderwerk is currently considered one of the earliest sites for controlled use of fire that has relatively good evidence, there are earlier sites that suggest fire use, including another cave in South Africa (called Swartkrans) that would put fire use at between 1 and 1.5 million years (but the evidence there is speculative).

The anatomical evidence of fire use, as has been discussed in the section, would suggest a possible earlier date still. The changes in jaw structure, cranium size, degree of flaring of the rib cage, and proportional width of the pelvis, along with changes in overall size of the body and loss of adaptations to arboreal life (i.e, living in trees) found in the arms, shoulders, and trunk, show the most extensive shifts around the appearance of *Homo erectus* (ca. 1.9 million years ago). The use of fire, in addition to sparking changes in hominid anatomy, could have been used to protect early people from large predators, meaning people could spend more time on the ground (including negating the necessity to sleep in trees for safety). Therefore, along with the changes in jaw structure, etc., archeological evidence also shows proportionally shorter arms (compared with the entire length of the body) in hominids as time progressed. While controlled use of fire, including the cooking of food, can explain all the anatomical changes that have occurred in the evolution of hominids, other suggested reasons (such as an increased proportion of animals foods) does not. These anatomical changes suggest the use of fire may date back to 1.9 million years. In any case, physical evidence in the form of ashes and fire-cracked stone that demonstrate multiple fires at a given location, dates back to around 1 million years, long before the appearance of anatomically modern humans. This evidence tells of a physical form that was highly influenced by the discovery of the use of fire. Said another way, we are a species that was molded, in part, by the use of fire.

But fire did not simply alter our physical form, it would have also shaped some of our behaviors. Fire-making and maintenance would require future-directed cognition. The act of waiting for food to cook would require inhibition of some normal responses (such as consuming food immediately). Also, cooking food from different sources (animal foods, plant foods) harvested by different people would potentiate group cooperation and interpersonal social skills. Certainly, the time our ancestors have spent around hearths cooking food has led to an ability to experience complex social interactions and collaborate with other people in our community. Cooking also freed time for communication as softened food requires less chewing and cooked food provides more energy (many wild animals, including primates, spend a significant proportion of the day eating food to acquire the necessary calories). At some point in time, the ability to share fire with others (through providing embers to initiate other fires) would have also strengthened bonds within the group. We are, in many ways, children of fire. Without this natural phenomenon (and learning how to both initiate and control fire), we would undoubtedly exist in a very different form today and likely without the large brains and capacity for high intelligence that we associate with modern humans.

DIETARY WISDOM

Our understanding of nutrition is in its infancy. With each passing decade and the addition of thousands of dietary studies, we become convinced that we have all the information at hand. And every passing decade, we are amused at some of things people believed regarding food and diet, but continue to make the same mistake (certainly we have all the information now—read with healthy sarcasm). Keep in mind, we (contemporary people) "discovered" vitamin C in 1907, though indigenous people knew how to prevent scurvy (i.e., vitamin C deficiency) long before this. Essential fatty acids were discovered in 1923, though all known wild and some traditional people had excellent ω6 to ω3 ratios without knowledge of these. We are still battling over the perceived effects of saturated fat and cholesterol (despite a long history of consumption of foods rich in these items by indigenous people—people who did not suffer chronic disease and could produce healthy, well-formed children). To believe that we, city builders, now must have nutrition completely understood because of numerous studies analyzing microscopic components of foods in isolation of the diet (i.e., without context) is really deluding ourselves. Further, to believe we can rate the quality of a food by adding up its known vitamins and minerals and subtracting out the contribution of its antinutrients is naive (no offense intended). It leaves out a discussion of life force, connection, and spirituality that are likely important contributions to health. But even keeping it very scientific, there is no doubt that unknown factors in foods will ultimately be discovered as critical for imparting health (this likely to come from a greater understanding of epigenetics).

Hunter-gatherers have been able to derive deep nutrition from their landscapes in every part of the world they have inhabited (which is very extensive). This is evidenced in the fact they showed far fewer signs of malnutrition than agricultural people and have been able to transmit health through the generations (until colonizers disrupted their lifeways). How did they accomplish this, especially in extreme environments where weather, topography, or limited resources (e.g., rainfall) constrained their activity? While I think the answer (or answers) to that question vary by indigenous group, there was definitely a dietary wisdom that was accrued by each culture from living in a location for many generations—a wisdom that allowed people to accomplish vibrant health. This wisdom was an integral part of the culture that was passed down to preserve the well-being and strength of each successive generation. Some authors have asserted that indigenous people simply were skilled at observing and interpreting cause and effect. Clearly, modern people have lost an ability to observe cause and effect or are apathetic about adjusting diet and lifestyle given the extremely poor health outcomes in our children.

The United States has long had a poor track record when it comes to nutrition. Even before the country was colonized by Europeans, the explorers who reached the continent's shores frequently suffered from vitamin C deficiency, which presented as lethargy, poor wound healing, gum disease, edema, and even death. These symptoms were a result of the kinds of foods they utilized during long voyages (primarily dried grains and salted/cured meats). Fruits and vegetables that would have provided adequate vitamin C were too perishable for trans-oceanic trips. Scurvy also afflicted sailors and voyagers when winter ice prevented them from returning to Europe, as happened to French explorer Jacques Cartier and his crew in the winter of 1536. In this famous story of scurvy, Jacques Cartier's crew was seriously reduced in number when their ship was frozen in the ice and they were forced to endure the winter in eastern Canada. The remaining crew members were ultimately saved by the local Native Americans who knew how to create vitamin C-rich teas from native evergreens that grew in the St. Lawrence River region. The tree, called anneda by the indigenous, is often believed to be northern white cedar (*Thuja occidentalis*), also called *arbor-vitae* ("tree of life"). However, historical details (particularly the size of the tree) point to the actual species of anneda as being eastern white pine (*Pinus strobus*), which modern tests demonstrate is rich in vitamin C (significantly more so than oranges). Jacques Cartier repaid the Native American's kindness by taking six of them captive and returning to France with them.

In the late 1800s and early 1900s, a large number of Americans in the southern states were afflicted with pellagra (vitamin B_3, or niacin, deficiency). Symptoms included sensitivity to light, altered mood, dermatitis, hair loss, weakness, diarrhea, and dementia (among others). While the US government considered this to be a disease spread by flies, it was ultimately determined to be a nutritional deficiency, which the government was forced to accept in light of overwhelming evidence. The problem was determined to be a reliance on corn (*Zea mays*) without proper processing. European colonists adopted the cultivation of corn from the indigenous of the New World, but failed to recognize the importance of their soaking in an alkali solution (a process called nixtamalization). This alkali soaking (accomplished by corn in water with added wood ashes) had the effect of making vitamin B_3 more bioavailable to the human body. The problem experienced by the Americans of the South (and some groups cultivating this species in Europe) was that they were relying heavily on corn for nutrition, to the extent that other foods that would have supplied niacin in sufficient amounts were not being consumed. Given the failure to utilize traditional processing of corn (and subsequent unavailability of niacin in that corn), the people were deficient in niacin and experiencing terrible symptoms. The story of pellagra in the United States is an excellent example of the need to adopt the traditional preparation methods of a food (and not just adopting the food itself).

The lack of deep nutrition in the United States is, unfortunately, ongoing. Part of the problem is the food we choose to eat, but part of the problem is that we have set very low standards. The Recommended Dietary Allowances (RDA) are values established to provide guidance with the intake of vitamins and minerals in the diet. The RDA is a daily intake level of a given nutrient to provide "sufficient" nourishment for 97.5% of the healthy individuals (by gender in different age groups). In the United States, we consider "sufficient" to be approximately 20% more of a nutrient than the level that satisfies the requirements of 50% of the population. These low standards, which many use to determine nutritional sufficiency, are so low as to prevent impeccable health and are a recipe for chronic disease and cancer. Case in point, the Food and Nutrition Board (FNB), a panel created in 1940 to, in part, establish principles and guidelines for good nutrition, recommends an intake of 600 international units (IUs) per day for vitamin D for young and middle-aged adults. An independent organization titled "Vitamin D Council" recommends 5000 IUs per day for the same age groups and has abundant research supporting their stance (a number that is more in-line with what Weston Price observed in intact indigenous cultures around the world). It is interesting to point out that the FNB considers the Tolerable Upper Intake Levels for vitamin D at 4000 IUs per day for people older than 8 years of age (a number that is below what the Vitamin D Council is recommending for daily intake). While it might be easy to leap to a conspiracy theory and suggest the FNB is trying to create patients for the medical industry, it may well be a case of incompetence based on a poor understanding of what actual human health is (especially as it relates to future generations).

Deep nutrition is accomplished by following the example of hunter-gatherers—it is not accomplished by consuming vitamins and other supplements. Many vitamins are synthetic and/or only part of the vitamin, meaning they often have significantly reduced activity in the body. For example, ascorbic acid, the commonly used chemical to supplement modern food, is not the entirety of vitamin C (vitamin C in food also includes flavonoids, rutin, the enzyme tyrosinase, and several other factors that benefit blood vessel strength and the oxygen carrying capacity of red blood cells). Numerous studies show that supplementing with vitamins does not extend life, avert heart disease, prevent memory loss, and so on (and studies that have shown benefit are largely observational ones and did not have controls—such as a group taking a placebo). And some studies even show high doses of vitamins can cause harm. Utilizing actual food is the way to nourish the body. Unfortunately, this causes a pause for many people who consider some of the hunter-gatherer practices (i.e., some of their foods) unappetizing or outright repulsive. Their minds immediately jumps to some of the most unappealing practices they have ever heard of—but keep in mind, I eat wild foods almost daily and my guests enjoy the foods I serve them. The idea of consuming organ meats or bone marrow (for examples) is simply too extreme for some folks. Liver certainly has a stronger flavor, but it is easily masked with simple tricks. And, liver is included on the menu of many high-end restaurants (as pâté), indicating our opinion of a particular food is entirely cultural (so start children early on these foods so that they are familiar to their palate). Further, these nutrient-dense foods were not (and do not have to be) consumed on a daily basis. The avoidance of traditional foods is, in part, one of the main problems with the Standard American Diet, a diet that leads to poor health outcomes. Avoiding time-honored foods merely because of their flavor generates the following question: do you like the "taste" of chemotherapy, or heart surgery, or insulin injections? I much prefer learning to prepare stronger-flavored (and health-promoting) foods than succumb to chronic disease and endure medical procedures. With this in mind, let's move into conceptual information that can be used to both create nutrient-dense foods and further understand their importance.

DIETARY DIVERSITY

One of the very important dietary strategies for acquiring deep nutrition is to consume a diversity of foods. Indigenous people (including their paleolithic ancestors) consumed a much greater diversity of foods than we do today, including both the organisms and the different portions of those organisms we ingest. This is perhaps best illustrated through plants. It is an often repeated number that about 30 species of plants are eaten by a typical American in one year. This number might seem low at first, but you have to consider some important things. First, many "species" you think you are eating are actually just different cultivated forms of the same plant. For example, broccoli, Brussels sprouts, cabbage, cauliflower, collard greens, kale, and kohlrabi are all the same species (*Brassica oleracea*). Another example, acorn squash, buttercup squash, Hubbard squash, and winter squash are all the same species (*Cucurbita maxima*). Another one, pattypan squash, pumpkin, spaghetti squash, summer crookneck squash, and zucchini are all the same species (*Cucurbita pepo*). Another one, black turtle beans (also known as black beans), green beans, kidney beans, navy beans, pinto beans, wax beans, and white beans are all the same species (*Phaseolus vulgaris*). And one more, beet root, chard, and sugar beet are the same species (*Beta vulgaris*). Therefore, when you create your list of plant species eaten in a year, do be sure you are tallying species and not merely different forms of the same species. When one considers the fact many apparently different plants that agriculturalists consume are actually the same species, it is likely that the estimated 30 species a year is not inaccurate for most people.

Counts of the number of species of food plants have been reported for various hunter-gatherer groups. The Hausa foragers of west Africa utilized 119 food plants (compiled from different sources). The !Kung of Africa ate 85 plants according to Sassaman in 2001. Given that these data were published in late 1960s, we can be fairly certain more species were gathered by the culture before agricultural societies had impacted their way of life. Also of note, the !Kung live in the northern Kalahari, a water-limited region (which constrains plant diversity). The indigenous of Tibet were documented to use 168 food plants (published by Ju and colleagues in 2013). From North America, Myra Perry interviewed members of the Cherokee Nation of the southeastern United States and estimated them consume approximately 80 species of wild plants. However, this figure is low because it was published in the 1975, at a time when much of the botanical knowledge would have been lost (this number reflects what the informants could remember). It also lumps together some species into aggregate groups (e.g., blackberries, hickories—which are genera that include multiple species). We can be certain the actual number from the intact culture would have easily exceeded 100. Even the Iñupiat of far northern North America consumed 40 species of plants, as reported by Anore Jones in "Plants We Eat" (beating out the average American in regard to plant diversity). None of these counts include medicinal plants that were also ingested and contributed to the phytochemical diversity experienced by humans. Nor do these counts reflect the diversity of animal foods in the diet (which are also substantially greater than that of American diets; see below).

Why is diversity in the diet important? Diversity in the diet protects against nutritional deficiencies as different foods contain different amounts and, equally important, ratios of vitamins, minerals, essential fatty acids, and kinds of fiber. In regard to plants, these organisms also contain suites of phytochemicals (i.e., plant compounds) that act on the physiology of our bodies. These actions include anti-inflammatory (reducing inflammation), anti-arrhythmic (promoting proper heart beat), hypotensive (lowering blood pressure), antioxidant (scavenging free radicals to prevent cancer, cognitive decline, and premature aging), blood vessel strengthening, antimicrobial (killing pathogenic bacteria, fungi, and viruses), antiparasitic (killing parasitic organisms in the GI tract), antineoplastic (shrinking cancerous tumors), immune system modulation, cleansing the human body through effects on lymph, urine flow, bile, and sweat, and many, many more actions. Most of the plant compounds are not produced by food animals. Further, many plant-derived antioxidants exert free-radical scavenging activity orders of magnitude greater than the vitamin antioxidants found in animal foods. None of this is to imply that plant foods are superior to animal foods, only that a diversity of plant foods is critical for health.

We could also perform this same exercise with animals, noting how indigenous people consumed a greater number of animal foods. The !Kung consumed 54 different species of animals, and all of these without long distance transport (Sassaman 2001). The Iñupiat ate 23 different species of just fish, again, all locally secured (Anore Jones, Fish That We Eat). They also consumed much of the animal, including skin, liver, and/or eggs from these fish. In the United States, people consume the vast majority of the animal food from a handful of species—chickens, turkeys, cows, pigs, and fish (the latter a composite category of wild and farm-raised fish and shellfish). Aside from eggs and dairy, Americans eat primarily the lean muscle meat of these animals (pork a notable exception), thereby reducing their intake of nutritional elements even further because another aspect of dietary diversity is full utilization of the organism being consumed. As far as animals go, lean muscle meat is a poor source of some items needed for optimal health that can be found in animal foods.

All of this discussion of food diversity is not a call to import more food from distant lands (with the resulting pollution, exploitation of resources, and development of transportation infrastructure). It is a call to increase food diversity at the table through growing and gathering more local species. Consider that from 1903 to 1983, approximately 93% of our crop seed diversity has been lost due to an over-reliance on relatively few popular cultivars (as reported by John Tomanio in National Geographic). Heirloom plant breeds, which are open pollinated, are those kinds that produce seeds that can be saved for future planting. They represent forms closer to the wild progenitor than most grown for the market and are an excellent way for people to increase plant diversity in the diet and bolster local food production and security. Equally important, there is a large diversity of edible plants that can be gathered from rural and relatively pristine landscapes throughout the United States. As a forager, I regularly consume over 100 wild species a year from northeastern North America (in addition to cultivated kinds), adding immensely to the diversity of plants I consume each year. Although local wild plants are not a viable option for everyone due to residence in an urbanized or industrialized landscape, it is an option for many people in the United States, one that offers more nutrition than the cultivated species we commit massive resources to planting, tending, harvesting, and transporting to market. Many authors prefer to discuss only those options available to everyone; however, this is a poor practice because each person lives in a different region that offers different possibilities (for various reasons). If someone has access to wild foods that grow in the necessary abundance to support collection, they should be prioritized in the diet because of the many nutritional advantages they offer (see Wild and Minimally Modified Plant Foods in this chapter).

THE RIGHT KINDS OF VITAMINS

This book is primarily about supplying concepts that can guide an individual, a family, or community toward a more natural and healthy lifestyle. Unfortunately, many people now are accustomed to following recipes and commands (e.g., do this, don't do this). They have a difficult time applying concepts and are more likely to seek out short sound bites, such as: "don't eat grain". This statement was one of the standard Paleo Diet mantras until relatively recently. Given that healthy cultures existed that consumed grain as a staple (and many cultures that included grains to a lesser extent), this statement is squarely contradicted by real world observations. Many people would consider a more accurate statement simply too complex: "choose wild and heirloom grains, restrict or (if necessary) avoid gluten-containing kinds, and eat less grain through diversifying the diet". I mention all this because this book will provide limited "recipes". It is more about supplying information that can be applied to any situation and on any landscape. Likewise, this book will not provide a detailed breakdown of macronutrients (carbohydrates, lipids, and proteins) and dictate what percentage you should consume. You should have a better understanding of your body and its dietary needs than anyone else. The complication that most encounter is not understanding what food cravings and aversions are biological and which are cultural (brutal honesty with yourself is one way to solve this dilemma). Likewise, we will not march though each micronutrient (vitamin or mineral) and provide a list of foods with the amounts that should be consumed on a daily basis. Knowledge of these items is not entirely necessary if a natural diet is followed. Keep in mind, indigenous and healthy traditional people did not have detailed knowledge of vitamins and minerals and enjoyed greater health (on average) than we do today. Therefore, I would rather one think of the writings here as ideas and guidelines (rather than doctrines and rules). With all this in mind, let us continue to explore different nutritional topics and how they relate to the aspiring neoaboriginal.

One of the critical items that must be understood is that certain vitamins occur in different forms, and those different forms exert different effects on our body. Said another way, different versions of the same vitamin present different levels of bioavailability and activity to humans. In the cases that will be discussed, we could name these different forms of vitamins as "plant forms" and "animal forms", and although this would not be the most accurate way to describe them, it would help with remembering where to acquire the most active forms of these vitamins.

Vitamin A

Vitamin A is a crucial, fat-soluble vitamin that is needed for a healthy immune system (including resistance to infections), for vital growth and development of bones and teeth, and for good eye sight. It also plays a role in the transcription of genes, is necessary for skin and mucous membrane health, and functions as an antioxidant, protecting the body from cancer and some environmental toxins. In the foods that humans consume, vitamin A occurs in two primary forms: retiniods and carotenoids. These two classes of vitamin A are both important for human health, but they differ substantially in their vitamin-A activity in the body.

Retinoids are the forms of vitamin A found in animal foods. These include retinol, retinal, and retinoic acid. These are also called "preformed vitamin A" because they do not require extensive conversion to active forms of this vitamin. In other words, these are the preferred forms of vitamin A for the body. Retinoids are most abundant in liver and some other organ meats (e.g., kidneys). They are also found in high amounts in ocean fish, shellfish, fish oils, eggs (specifically the yolks), and butter, and occur in lesser degrees in other animals foods. Hunter-gatherers received much more active vitamin A in the diet than most contemporary people because they fully utilized the animals they consumed as food. Many Americans (and others in affluent countries) rarely consume organ meats, eliminating a very nutrient-dense source of food in the diet.

Carotenoids are the forms of vitamin A found in plant foods. These include α-carotene, β-carotene, γ-carotene, and β-cryptoxanthin, all of which are pigments, and the first three are photosynthetic pigments (the Greek symbols used in this sentence are read as alpha, beta, and gamma, respectively). Cultivated foods rich in carotenoids include those fruits with orange and yellow pigments (e.g., carrots, squash, sweet potatoes, mangos) and dark leafy greens (e.g., kale, spinach). Carotenoids are also called "pro-vitamin A" because they cannot be used by the body as vitamin A without extensive conversion to the active forms. To be very clear about this, there is no plant on earth that actually contains vitamin A, instead, they all contain precursors which must undergo conversion before the body can use them. For each microgram (μg) of retinol (from animal foods) consumed by a person, it would require (on average) the ingestion of 12 μg of β-carotene and 24 μg of the other carotenoids to be equivalent. This means that plant forms of vitamin A are considered to possess from 1/12 to 1/24 the activity in the body as the animal forms. This is due to the lengthy and inefficient conversion process that must occur. Given this understanding, it is a mystery as to why the Food and Drug Administration allows companies to list carotenes as vitamin A (i.e., as having equal activity as retinol). It is highly misleading and contributes to many plant foods being listed as excellent sources of vitamin A, when in fact they are poor to moderate (at best) sources. Important to this discussion is that lipids (i.e., fats) are needed to make the conversion from pro-vitamin A to active forms of vitamin A; therefore, low fat diets impair the body's ability to create vitamin A from plant foods. Studies have shown that some people do not make this conversion at all, especially (but not limited to) those who are elderly, in infancy, with compromised thyroid function, with reduced bile production, and who are diabetic. The point of this entire paragraph is that plant forms of vitamin A, although still very healthful to us (especially due to their antioxidant ability), may not provide enough of this vitamin for optimal health. Keep in mind, one should not be trying to merely reach the FNB's recommended levels—which is merely 700 or 900 μg (female vs. male) for young adults and adults who are not pregnant or lactating—but exceed these levels multiple times for optimal health (note: that is not a call to take supplements, rather to include vitamin A-rich food sources in the diet to prevent possibly toxicity).

Take home message: consume an omnivorous diet that is rich in wild and pastured animal foods AND includes lots of orange, yellow, and green fruits and vegetables. Note that many wild leafy greens far exceed cultivated leafy greens in pro-vitamin A content.

Vitamin D

Vitamin D is another fat-soluble vitamin (though perhaps better described as a hormone because it can be produced by the body) that has many important functions in the body. These include immune system and cardiovascular system function, the absorption of certain minerals needed for optimal bone and tooth health (e.g., calcium, magnesium, phosphorus), gene expression, and proper growth (including brain development). Vitamin D may be one of the most important vitamins in regards to the body's defense from cancer. There are several forms of this hormone-vitamin, with vitamin D_2 and vitamin D_3 perhaps the best known. The former is called ergocalciferol and is found in plants and fungi. The latter is called cholecalciferol and is found in animal foods and is produced by the body when ultraviolet light (specifically UVB) irradiates the skin. While both forms are useful in raising the levels of the metabolically active form of vitamin D in our body (called calcitriol), they are not the same. Further, oral vitamin D_3 and dermally produced vitamin D_3 are not the same (even though most health authorities consider them so).

When you consume vitamin D (in any form) it must go to the liver where it is converted into an intermediary form (the exact form depends on the source of the vitamin D). These intermediary forms can be stored for later use or transported in the body by cholesterol molecules for conversion to calcitriol. When any of the intermediary forms are sent to the kidneys (or other tissues), they are converted into calcitriol, which is the version of vitamin D that manages calcium levels in our blood. Research suggests that vitamin D_3 is 87% more potent than vitamin D_2 in raising vitamin D concentrations in the body and is stored much more efficiently. Further, vitamin D_3 is converted into calcitriol 500% faster than vitamin D_2, all of which clearly points to the fact that vitamin D_3 (cholecalciferol) is the better form of this vitamin to receive. While this is not to say we should avoid ingesting naturally occurring vitamin D_2, such as that found in sun-dried mushrooms, we should prioritize animal foods for acquisition of oral vitamin D. Good animal sources include fatty fish (e.g., salmon, trout, mackerel), fish oils, duck and goose eggs (which are substantially better than chicken eggs), and fish eggs (i.e., roe).

While identifying that vitamin D_3 is the superior form of vitamin D, there are two forms of cholecalciferol: that acquired through ingesting food and that acquired through sunlight shining on the skin. The main difference is that the latter form is sulfated (i.e., has a sulfate molecule attached to it). So, when vitamin D_3 is made by sunlight, it is actually vitamin D_3-sulfate. This form of vitamin D is water soluble, so it is easily transported in the blood stream and does not need to be packaged up inside a cholesterol molecule. It is not possible to overdose on this form of vitamin D because your body effectively self-regulates how much is made. Vitamin D_3-sulfate is ineffective at regulating calcium in the blood, but some researchers consider this form (along with cholesterol sulfate, which is also produced when sunlight shines on the skin) to be what benefits the immune system, protects against cardiovascular disease, is beneficial for the brain, and helps elevate mood (i.e., protects against depression). Vitamin D_3-sulfate may serve as a messenger molecule telling the body that cholesterol sulfate is widely available. While vitamin D_3-sulfate can lose its sulfate molecule and become "normal" vitamin D_3, the reverse may not occur readily. Therefore, we want both forms of cholecalciferol in our "diet", because they appear to have different functions. To do this, we must consume animal foods (in part) and practice conscientious sun exposure (more on this later in the chapter). Of particular note is that the form of vitamin D_3 found in raw milk (including human breast milk) is the sulfated form.

Take home message: When it comes to food forms of vitamin D, while both are helpful, the animal food forms are more potent, are stored more easily in the body, and converted to the hormone form of vitamin D the fastest. However, the form of vitamin D made from the sun is different and plays other roles in the body. We need both forms (i.e., vitamin D from food and sunlight) to be optimally healthy.

We could go on at great length with this discussion, including paragraphs of vitamin B_6, vitamin B_{12}, and vitamin K (there are substantial differences between the plant and animal forms of these vitamins). While the examples used here described animal food forms as the superior forms, this is not meant to be taken as a message that we should consume only animal foods. There are plenty of vitamins and beneficial chemicals that are found solely or much more abundantly in plant foods. My intent with the last paragraphs was to help people realize that the science of nutrition is difficult to simplify to a couple of short, blanket statements (as many authors do) and help people realize that what they receive for nutritional information is sometimes (unfortunately) incorrect. We must remain truly open to information; it is openness that will remove the blinders produced by certain cultural memes. We have all been influenced by the messages of politically correct nutrition, which often prioritize foods that are abundantly produced rather than those that are the most nutrient dense. Fortunately, much of the need to study the minutiae of nutrition disappears as we undo domestication in our life because the foods and the practices associated with a truly natural diet produces health (through the generations). Said another way, the more your diet emulates hunter-gatherers, the less nutritional minutiae you need to know.

THE INTERACTION OF VITAMINS AND MINERALS (THINK SYNERGY)

The human diet has primarily consisted of the bodies or portions thereof of living organisms (usually after the death of the organism and sometimes also after some amount of preparation and processing). While this may seem to be a crude way to describe what we now call food, this term ("food") conceals what we actually consume—life. We have been consuming a diverse array of life throughout human history and incorporating other organisms' bodies and energy into our own being. Eating in this way, we always consumed vitamins and minerals together (i.e., with each other)—we did not ingest them in isolation as a single vitamin or mineral. Our bodies are designed to extract nutrition from other beings and use the vitamins and minerals (in concert) to build, maintain, and repair our own bodies.

Much of the nutritional research has sought to isolate a single vitamin or mineral's role in promoting health and defending from various ailments. This strategy has obvious strengths and weaknesses. But what this has done is to convince a populace of people that supplementation with a single vitamin or mineral is an effective strategy for correcting health issues or maintaining health. As such, people now seek the "magic bullet", the one item that will correct the ailment they are experiencing. And while this method may produce a result that is considered successful, it will never be as productive as adjusting the diet and lifestyle to incorporate better overall nutritional practices. That is because the latter method has several strengths, one of which is providing not only the vitamin (or mineral) of interest but also its necessary cofactors of that nutrient, allowing it to perform optimally in the body. Vitamins and minerals do not work in a vacuum but, rather, interact in a complex manner. Sometimes the problem is not nutrient X but that the body has insufficient stores of nutrient Y that is essential for the proper utilization of nutrient X. An example will be useful here in understanding how extensive the interaction is between vitamins and minerals.

Calcium is an essential mineral that has great importance in muscle growth and contraction, nerve transmission, proper metabolism, heart and hormone function, and strong bones and teeth. It is also one of the best examples of the problem of supplementing with a single nutrient. Many people, especially older women, are concerned with bone health, or, more specifically, the loss of bone density (osteoporosis). They supplement with the mineral calcium in an attempt to strengthen their bones. Unfortunately, the problem for some people was never a limitation of calcium but a limitation of the necessary cofactors of calcium. What occurs is that the calcium is directed to the incorrect locations and ends up being deposited in the joints, the blood vessels, and, potentially, the lens of the eye. It requires several items to direct calcium to the bones where it can be useful (and not detrimental).

First, strong bones require stress. Not the emotional kind of stress, but physical stress that places a mechanical load on the skeletal system. Such stresses create small electric signals that attract osteoblasts (bone-building cells) that ultimately deposits minerals (primarily calcium) on the stressed areas of the bone, increasing the density and strength of the bone. Therefore, a sedentary lifestyle is unfavorable to bone building. Second, vitamin D is necessary for the metabolism and transport of calcium (it creates specific proteins responsible for moving calcium around in the body). Without adequate vitamin D, calcium will not reach the bones. Third, vitamin K_2 is needed activate the proteins that move calcium around. So, again, without adequate amounts of this vitamin, calcium will not reach the bones. Fourth, magnesium is needed to activate the hormone thyrocalcitonin, which sends calcium to the bones. And again, without adequate amounts of magnesium, calcium does not reach the bones (by now, you can see the pattern). Interestingly, supplementation with calcium can create a surplus of calcium, capable of impairing magnesium's ability to activate the aforementioned hormone, meaning the calcium ends up in the wrong place (this is important: it is not just the amount of vitamins and minerals but also their ratios that affect their function in the body, and supplementation can distort healthy ratios). And there are even more minerals needed for bone health, including phosphorus, silicon, and others. Without all these vitamin and minerals, along with movement, working in concert, bones do not get denser and stronger.

There are many other examples that could be discussed here, including the ability of vitamin C to regenerate vitamin E so that it can continue to function as an antioxidant that protects lipid membranes, polyunsaturated fatty acids, and nutrients from being harmed by free radicals. Discussion could also include the close interaction of vitamin B_9 and vitamin B_{12} to make red blood cells, support the function of iron in the body, and control blood levels of homocysteine. And so on. We are meant to derive nutrition from food (i.e., life) so that we receive the vitamins, minerals, fats, fiber, amino acids, phytochemicals, and other components of a healthful diet together. Supplementation (aside from its use in healing acute and chronic ailments) is an admission of a nutrient poor diet. When you supplement, you are admitting that your diet is deficient. Said another way, you are acknowledging that your diet is substandard in one or more vitamins and/or minerals. Of course, the logical question becomes (for those who have a choice): why would you willingly choose to consume a substandard diet? This question is especially pertinent when you consider that diet is one the major ways that your genes are regulated. Poor regulation of genes leads to poor expression of genes, and poor genetic expression leads to poor health and/or poor physical form.

EPIGENETICS

We are frequently told that our genome, the sum total of genetic information coded in our deoxyribonucleic acids (DNA) and ribonucleic acids (RNA), is a major governing factor of our health. The idea is that once our genetic code has been laid down after conception, our fate is sealed and the illnesses we experience are part of our destiny. People believe this idea to such an extent that some, due to the fear they experience, undergo prophylactic surgeries to remove parts of their body due to "family history" of disease (e.g., breast cancer). While it is true that our genetic information is a vitally important piece of the health we will experience in our lifetime, it is not important in the way most people believe it to be. Health professionals are, unfortunately, doing a major disservice to the public at this point in time by failing to empower people with an understanding of epigenetics. I cannot stress to you enough how important the following discussion is to your vitality and how you should approach healthful, nature-connected living.

First, we must provide a little bit of background to fully appreciate just how powerful an understanding of epigenetics is. Briefly, epigenetics is a term for all of the factors that influence our genes ("epi" is a Greek prefix that means over, outside of, around). The term epigenetics includes the word "gene", which is a sequence of genetic information that provides a code for a particular trait. Keep in mind, we are not just discussing physical traits, such as eye color. While many people realize that our genes contain hereditary information that we pass on to the next generation, many do not appreciate that our genes are functioning within our bodies every day producing polypeptides. These polypeptides are amino acids linked together to form proteins that perform the various functions coded within our DNA, such as catalyzing chemical reactions in our body (enzymes), cell signaling, antigen binding, providing cell structure, enabling cell transport, and influencing DNA processes (e.g., repair, replication, transcription). Therefore, genes do not simply code for physical traits, but also physiological actions that are occurring within our body billions of times each second. But, for these events to occur, a gene must "express" itself, which involves a suite of enzymes and other chemicals that orchestrate the unwinding and transcription of the DNA molecule. If the gene remains silent (which could occur by the DNA molecules remaining tightly wound), no proteins are made. Only on expression are proteins made that are utilized in the biological functioning of our body. The crux of this entire discussion is this: what you experience in your lifetime (including *in utero*) affects the expression of your DNA.

Your genes require you to interact with your environment to perform properly. Part of this interaction includes what you ingest for food. Through diet, you literally bring fragments of the environment into your body and incorporate them into your tissues. Your diet has profound effects on how well your DNA express themselves (i.e., influence when they "turn on" or "turn off" protein synthesis). Poor diets rich in refined carbohydrates, oxidized fats, and synthetic ingredients interrupt proper DNA expression and cause genes to turn on or off at the wrong time, producing too many or too few of important proteins. But it is not simply the food you ingest, but also other aspects of your environment. Exposure to the elements is a major factor influencing epigenetic expression. Through elemental exposure, you have the potential to breathe clean air and expose your skin to sunlight. You also have the opportunity to receive exposure to environmental toxins. The kinds of social interactions and other factors that contribute to your emotional well-being are also important. Experiencing love and support from your community, the embrace of a loved one, and feelings of contentment are powerful positive influences on your epigenetic health. Likewise, being abused or ridiculed, always in a state of chronic stress, and living with feelings of uselessness would contribute to poor functioning of your DNA. Almost anything you do, from physical movement to addictive smoking to eating phytochemical-rich wild plants to contact with toxins in your bathroom products, affects the expression of your DNA. Poor health and poor living conditions ultimately will compound upon the health issues you may already be experiencing.

For many years, genetic and health authorities have assumed that your underlying genetic code (i.e., the base sequences of your DNA) were the primary actors governing your health. It turns out that, in most cases, this is simply untrue. In fact, many diseases considered to be genetic in origin are not genetic at all. It turns out that people don't just inherit genes, they inherit a lifestyle, which includes similar diet and similar social and environmental exposures as the parents. Therefore, when parents experience an illness, it is often true that their children are at risk, but the risk is based on experiencing the same factors that produce the same genetic expression. If the children instead consume a more natural diet, belong to a supportive community, and experience frequent immersion in natural places, they do not necessarily experience the same health problems. In fact, it is only about 10% of diseases that are truly genetic and, once inherited, the children will experience those diseases regardless of the changes they make to their diet and lifestyle.

As Alschuler and Gazella write in their book Five to Thrive[4]:

"All of this is really cause for celebration. Our genes are not our destiny. We have the opportunity, through the choices we make, to change our genetic expression. Much like the musical notes on a page, the music that is us depends entirely upon how the notes our played. While we cannot change our internal notes, we can play some loudly and others softly, and we can repeat some and skip others, changing the song completely. This gives us tremendous opportunity to alter our genetic destiny".

Epigenetics is especially important when it comes to cancer. Cancer can be (in very simplified terms) described as either normal expression of mutated genes or mutated expression of normal genes. Both of these scenarios are (usually) the result of factors that are external to our DNA (i.e., they represent epigenetic influences on our genome). Mutations can occur by exposure to mutagenic substances in our environment (e.g., industrial chemicals, cigarette smoke) or those produced by our body (e.g., certain estrogen breakdown products). All of these factors can be positively affected by diet. Fortunately, diet is also one of the most easily adjusted aspects of our lifeway and can profoundly impact our health even when exposure to environmental toxins cannot be avoided. Unfortunately, for Americans, the standard diet is deficient in many vitamins, minerals, and other nutritional elements (e.g., phytochemicals, essential fatty acids, fiber). For example, studies have shown that over half of American adults are deficient in vitamin A, a micronutrient that influences DNA methylation (one aspect of epigenetics) and susceptibility to cancer. Recent studies have suggested that ¾ of American teens and adults are deficient in vitamin D. When you consider that research shows that up to 10% of our genes are waiting on a second by second basis to be told what to do by vitamin D, this makes this vitamin-hormone vitally important to receive in adequate amounts (see The Right Kinds of Vitamins earlier in this chapter). Examining another micronutrient, a recent study suggested that just over 90% of Americans were deficient in Vitamin E, which is yet another important vitamin that affects the expression of certain RNA molecules. And we could go on, marching through the list of vitamins and minerals, demonstrating high rates of deficiency and their roles in epigenetics. Given that diet is probably the most profound way we influence our genetic expression (and protect ourselves from cancer), not only through the nutrition we receive but also the chemicals we expose ourselves to (from industrial agriculture), it is not really surprising that cancer is so prevalent in the United States. (And if you are thinking that you can just supplement with multivitamins, you haven't yet understood what constitutes a good diet.)

One of the very important things that we now know about epigenetics is that the quality (or lack thereof) of gene expression is (in some cases) heritable for one or more generations. While this too goes against the traditional understanding of genes, it has been confirmed in many studies. It used to be thought that our egg and sperm cells were "blank slates" in that they were devoid of epigenetic tags that influence gene expression. These tags are created by various processes in the parents as a result of their environment. They are usually removed through several mechanisms in reproductive cells; however, some are not removed and pass on to the offspring. There are different ways by which these tags are placed on the genes (e.g., DNA methylation, RNA silencing, histone acetylation). It is not important that you understand how this happens, but that

[4] Lise Alschuler and Karolyn Gazella. 2011. Five to Thrive: Your Cutting-edge Cancer Prevention Plan. Active Interest Media, Inc., El Segundo, CA.

it does occur (i.e., one can pass on a given quality of genetic expression to their offspring). So, when parents-to-be are in poor health, they not only give life to an infant that may be deficient in nutrition, but also an infant that begins his or her existence with poor genetic expression (which sets the infant up for a lifetime of health issues unless diet and lifestyle are corrected). Once this fact is known, it becomes an ethical issue for how parents-to-be choose to eat and live (because those factors affect their offspring in ways that can remain with the child for a lifetime). Fortunately, at least some of the epigenetic expression we inherit from our parents can be maintained (positive ones) or improved (negative ones) by making beneficial alterations in our environment and our interaction with that environment.

Though we have been told that our genes determine our destiny, this assertion is patently false. It is obvious through examining identical twins. Despite having the same genome, their individual experiences have made them into unique beings that, despite many similarities, look and act somewhat differently and can experience different health outcomes. Epigenetics helps us understand that we are more than just our genome, we are how our genome expresses itself. Therefore, our epigenome (the sum total of the changes to our DNA expression) is, to an extent, under our control because all the factors that alter genetic expression (our exposome) are within our power to alter during our lifetime. Certainly, not everything can be changed overnight, and some things cannot be corrected by diet and lifestyle. For example, you cannot repair the crowding of your teeth as an adult by improving your diet. But many, many ailments can be positively and permanently affected through changes (and the changes we are discussing here are not pharmaceutical drugs). It is your choice (at least to some extent) what you consume, where you live, how much you move, the quality of sleep you receive, and who you socialize with. Keep in mind, genetics load the gun, but it is the chosen diet and environment that pull the trigger. Your health (and that of your children) is under more of your control than you may believe. Be aware that positive thoughts are also important for epigenetic health (e.g., even the belief in a remedy alters genetic expression, as evidenced by the placebo effect).

Following is a short list of items that can beneficially influence epigenetic health (listed in no particular order). Note that we must think of "nutrition" as more than just food. *Homo sapiens* is nourished by many things, some are ingested, and some must be experienced through immersion. As such, our idea of diet requires expansion in order to include all the things that impart health.

1. Deep nutrition. While I stated this list was not arranged in a particular order, I do consider diet to be the most important element in achieving epigenetic health. The nutrition you receive is vital for healthy genetic machinery. Numerous studies demonstrate the role of various vitamins and minerals correcting and maintaining various aspects of proper genetic function. I would also add to this the phytochemistry and other items we receive when we ingest plant foods (e.g., micro RNAs that are known to silence gene activity). Keep in mind that through most of human evolution (save for the last piece of history), it has been wild foods that have nourished people and shaped their epigenome. Most fad diets depart radically from the original human diet (and by that, we are talking about the traits these diets had in common), and they are often lacking in several (or many) nutritional elements. Only through returning to a nutritional intake that emulates hunter-gatherer diets can we hope to experience excellent genetic expression.

2. Supporting your microbiome. One of the most neglected areas of human health is the microbiome that inhabits the body. Given the vast numbers of organisms that live on and inside the human body and their crucial role in our health, it is more appropriate to think of humans as symbiotic organisms than as a single individuals. Emerging research shows that the quality of our microbiome and the metabolites they produce influence genetic expression (and the prevalence of certain kinds of cancers). Our probiotic flora is also responsible for creating vitamins that we benefit from. To promote our symbionts, we must eat a natural diet that is rich in foods that feed our probiotic flora (such foods are called prebiotics), reduce food intake that feeds pathogenic bacteria and fungi (such as refined grains and sugars), seriously curtail pharmaceutical antibiotic use (which indiscriminately kills our flora), consume fermented foods rich in living organisms, and avoid ingestion of chemicals that harm our probiotics (e.g., chlorinated and fluoridated water, antibiotic residues in industrially raised animals, residues on plants grown by chemical agriculture).

3. Avoiding GMOs. There are several reasons it is important to avoid genetically modified organisms when it comes to epigenetic health. Keep in mind we are primarily targeting transgenic modifications here. However, cultivated plants are also genetically modified (through breeding) with substantive changes to the nutrition and phytochemistry they supply to the body. Genetically modified organisms expose us to novel chemicals and DNA molecules, which can affect our own genetic expression. These are new foods and we simply don't know their long-term effects to humans. But leaving hypothesis aside, "Roundup Ready" plants that utilize Glyphosate as an herbicide expose humans to chemical residues that, in this case, interfere with the biochemistry of the bacteria in our gastrointestinal tract. This interruption results in harm to our microbiome (see number 2 in this list).

4. Frequent movement. It is well established that physical movement alters genetic expression, influencing some genes to become more active, others to be less active. Movement is shown to alter methylation patterns, one of the mechanisms by which genetic expression is affected. Studies have demonstrated that movement enhances beneficial expression of genes, upregulating protein synthesis and providing benefit to inflammation, insulin response, and metabolism. Physical exercise is also known to lead to expression of genes that suppress cancerous tumors (more on this in chapter 8). Movement is another cornerstone of healthy genes.

5. Occasional intense activity. Humans are not just meant to move with great frequency on the landscape, they are also well suited to bouts of intense physical activity, whether that be sprinting, lifting heavy objects, climbing difficult routes, or even defending themselves from physical assault. Much like with lower intensity movement, studies have shown that intense activity upregulates beneficial expression of genes (in fact, the more intense the movement, the greater the expression of certain genes). Such genes include those that boost metabolism and protect against chronic inflammation.

6. Meditation. Meditation has been shown to positively influence epigenetic health in a number of ways. Research has demonstrated that meditation promotes rapid recovery from stressful situations and down regulates pro-inflammatory genes. The recovery from stressful situations involved faster cortisol recovery, subsequently benefitting mental calculations, public speaking, and responding to unrehearsed situations. Pain reduction has also been documented in people practicing meditation. This rarely used practice has tremendous value to offer in recovering health and promoting proper genetic expression.

7. Elemental exposure. Exposure to the outdoor world (i.e., stepping outside of the home) has more advantages for human health than can be described in this book. Through elemental exposure, one has the ability expose the skin to ultraviolet light, helping the body produce more vitamin D (note: optimizing vitamin D levels may be one of the single most important features for improving epigenetic function). Outdoor time can allow access to air much cleaner than inside our homes (which are often quite toxic due to carpets, paints, solvents, cleaners, etc.). However, if you are from a highly urbanized area, be aware that breathing factory discharge, car exhaust, and other air pollutants negatively affect genetic expression. You cannot become adapted to your local environment without spending time in it, experiencing the wind, water, soil, temperatures, and other aspects of that landscape. All these features change the expression of our DNA so that we become better adjusted to our natural world (rather than the indoor setting). Elemental exposure (to bright light) is also implicated in quality sleep (see number 8).

8. Quality sleep. Without sleep, our functioning during awake hours is severely compromised. Sleep is necessary for a host of items, including learning and memory consolidation. But research has also shown that sleep affects epigenetic mechanisms with a host of ramifications. Quality sleep improves the functioning of the immune system and enhances defense against infections and diseases (including cancer). While many are aware that we need a dark environment for quality sleep, realize that we also need a bright day-time environment for quality sleep—something indoor lighting does not produce (outdoor brightness is often orders of magnitude brighter than indoor settings). Without bright outdoor lighting, our circadian rhythms are compromised and our health (including metabolism, cardiovascular system, and genetic expression) suffers.

9. Managing stress. Human stress patterns have changed from primarily infrequent short-duration stress (in our hunter-gatherer ancestors) to frequent or continual chronic stress (in modern people), a pattern the human body is not evolutionarily designed to tolerate. Chronic stress is implicated in exacerbating numerous diseases and compromising epigenetic function through production of glucocorticoids, which are hormones that affect key organs in our body and the functioning of their genes. Through meditation and quality sleep, the severity of health effects from stress can be somewhat mitigated. However, ultimately people must be willing to alter stressful interactions or outright remove themselves from stressful environments (e.g., work place, social, living situation). Avoiding stress is not the same as avoiding a problem—removing one's self from non-necessary situations that promote stress is a wise practice.

10. Avoiding toxins and synthetics. Human-produced environmental toxins and various synthetic compounds have been shown to alter genetic expression in people exposed to these materials. Pollutants in our environment can enter the cells in various tissues and interface with genetic material or alter the function (i.e., the expression) of those genes. Pollutants include metals (e.g., aluminum, arsenic, cadmium, mercury), endocrine disruptors (e.g., bisphenol A and related compounds, dioxins, phthalates), air pollutants (e.g., benzene, particulates), and many other classes of compounds. Research has shown that toxic exposures can affect epigenetic expression several generations later. Even aside from their affects to our genetic functioning, environmental toxins are responsible for over 13,000,000 deaths each year. Therefore, finding ways to live more naturally and limit your body's exposure to these new materials is crucial. Given that we all spend part of our time indoors, this is also part of the environment we inhabit, and cleaning up this space is also important to our health.

11. Supportive community. The social environment that people experience is an important piece in determining the overall health and the quality of our genetic function. Neglect, mistreatment, stress, and depression are features that can be found in people who live without supportive community (i.e., those who live with uncaring and/or abusive parents, relatives, and neighbors). While it is well known that poor environments can dramatically alter children's ability to learn and both express and control emotions, these situations also affect adults and inhibit beautiful health (in part, through its effect on genetic function). Community practices such as celebration and offering gratitude are important elements of well-being. Engaging, caring, and supportive communities are a necessary piece for vibrant health.

12. Optimistic mood. A person's attitude toward life will play a strong role in their health. There is much to be pessimistic about in this time of human existence; however, constant grief and continual complaining (i.e., "throat choked with the dust of death") only serves to amplify feelings of depression and hopelessness, further compounding on existing health issues. Depressive moods and the stress they can generate ultimately effect the very functioning of our DNA. While contemplating issues to identify positive solutions is helpful, it is very different than dwelling on them for no constructive purpose. Every issue we face has a solution—you must not simply believe this, but you must practice this. Keep your internal fire glowing bright; do not let anything in this world extinguish it. You are not defined by the events that create grief, you are defined by the manner in which you choose to witness and celebrate creation (something that is always within your power to alter).

13. Positive spiritual practices. Your religion and the thoughts and moods it produces have the capability to influence genetic expression. Spiritual practices form part of the environment in which you exist. Practicing shame, intolerance, guilt, fear, and hatred (features that are common to some modern religions) are not a path to health. They create ill moods that would not be described as optimistic (see number 12). Further, some domesticated religions describe humans as having dominion over the natural world, which certainly stands in the way of people reconnecting with nature and feeling a deep love for all of creation (one of the most powerful healing sensations that humans can experience). The people that share your spiritual practices form part of your community—be sure these people possess the characteristics of a mature, supportive community.

14. Limiting addictive behaviors. "Reaching for the poisonous plants", one manner of describing addiction to various substances, is extremely harmful to genetic health as it exposes the body repeatedly to injurious chemicals and has profound effects on mood. Cigarette smoking and alcoholism have been linked to deleterious genetic changes in the body. Worse still, these alterations to gene expression are heritable; therefore, the compromised genetic expression one experiences as a result of exposure to these chemicals is passed on to their children and grandchildren. Therefore, addictive substances do not just harm the individual partaking in this behavior, but subsequent generations. Eliminate your use of addictive substances—it is not just your health that is at stake.

15. Experiencing happiness. Joy and bliss are highly influential to health. Happiness is related to mood and positively affects genetic expression. Spending time with people who create cheerful moods through humor, celebration, uplifting stories, and constructive actions generates a powerful environment that can support an optimistic frame of mind. Happiness is a critical piece of community and is implicated in people's ability to heal and defend themselves from disease.

16. Engaging in loving relationships. Caring relationships are vital to human well-being. Experiencing a strong and deeply loving partnership (or partnerships) promotes happiness and beneficially influences mood (all of which affect genetic expression). Intimate union that provides pleasure and gratification are supportive of a positive outlook on life and can be accurately described as medicine for the soul.

17. Practicing forgiveness. Holding ill feelings toward another being or object contributes to poor mood. Practicing forgiveness has been shown to improve traits such as anger, depression, and anxiety, all of which represent improvement to mood. Therefore, forgiveness both reduces emotional pain resulting from a stressful event and generates positive feelings. Forgiveness is a necessary skill today when so much hatred and violence permeates society, social media, and religion. It is important for people to realize that many people that perpetrate horrible acts of violence (on people, animals, and environment) are not well—they have a lifetime of dietary and lifestyle factors that have taken away any chance of well-being (i.e., they are simply acting as mentally ill individuals do). While I am not attempting to present that they have no choice in the decisions they make, I do recognize that the acts we witness are the inevitable outcome of a sick society. Remember, it is not personal, these people are emotionally damaged and, when forgiveness is practiced, they too can benefit.

18. Spending time in natural settings. Spending time in nature does more than merely provide exposure to the elements (number 7), it provides humans with a host of health benefits through immersion in our ancestral setting. Natural areas are geometrically more complex than urbanized area, providing beneficial stimulation to our central nervous system. Further, the sensations experienced in that environment (e.g., sounds, sights, smells) generate optimal moods for healing, creativity, compassion, and cooperation. Time in nature (as wild a setting as we can access) is crucial for physical, emotion, and spiritual health.

It is (hopefully) very clear at this point that (1) what nourishes humans is more than just the food items we consume and (2) ignoring our daily experiences as important causes of health or illness is not wise. Everything we experience in our environment changes our genetics. While diet and lifestyle do not rewrite our genetic code, they do change the expression of our genes and influence which ones are active and which are not. This is an amazing revelation which gives us tremendous opportunity to rewrite the stories of our health and well-being. To summarize, humans need to "consume" food from six categories or "kingdoms" in order to experience health and well-being. These kingdoms are (in no particular order): **animal foods**, **plant foods**, **fungal foods**, **bacterial foods** (e.g., probiotics), **elemental foods** (e.g., sunlight, soil, water), and **experiential foods** (e.g., happiness, spirituality, celebration, movement). The realization that our health is affected by more than just what is served on a plate necessitates a redefinition of nutrition. While many people go to great lengths to secure and prepare nutritious foods, those same people do not necessarily make time each day for the other forms of nutrition people need. This is imperative. For example, we need to make time for sun exposure on most days when the season allows such activity.

Finally, to reiterate, changes in gene expression (which can include silencing of genes) are now realized to be heritable for one or more generations, making it very important how one treats their body. Americans have stewarded their genomes as well as they have stewarded the environment (i.e., dismally poor). It is time create awareness around this issue and change our practices—it is completely selfish (and immoral) to participate in practices that negatively affect the health of generations yet to be born.

PLANTS AND THEIR NUTRITIONAL ELEMENTS

Plants are an important foundation for healthful living and nutritional intake. They were consumed by all cultures and, in many regions of the world, formed staples in the diet. Even in the far north, where plant foods were not available for much of the year, hunter-gatherers consumed a diverse array of leaves, shoots, roots, berries, and other plant portions. Consider the Iñupiat of extreme northwestern Alaska, where it is estimated that only 1% of their yearly calories were from plant foods, but 50% of the vitamin C was derived from this 1%. While we could cover many aspects of plant nutrition, the discussion here will center primarily on micronutrients, phytochemistry, essential fatty acids, and dietary fiber. These topics allow us to highlight the differences between wild and cultivated plants, the latter of which have been genetically modified through breeding. While many people are comfortable with this version of genetic modification, it is likely this acceptance is based, in part, on a poor understanding of what has happened to the plant foods usually ingested in affluent countries. The next paragraphs will detail the modifications (which are sometimes extensive) that have occurred to modern plant foods.

Plants provide certain **micronutrients**, which are needed by the body in various amounts (depending on the specific nutrient and the lifestyle demands) to coordinate physiological functions and fulfill structural requirements. For purpose of this discussion, micronutrients will include all minerals, including those sometimes referred to as macrominerals because they are used by the body in larger amounts than trace minerals. In general, plants are important sources for pro-vitamin A (i.e., carotenoids), certain B-complex vitamins, vitamin C, vitamin E, vitamin K_1, and many minerals. On average, wild plants are a better source of vitamins and minerals than cultivated species. This is born out in many studies (a good summary of the studies was printed in the third chapter of Ancestral Plants volume 2 published in 2015). To illustrate the nutrient density of wild plants, let us first examine vitamin C, sometimes incorrectly called ascorbic acid (vitamin C is this aforementioned organic acid, along with flavonoids, rutin, the enzyme tyrosinase, and several other factors that benefit blood vessel strength and the oxygen carrying capacity of red blood cells). Vitamin C is required for several enzymatic reactions, including the synthesis of collagen, is an antioxidant, and is important in the functioning of the immune system. In the United States, we have been led to believe that oranges (*Citrus ×sinensis*), a cultivated fruit derived through many generations of breeding wild fruits, are a good source of this vitamin. Most sources report a value close to 50 mg of vitamin C per 100 grams of tissue for this nothospecies (i.e., hybrid), though it should be noted that some measured oranges contained no vitamin C at all—it depends on their growing conditions and other factors. If we examine the wild food literature, we can identify many sources of plants that far exceed this fruit in vitamin C content. For example, Zennie and Ogzewalla studied wild plants in Ohio and Kentucky (publishing their work in 1977). Some of the plants they assayed follow (in alphabetic order).

garlic mustard (*Alliaria petiolata*) leaves: 190 mg/100 g
crow garlic (*Allium vineale*) leaves: 130 mg/100 g
garden yellow rocket (*Barbarea vulgaris*) leaves: 130–152 mg/100 g
shepherd's purse (*Capsella bursa-pastoris*): 91 mg/100 g
eastern redbud (*Cercis canadensis*) flowers: 69–82 mg/100 g
highbush-cranberry (*Viburnum opulus*) fruits: 100 mg/100 g
woolly violet (*Viola sororia*) leaves 130–264 mg/100 g

If we were to take a simple mean of the 24 values they report (some species were tested multiple times at different points in the growing season), we find the average vitamin C content of the plants in their study to be approximately 81 mg of vitamin C per100 g of tissue. While clearly a sample size of 16 species of plants cannot be considered a large sample, note that the average content of these plants surpasses that of the orange. The only intent of these rudimentary statistics is to suggest that the orange may not be a "high" source of vitamin C. The work of Halásová and Jičínská (published in 1988) further illustrates where oranges actually rank. They studied one of the true standout species in regards to vitamin C, roses (genus *Rosa*). Some of the more noteworthy figures they reported follow (in order of vitamin C content).

beach rose (*Rosa rugosa*): 2730 mg/100 g
small-flowered sweet-briar rose (*Rosa micrantha*): 2828 mg/100 g
dog rose (*Rosa canina*—reported as *Rosa corymbifera*) 4571 mg/100 g
red-leaved rose (*Rosa glauca*) 5108 mg/100 g
cinnamon rose (*Rosa cinnamomea*) 5300 mg/100 g

These figures range up to 106 times the vitamin C content of oranges, and are equal to or exceed other exceptional sources of vitamin C, such as kakadu-plum (*Terminalia ferdinandiana*) and camu camu (*Myrciaria dubia*). As these numbers illustrate, oranges are not particularly rich in vitamin C, but Americans have been convinced of such by a continuous marketing campaign. The Standard American Diet is relatively poor in nutrition due, in part, to its over-reliance on excessively modified produce.

For a second example of the nutrient density of wild plants, we will examine the mineral calcium. This mineral is one of the most important micronutrients used by the body, and is vital for cell signaling, muscle contraction, and skeletal and dental integrity (among other purposes). Plants can be valuable sources of bioavailable calcium, and while they do not rival certain unpasteurized dairy products, plants can be better sources than many animal foods. For comparative statistics, we look back to 1966 and the work of Euell Gibbons, where some of the first nutritional assays on wild plants were performed. What was interesting about his work is that he compared the nutrition of wild plants with cultivated plants to provide the reader with a relative measure of nutrient density. In two comparisons that were made, he first listed nine wild edible plants, including the leaves and/or shoots of American pokeweed (*Phytolacca americana*), "green" amaranthus (genus *Amaranthus*), and common dandelion (*Taraxacum officinale*), which were compared with nine cultivated plants, including celery (*Apium graveolens*), spinach (*spinacea oleracea*), and Swiss chard (*Beta vulgaris*). The mean calcium content of the wild plants was 152.8 mg per 100 g. The mean calcium content of the domesticated plants was 61.1 mg per 100 g. Therefore, the wild plants contained more than twice the calcium as the included cultivated plants (some of which are considered to be very nutritious produce). Of the nine species of wild and cultivated plants assayed, the range of calcium content per 100 g was 53–309 mg for wild species and 9–93 mg for the cultivated species.

Gibbons then compared nine wild fruits with seven cultivated fruits. In this case, the plants chosen were mostly those that follow the lay definition of fruit (i.e., a relatively sweet, fleshy fruit). The wild plants included species such as black elderberry (*Sambucus nigra*), blueberries (genus *Vaccinium*), and black raspberry (*Rubus occidentlis*), whereas the cultivated species were familiar fruits such as apple (*Malus pumila*), orange (*Citrus ×sinensis*), and peach (*Prunus persica*). In this case, the mean calcium value (per 100 g) for the wild plants was 29.5, compared with 13.9 for the cultivated species. The range of reported calcium values was 9–81 for the wild species and 6–41 for the cultivated species. While the sample size (n=18 and 16) is not large, similar results are borne out in other studies that compare wild vs. cultivated plants. There is variation in wild and cultivated plants regarding their nutritional content; however, on average, wild plants do supply greater amounts of vitamins and minerals. This is an important fact because it allows people to achieve optimal nutrition while consuming fewer overall calories than cultivated species.

Perhaps where plants shine the most (from a nutritional perspective) concerns the **phytochemicals** (i.e., plant compounds) that they supply to those who consume them. Unfortunately, most people don't realize that plant chemistry is extremely important for human health. Further, the plants that most people consume have lost some or much of their phytochemistry due to the breeding that they have experienced. Unlike domesticated animals, which we genetically modified to produce traits like tameness and greater mass, in plants we intentionally (in some cases) and unintentionally (in other cases) bred out the phytochemistry (read medicine) to produce plant foods that were less bitter and more sweet. What was lost during this process were compounds that produce an array of benefits in the body, including the following actions: analgesic, anti-allergenic, anti-arrhythmic, anti-diabetic, antihypotensive (i.e., lowering elevated blood pressure), anti-inflammatory, antimicrobial, antineoplastic (i.e., combatting cancerous tumors), antioxidant, cardiotonic, genoprotective, immune system modulation, and nervine (i.e., benefitting the central nervous system). The loss of these medicinal benefits in our foods is one (of many) reasons the Standard American Diet produces such poor health outcomes.

Phytochemicals come in a diverse array of forms and biological activity. Some are highly beneficial, others are toxic in sufficient doses. However, some of those "poisonous" phytochemicals are used as herbal medicines in smaller amounts, indicating we need to rethink how we classify plants—the difference between food, medicine, and poison is the dose (you already realize this, take a couple ibuprofen and you experience relief of inflammation and pain, eat the entire bottle of tablets and you will experience a completely different result). Plant compounds not only vary in their physiological effects on the body, they also vary in their tastes and flavors (e.g., bitter, acrid, aromatic, spicy). Overall, we know that wild plants contain higher levels of beneficial phytochemicals. This has been borne out in numerous studies and is another piece of evidence indicating wild plants are nutritional superior to cultivated plants.

There are several examples from the literature that can be used to support an assertion that wild plants possess greater levels of beneficial phytochemicals than cultivated plants. Perhaps of most use are comparisons using wild and cultivated kinds of the same type of plant food. For example, one study from Turkey performed by Yilmaz and colleagues examined blackberry (genus *Rubus*) fruits from nine cultivars and 16 wild species. While the cultivated species had (usually) larger fruits, the wild species had greater phenolic content and greater free-radical scavenging capacity. Phenols belong to a class of organic compounds called polyphenols, which are are a large group of water-soluble biomolecules, some of which are responsible for significant positive health effects in humans. These effects include reducing inflammation, strengthening of blood vessels, suppression of tumors, and quenching free-radicals (i.e., charged molecules) that damage DNA, cell membranes, and the interior of blood vessels through their ability to steal electrons (which contributes to disease and premature aging). In this study, the mean phenolic content was over 40% higher in the wild fruits and the mean free-radical scavenging ability was nearly 7% higher. In another study comparing wild and cultivated blackberries (by Koca and Karadeniz), the wild species possessed, on average, 25% more free-radical scavenging ability than cultivated ones (and some wild forms had nearly 80% more antioxidant capacity than the average cultivated blackberry. Results similar to these are frequently borne out in other studies examining other fruits.

Humans require two kinds of **essential fatty acids** called ω6 and ω3 fatty acids (remember, the Greek letter ω is read as "omega"). Humans cannot manufacture these lipids in their body; therefore, they must be acquired in the diet. While both of these lipids are essential for health, they have opposing biochemical effects, which means they must be ingested in roughly similar amounts (in a ratio of 1:1 to 3:1 ω6 to ω3). Unfortunately, most modern diets actually range much higher in ω6 fatty acids (as much as 24:1), this owed in large part to our use of modern grains as staples and our high use of extracted seed oils, such as corn, soy, cotton, and safflower oils, all of which are typically high sources of ω6 fatty acids. For example, these seed oils are approximately 50 to 100 times more rich in ω6 fatty acids than ω3 fatty acids, contributing to inflammation and suppressing the functioning of the immune system. Wild foods, including plants, are, on average, foods that supply a more balanced ratio of essential fatty acids.

Bere (2007) performed a small study to examine three wild fruits found in Norway and three cultivated fruits that were commonly imported into the country. The three wild fruits were mountain bilberry (*Vaccinium myrtillus*), baked-apple-berry (*Rubus chamaemorus*), and mountain cranberry (*Vaccinium vitis-idaea*), which were compared with cultivated apples, bananas, and oranges. What Bere found was that the wild fruits possessed more ω3 fatty acids (both actually and relatively) than the cultivated fruits. The mean value of the ratio of ω6/ ω3 fatty acids in the wild fruits was 0.9 vs. 1.8 in the cultivated fruits. The mean content of ω3 fatty acids was 0.25 grams per 100 grams of tissue in the wild fruits vs. 0.02 g/100 g in the cultivated fruits (note that the wild fruits supplied 12.5 times the ω3 fatty acid content of the cultivated fruits). This study was interesting in that it supported the consumption of wild fruits present on the Norwegian landscape as a method of attaining health and dealing with a surplus of ω6 in the contemporary diet of that country.

Wild plant foods are rich sources of **dietary fiber** and, as a corollary, provide fewer calories per unit mass than cultivated foods. Fiber is an important component of wild diets and has been shown to increase satiety without increasing calorie ingestion, lower cholesterol levels, regulate blood sugar through an increased glycemic response, promote insulin sensitivity, and reduce certain kinds of cancers through the production of specific fermentation products (e.g., short-chain fatty acids) in the colon. In fact, through epigenetic mechanisms, diets rich in certain kinds of fiber, such as resistant starches (called prebiotics) that pass through the small intestine without being digested to the large intestine, improve the glycemic health of the next generation through epigenetic mechanisms. Boyd Eaton (in a couple of publications) has estimated that modern produce contains almost three times the calories (read sugars) than the wild foods they were derived from (when a broad selection of foods is examined). An increase in sugars is the result of a lower density of dietary fiber within the foods. Higher caloric intake (and the corresponding lower nutrient intake, which includes losses in dietary fiber) is a recipe for poor health and cancer.

Given that the plant foods we have access to on this planet are not equivalent sources of calories (based on their nutrient density and other factors), it makes sense to group the plant foods and provide a means of prioritizing which ones should be consumed in the diet (when possible). Categorizing plant foods based on their nutritional value (which would also include their plant chemistry) and how harmful they are to our physical and ecosystem's health is a simple but powerful way to rank plant foods. The following list includes four categories of plant foods. You should strive to eat as high on this list as often as possible. It includes a brief synopsis of the reasons for the value or harm these plants cause.

Wild Plants. These are species that grow outside of cultivation and their genomes have not been intentionally manipulated by humans (save for rare cultivated species that can naturalize). They are documented as the most nutrient-dense plants on the planet. Because they have not been genetically modified through breeding, they possess unmodified levels of phytochemicals (i.e., plant compounds) that present potent medicinal actions in the body, including protection from cancer. Their growth occurs outside of intentional landscape manipulation by humans (though they may take advantage of human-caused disturbance). No pesticides, no herbicides, no fungicides, and no fossil fuels are needed for their growth. Wild plants are a resource that humans and wild animals compete for; therefore, conscientious collecting is a must to sustain wild plant populations and share foods with the other-than-human persons we live alongside. Wild plants represent the most eco-conscientious foods on the planet.

Organically Raised Plants. These are cultivated plants that have, to some degree (sometimes extensively), been modified by people to present desired qualities (e.g., sweetness, flavor, shelf-life, greater size, shortened period to maturation, seedlessness). As a result, there have been documented losses in nutrition, phytochemistry, and fiber in these plants. Their growth often requires dramatic alterations to the landscape to clear forests, drain or alter wetlands, and plow the soil; however, those grown in perennial polyculture require less. In large scale agriculture, organically raised plants require huge amounts of fossil fuels to perform a variety of actions on the farms (e.g., tilling, planting, fertilizing, burning weeds, harvesting). Fortunately, these plants still need to defend themselves against insect herbivores and pathogens, so they do produce various phytochemicals to protect themselves. In regard to these types of plants, the more the plant resembles its wild progenitor in form and flavor, the more healthful it is likely to be.

Conventionally Raised Plants. These are species that have all of the drawbacks of organically raised plants, plus they are raised in a chemical-laden fashion that pollutes the soil, water, and air. Chemical herbicides, fungicides, and/or pesticides are used to grow such cultivars. Industrially created fertilizers (from fossil fuels) may be used to enrich soils in a few key nutrients; however, many minerals are known to be depleted in the soils using this practice alone. Because these plants do not need to protect themselves from insect herbivores and pathogens, their already muted levels of phytochemistry (due to breeding) are further suppressed by the absence of need to defend themselves (human growers take care of this). Conventionally raised plants supply less nutrition to humans directly, less nutrition to animals who are fed these plants (hence, less nutrition to humans indirectly), and pollute the landscape (sometimes at great distances from where the chemicals are used).

Roundup Ready GMO plants. These represent the least healthy and most damaging plants on the planet. They have all of the drawbacks of organically raised plants and conventionally raised plants, plus they provide even less mineral nutrition, harm the health of the people who consume them, and genetically contaminate other species of plants. Compounds in the herbicide Roundup bind with soil minerals and prevent plants from taking them up, which means the plants can't supply them to the animals (including people) who consume them. Building evidence suggests these plants may not be substantially equivalent, in regard to health, as non-laboratory GMO plants (as stated by the companies that create them). Further, these species ultimately contaminate nearby fields of plants because the pollinators (e.g., wind, flying insects) do not limit their travels to fields where Roundup Ready plants are grown, transferring genetic material to closely related plants. Given all of the drawbacks, one has to wonder why anyone would consume these plants or feed them to animals.

BREEDING THE MEDICINE OUT OF FOOD AND HOW TO RECOVER IT

We have already discussed the fact that wild plants contain higher levels of beneficial phytochemicals that have a host of positive actions in the body. Here, we will discuss a few examples to expand our awareness of this concept and further support that modern produce (as a whole) has drawbacks for a life free of chronic disease. Fortunately, there are solutions that we can employ, regardless of where we live. Those solutions will be presented later in this section.

One of the great examples of breeding the medicine out of food can be told by the story of grapes (genus *Vitis*). Wild grapes typically contain 2–4 seeds that are firm (but can be chewed up), slightly fibrous, and are not pleasant tasting like the flesh is. For this reason, most modern cultivars of grapes sold for food in supermarkets are seedless. While the seeds may be considered an annoyance to contemporary people, they are a treasure trove of nutrition and medicine. Grape seeds contain vitamin E, a powerful antioxidant vitamin that protects cell membranes from oxidation (i.e., the process of biological molecules being harmed by oxygen radicals). Grape seeds also contain substantial amounts of proanthocyanidins, a group of polyphenol plant chemicals that have 20 times the free-radical quenching ability of vitamin E. Antioxidants in food help to protect our bodies from damage caused by environmental toxins, refined foods with oxidized lipids, sunlight, normal metabolic activity, and aging. In fact, antioxidants are one of the body's first lines of defense against damage that can (ultimately) lead to cancer. The proanthocyanidins are also benefit vascular health and can improve circulation and protect against (and heal) varicosities. Animal studies even have demonstrated that proanthocyanidins exert an antidepressant action. Be aware that grapeseed oil, sold as a health food, is devoid of most of the medicine described in this paragraph due to the extraction and processing it has received (i.e., you need to go to the source for health, not a commercially constructed form of the food).

Given all these benefits, one has to wonder why people would consume seedless grapes. This modern version of grapes, while tasty, has been robbed of much of its medicine through genetic changes due to breeding. Today, some people who seek "natural remedies" for various problems they are experiencing purchase extracts (i.e., supplements) of various plants in an effort to heal ailments without resorting to pharmaceutical drugs. Grape seed extract is a common supplement sold in health food stores that is used to treat varicose veins, enlarged and swollen veins as a result of faulty valves that prevent the reverse flow of blood. If you think about this practice critically, this is what is occurring: we (i.e., humans) take a wild food that is rich in health-promoting compounds, we genetically modify the food to substantially reduce its medical value, and then purchase the medicine from various companies to make up for the lack phytochemistry in the cultivated version. While the lack of seeds in grapes is not the cause of the high rates of cancer city builders experience, the process of changing our foods to present muted levels of phytochemistry and other medicinal compounds (such as conjugated linoleic acid in grazing animals) is one of the critical factors for the cancer epidemic today.

While losing the seeds from grapes may not appear, on the surface, to be a major modification of a plant food (because it does not represent a major change in the form of the food), the following examples may better explain the changes that have occurred to modern cultivated produce. Pictured below is prickly lettuce (*Lactuca serriola*; figure 3.1), the wild progenitor of cultivated lettuce (*Lactuca sativa*; figure 3.2) that is native to Europe, Asia, and northern Africa. Prickly lettuce, despite its name, is an edible plant that contains polyphenols and another group of phytochemicals called terpenes. Collectively, these phytochemicals produce a slight bitter flavor. They also supply mild sedative, analgesic, and antispasmodic activity. As a result, consumption of this wild plant (and others like it) held to calm the human body, mildly suppress pain, and allay coughing and intestinal pain. The significant loss of these phytochemicals in cultivated lettuce is evidenced by the fact this produce does not taste bitter. Bitters, unbeknownst to many people, have an array of benefits for human health, including bolstering production of enzymes and bile used to digest foods, increasing absorption of fat-soluble vitamins, supporting the function of the liver, promoting regularity of bowel movements, and assisting with some gastrointestinal issues (e.g., bloating, flatulence, upset stomach). In other words, the mild taste found in farm-grown lettuce is correlated with both the loss of medicine and a loss in digestive health. Further, the dramatic change in morphology from the wild to the cultivated form offers (generally speaking) an understanding of the degree of genetic change that has occurred in this produce. If you plan to still consume lettuce, I would encourage you to focus on leaf lettuce over romaine lettuce over iceberg lettuce, as leaf lettuce is the older form and contains more of the original nutrition found in prickly lettuce.

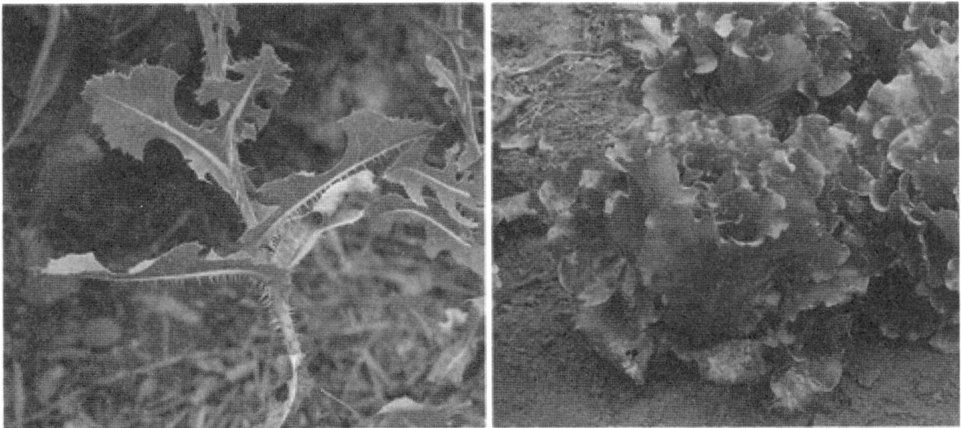

Figures 3.1 (left) and 3.2 (right). Figure 3.1—Prickly lettuce (*Lactuca serriola*) by Arthur Haines. Figure 3.2—cultivated lettuce (*Lactuca sativa*) by Dwight Sipler (Wikipedia Commons).

One more example of the loss of medicine from wild plants concerns a native of Africa and Asia called gray bitter-apple (*Solanum incanum*; figure 3.3), the wild progenitor of eggplant (*Solanum melongena*; figure 3.4), both of which are pictured below. Gray bitter-apple is a harshly prickly plant with a small, roughtly spherical green to yellow fruit that is seeded and very bitter (i.e., unpalateable). The bitterness is produced from a suite of alkaloids, a pharmacologically active class phytochemicals that are found in some plant medicines. Gray bitter-apple was traditionally used for several forms of medicine, including pain relief, treatment of infections and parasites, and to aid in healing wounds. Modern research demonstrates is has potent antibacterial activity against some pathogenic bacteria and fungi, produces improved glycemic health, and may be useful in the treatment of several cancers. Historical cultivation primarily sought to change three features of this plant's fruit—size, shape, and taste. Along with these changes, the medicinal content of the leaves and the prickliness of the plant were also altered during its genetic modification. Ancient Chinese texts document the gradual increase in fruit size and length, and loss of bitterness through the centuries (as chronicled in the research of Wang and colleuges, published in 2008). Today, the eggplant is a large, elongate, and very mild-flavored sterile fruit (i.e., without viable seeds) with a dark exterior color. At this point, you might be thinking that this genetic modification must have been a good thing because the wild progenitor wasn't a food at all, and now we have an additional kind of cultivated produce. To that, I would answer yes, but we should have stopped the genetic modification earlier in the history of this fruit, at a time when some of its medicine was still present. We should have stopped at a point when the fruit size was not substantially large and when seeds were still present. We shouldn't have tried to breed most of the medicine out of this plant (which has occurred today with the forms we consume).

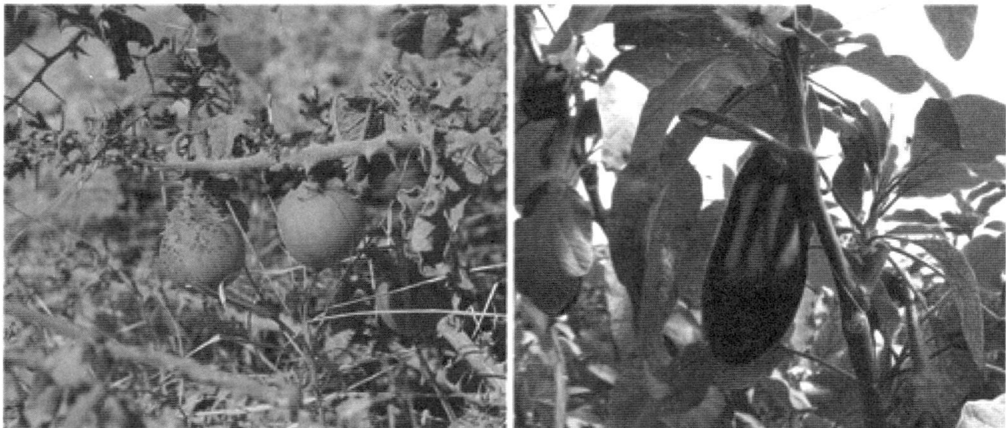

Figures 3.3 (left) and 3.4 (right). Figure 3.3—gray bitter-apple (*Solanum incanum*) by Nepenthes (Wikipedia Commons). Figure 3.4—eggplant (*Solanum melongena*) (Wikipedia Commons).

Despite that fact that wild plants are the most nutrient-dense plant foods available to humans, most people are not able to consume them as often as they would like to (or not all all) for various reasons. Some people do not have easy access to wild plants, due to the location of their residence. As often the case, people do not have the knowledge to locate, identify, gather, and process wild plants. This lack of knowledge effectively prevents access to the original plant foods of our ancestors. For some people, it is simply lack of motivation given how little work is required to source foods at the local supermarket. For those that can't consume ample wild foods in the diet (for whatever reason), there are two solutions that they can employ to deal with the loss of medicine from our cultivated foods:

1. eat plants that have lost much of their medicine and then purchase medicine (in the form of pharmaceutical drugs) from local pharmacies; or
2. eat plants that still contain their medicine and (in conjunction with a natural lifestyle) live lives that are relatively free of health ailments.

Actually, solution number 1 doesn't work that well for many people because that is the Standard American Lifeway. Given the abundant health issues faced by Americans, it is clear that the medicine we purchase doesn't prevent ailments from appearing—it only treats the symptoms once our health is compromised. Prevention of a disease is always preferred to contracting a disease and then trying to treat it. So, let's recognize that wild plants are fundamentally more nutrient dense than cultivated plants, especially when we consider nutrition to represent not just vitamins and minerals, but also beneficial compounds (i.e., the medicine), essential fatty acids, dietary fiber, and a host of items we haven't even identified yet.

Fortunately, there is a "next best option" for bringing nutrition (in all its forms) into your life. This option is to focus on **minimally modified plant foods** that you can purchase at the farmer's market and in supermarkets. Minimally modified plants are those that resemble their wild progenitors more closely in form, flavor, nutrition, fertility, and/or vigor. Given that the supermarket produce has been created by genetically modifying wild plants, early in this process (i.e., thousands of years ago in some cases), the cultivated plants were more similar to wild plants in their nutrient content. These heirloom versions are older forms of cultivated plants that can be still grown and purchased today. Some of the produce we find in stores today has little similarity to wild plants. These are the forms you would want to avoid because they have lost much of their beneficial phytochemistry. Below are four criteria I use to help guide my cultivated plant purchases.

1. Does the cultivated plant food in question resemble that of the wild plant?
In other words, does the leaf or fruit look like that produced by the wild plant (in terms of morphological similarity). Good examples of cultivated plants that produce fruits that look very similar to their wild progenitor include blueberries, blackberries, and raspberries. Examples of cultivated plant fruits that don't look at all like their wild progenitor include sweet corn, eggplant, and watermelon.

2. Do the cultivated shoots or greens have a robust flavor?
By this, I'm referring to a stronger flavor, whether that is some bitterness, spiciness, or aromatic qualities. All of these traits indicate that the plants are still phytochemically potent. There are many examples of cultivated plants that have these traits. Bitterness can be experienced with endive and cultivated chicory greens. Spiciness is found garden rocket and other mustard greens, horse-radish roots, and spicy peppers. Aromatic plants include many mints (e.g., basil, oregano, spearmint), members of the onion family, and spices from the celery family (e.g., anise, dill, and cumin).

3. Does the cultivated fruit still contain its seeds?
Fruits that contain viable seeds are still able to perpetuate themselves. The loss of seeds from fruits represents both a further modification from the wild form as well as a loss of nutrition (some seeds are edible and contain essential fatty acids, vitamin E, and additional phytochemicals). Fruits that still contain their edible seeds include blueberries, seeded figs, and seeded grapes.

4. Can the cultivated plant escape the tended garden setting and grow wild?
If a wild plant has been modified extensively enough, it often loses its ability to grow in the wild (i.e., outside of cultivation where it is propagated and tended by humans). The inability to grow in the wild demonstrates that a plant has lost its adaptations that allow it to survive the stresses it must endure, such as water shortage, insect herbivory, and fungal pathogens. Different regions will have cultivated plants that are capable of growing in the wild. For example, in the northeastern United States, species such as asparagus, parsnip, and turnip can (and often do) escape the garden setting and grow in the wild.

To further provide an understanding of the idea of minimally modified plant foods (including wild plants that are available at markets), the following list in provided. Keep in mind, this list is, by no means, comprehensive. It is only meant to further illuminate the idea of what a minimally modified plant foods are (use it to understand the concept of minimally modified plants).

BULBS, TUBERS, AND OTHER UNDERGROUND ORGANS

beets (*Beta vulgaris*)
burdock (*Arctium lappa*)—taproots are often available in stores
garlic (*Allium sativum*)—with a host of medicinal uses
ginger (*Zingiber officinale*)
horse-radish (*Armoracia rusticana*)
onion (*Allium cepa*)
parsnip (*Pastinaca sativa*)
purple carrots (*Daucus carota* subsp. *sativus*)—the original cultivated carrot was purple, not orange
tuberous sunflower (*Helianthus tuberosus*)—often referred to as Jerusalem-artichoke
turmeric (*Curcuma longa*)—well-studied for its cancer fighter ability

FLESHY FRUITS

avocado (*Persea americana*)
blackberry (*Rubus* hybrids)—cultivated forms have complicated parentage
blueberry (mostly *Vaccinium angustifolium* and *V. corymbosum* in North America)
cranberry (*Vaccinium macrocarpon*)
currants (*Ribes rubrum*)
matrimony-vine (*Lyceum barbarum*)—also referred to as goji-berry.
mulberry (*Morus alba*)
Peruvian ground-cherry (*Physalis peruviana*)—often sold under the name goldenberry
prickly pear (*Opuntia ficus-indica*)—also called Indian-fig
red raspberry (*Rubus idaeus*)

LEAVES AND SHOOTS

asparagus (*Asparagus officinalis*)
beet greens (*Beta vulgaris*)—this is also called chard
chicory greens (*Cichorium intybus*)—sold as "dandelion" greens
dill (*Anethum graveolens*)
endive (*Cichorium endivia*)
fennel (*Foeniculum vulgare*)
garden rocket (*Eruca vesicaria*)—also called arugula
kale raab (*Brassica oleracea*)—some forms of this species (e.g., cauliflower) are very modified
leaf lettuce (*Lactuca sativa*)— iceberg and Romaine kinds are less nutritious
oregano (*Origanum vulgare*)—also known as wild majoram
sage (*Salvia officinalis*)—also known as West Indian sage
spearmint (*Mentha spicata*)
spinach (*Spinacea oleracea*)
sweet basil (*Ocimum basilicum*)
two-rowed water-cress (*Nasturtium officinale*)

NUTS, SEEDS, AND OTHER DRY FRUITS

amaranth (*Amaranthus caudatus*, *A. cruentus*, *A. hypochondriacus*)
Brazil nuts (*Bertholletia excelsa*)—mostly collected from wild trees
coconut palm (*Cocos nucifera*)
chia (*Salvia hispanica*)
hazel nut (*Corylus avellana* and others)

hemp (*Cannabis sativa*)—the small, seed-like fruits are highly nutritious
pecan (*Carya illinoinensis*)
pine seeds (*Pinus edulis* and others)—usually, and incorrectly, referred to as "pine nuts"
quinoa (*Chenopodium quinoa*)
sunflower (*Helianthus annuus*)—the fruit is often referred to as "sunflower seeds"
wild rice (*Zizania aquatica* and *Z. palustris*)—find wild-harvested kinds, avoid paddy-grown versions

Consider a few items before we leave the topic of minimally modified plants. First, essentially all spice plants can be included on this list. They are rich in phytochemistry (which provides their aromatic qualities). Many spice plants are also more capable of surviving outside of the garden setting as they have not been genetically altered as much because we (humans) wanted to maintain their phytochemistry, not remove it. Two, there are companies that offer wild-collected seaweeds, such as dulse (*Palmaria palmata*) and kelp (*Saccharina longicruris*). These are additional examples of plants (algae) that contain their potent nutrition. And three, consider reviving an appreciation for bitter tastes. Bitters benefit digestion by stimulating the flow of digestive fluids. Regular consumption of bitters has been shown to assist with supporting liver function, increasing the absorption of fat-soluble vitamins, relieving symptoms of heart burn and excessive gas, easing constipation, and reducing the cravings for sweet foods. Bitter tastes also indicate that the plant food in question still contains some of its phytochemistry (i.e., its medicine) and is one the evolutionary mechanisms that humans use to determine the antioxidant quality of certain foods (because many antioxidant compounds impart a bitter flavor to the food—Drewnowski and Gomez-Carneros published a nice review of this in 2000). In other words, the bitter taste your tongue is designed to detect is, at least in part, there to help you identify high antioxidant foods. But, if you think about it, the Standard American Diet is practically bereft of bitters, indicating a general loss of medicinal food in the cuisine.

In conclusion, wild plants are the versions of plants that have nourished anatomically modern humans for over 95% of their existence, it makes sense to think of our bodies as being adapted to the nutrition found in those wild organisms. Said another way, we need the levels of nourishment found in non-cultivated plants or our genetic expression can be compromised and our health can falter. If you are willing to examine your plant food purchases and make adjustments, it is possible to step up your nutrition, not just in terms of vitamins and minerals, but also in amounts of beneficial phytochemicals, essential fatty acids, and dietary fiber. Large, seedless, incredibly sweet versions of plants are not a foundation to build health upon (especially when the wild progenitors were small, seeded, and bitter). Such cultivated fruits provide more fructose, less fiber, and less medicine than the species from which they were derived. Seek out plants that are not twisted into bizarre forms. For example, cabbage is very different from the wild mustard (*Brassica oleracea*) it hails from. Therefore, I would much prefer kale and kale raab (also from this same species) if the choice was available. Another way to achieve this goal is to identify the older versions of cultivated plants (the heirloom breeds mentioned previously). Using this search criterion, I would seek out heirloom flint corn over a modern sweet corn (if I were to purchase corn). I do this for the simple reason that the more human-modified a plant becomes (i.e., the further it is contorted from the natural form of its wild ancestor), the more new it becomes as a food. The newer it becomes, the less understanding we have of how it affects our health and the health of the next generations. Further, the newer it becomes, the less nutrition (usually) it provides. Food's purpose isn't just to supply calories, it is to power our physical, emotional, and spiritual bodies so that we may achieve our full genetic potential.

PLANT ANTINUTRIENTS

Animals have many methods of protecting themselves from predation. Some can fly away at the first hint of perceived danger, others can run very fast. Some species defend themselves with teeth, claws, hooves, or antlers. Others produce foul smells to deter predators from chasing, killing, and eating them. But plants are sedentary. They cannot run away when their predators approach them. Some species do arm themselves with prickles, spines, or thorns, but these are not a defense against all species. Therefore, plants have developed an elaborate system of chemical defenses to make their organs unpalatable, cause sickness, reduce growth and fertility in herbivores, or even stupefy (through intoxication) the animals that feed on them (making those who consume them easier to capture by their predators). However, humans are incredibly intelligent and very resourceful. They have developed ingenious ways to overcome the phytochemical defenses of plants. These were developed primarily by the indigenous of the world (and some of the traditional cultures who followed them). Antinutrients are hardly mentioned anymore in American cuisine—and it shows in the health of the people.

Following is a brief discussion of a few of the most important antinutrients that are encountered in wild plant foods. Knowing about these and learning proper food processing can make profound differences in the actual nutrient absorption from one's food. Included are concepts that can be used to reduce or remove the antinutrients. Ignorance of this topic contributes to a number of health issues, including osteoporosis, anemia, delayed growth, poor immune system function, slow wound healing, depressed thyroid function, dysregulation of blood glucose, and learning disabilities. Recipes that incorporate proper processing can be found in "Nourishing Traditions" by Sally Fallon.

Phytic acid is an antinutrient found in a suite of fruits and seeds, including grains, legumes, nuts, and achenes (the last are seed-like fruits, a good example is quinoa). The biological role of phytic acid is to hold on to phosphorus until a fruit or seed sprouts, at which time it releases the phosphorus for the seedling to utilize (phosphorus is an important mineral for seedling growth). When phytic acid is bound to a mineral, it is referred to as phytate. The problem is that phytic acid can also hold on to other minerals, blocking their absorption by the body and rendering a particular food less nutritious. Calcium, iron, copper, manganese, magnesium, potassium, zinc, and other minerals can be held tightly by phytic acid, and these minerals pass through the digestive system without being utilized by the body. Evidence indicates that vitamin B_3 can also be bound to phytic acid. A lifetime of consuming phytic acid-rich foods can leave a person in a state of nutrient depletion.

In nature (or in the garden), a seed that begins to germinate (i.e., is sprouting) goes through several changes. One of those is that an endogenous enzyme, called phytase, is produced. Phytase deactivates phytates (i.e., phytic acid with phosphorus or any other mineral bound to it). In other words, the enzyme causes a chemical change to the phytic acid and reduces its ability to hold on tightly to minerals. Therefore, the consumption of sprouted grains, legumes, nuts, and achenes means less phytates are consumed in the diet. Said another way, consumption of sprouted foods provides more mineral nutrition because some of the phytates are deactivated and the body is free to absorb those minerals in the gastrointestinal tract.

Of course, one does not need to collect sprouted seeds out of the soil to take advantage of this method of food preparation. One can sprout grains, nuts, etc., prior to their consumption. The process is relatively straightforward. It involves soaking these foods for 8–12 hours in water and then draining the water and placing them so that the fruits/seeds remain moist (but not inundated) for 2–4 days (depending on the food). Some items require that they are spread out inside a container to sprout properly, others do just fine when clumped in a pile. Sprouting at room temperature leads to approximately 25–50% reduction in phytates for most foods, though this can be increased by extending the time and increasing the temperature, such as ca. 25–30 degrees Celsius (approximately 80 to 90 degrees Fahrenheit). Though the details vary for each food, such as what exact temperature works best, using extended sprouting time at higher temperatures can result in phytate reduction of 75–92% (again, depending on the food and exact methods used). The point is, sprouting via any method will result in greater levels of nutrition being derived from the food one consumes.

Sprouting (i.e., germinating) can work for intact fruits/seeds. However, sometimes we are dealing with a food that has been ground to fine particle size for various reasons, such as flour. In this case, the food cannot be sprouted. Therefore, other methods must be used (and these same methods can also be used with intact fruits/seeds). One of those is soaking, where the food (whole or ground) is placed in water and allowed to soak for 12–24 hours. It generally works best if the soaking water is slightly acidic, which can be made so by the addition of some vinegar, yogurt, cream, sour milk, sour fruit juice, etc. I usually add 30–45 cc's (ca. 2–3 tablespoons) of an acidic agent per liter (barely more than a quart) of water used in soaking. Assuming the food is intact or is made up of whole ground material, the endogenous enzyme phytase can still be activated to deactivate the phytates. Soaking varies in its efficacy for reducing phytates. Again, depending on temperature and time, this method has been shown to reduce phytates by 4–51% (the addition of fermenting organisms increases this greatly; see below). Soaking won't deactivate phytic acid in foods like white flour and white rice because the bran has been removed (where most of the phytates and the phytase are located). So, these kinds of foods, while robbed of their nutrition (including phytochemicals, micronutrients, and fiber), do not present the same levels of antinutrients.

The most effective way of reducing phytates is through fermentation. There are many different methods of fermentation, one of the most well-known is sourdough leavening of bread. With this method of leavening, micro-organisms (bacteria and fungi) are allowed to use the dough as a growth medium and they convert carbohydrates into gases that create small pockets of air, causing the bread to rise. Beneficially, these micro-organisms also deactivate phytic acid. In fact, studies show that this method of preparing grains can result in near 100% phytic acid reduction, creating one of the most healthful breads available to humans (assuming the use of whole grains grown in a conscientious fashion). Today, people want quickly produced foods, and the use of yeast is frequent in bread making. However, this method does not reduce phytic acid anywhere near the levels found in a slow fermentation, such as a sourdough bread allowed to slowly rise over the course of the day. Fast foods means improperly prepared foods, which equates to greater levels of antinutrition and the subsequent decline of health in the organism that consumes such food, including our non-ruminant livestock, such as birds, pigs, and fish, who do not have resident bacteria to produce phytase. They too suffer nutrient deficiencies and pass these on to the humans who consume them.

With the mention of fast food, everyone realizes that even the most conscientious food preparer sometimes finds themselves in a situation where time is limited. For some foods, like nuts, which are often gathered or purchased in a raw state, one quick way to help reduce phytic acid content is to roast them. Roasting does cause an appreciable level of reduction in phytic acid. Tests demonstrate a reduction by up to 40%. Roasting does, unfortunately, also destroy the phytase enzyme, so additional soaking will not further reduce phytic acid content (unless a source of phytase is added). Roasting is easily accomplished in a pan over a fire or on a modern stovetop or in the oven. Keep in mind that roasting does not mean scorching and burning (these indicate a damaged food). Of interest is that an almond is not a nut, but the seed of a plant (*Prunus dulcis*) related to peaches, cherries, and plums. Roasting almonds above 54 degrees Celsius (130 degrees Fahrenheit) can create relatively high levels of acrylamide (a carcinogen) due to their high asparagine content. Also, nuts that are rich in ω3 fatty acids, a polyunsaturated fatty acid, should not be roasted. These PUFAs are prone to damage (oxidation) from high heat, making them detrimental to one's health. Good examples of such nuts include species of walnuts (genus *Juglans*), such as white walnut (*Juglans cinerea*) and the cultivated English walnut (*Juglans regia*) found in supermarkets.

Oxalic acid is a naturally occurring compound in many plants. It is capable of binding to (i.e., chelating with) certain minerals, such as calcium, magnesium, and iron, and then becomes called an oxalate. Oxalates are important in modern diets because they can create health problems. For example, oxalates precipitate as small crystals that are excreted in the urine. However, larger crystals can form in the kidneys (as kidney stones) and obstruct kidney tubules. Large crystals can form also in other locations, such as the urinary tract (urinary tract stones), which create pain as they pass through the urethra. Most stones in the urinary tract are formed with the mineral calcium (but other mineral crystals can also occur).

Oxalates are found in so many plant foods that their avoidance is difficult. Following is a list of some plants (wild and cultivated) that are rich in oxalates:

amaranth foliage (*Amaranthus* species)
black pepper (*Piper nigrum*)
broccoli (*Brassica oleracea*)
Brussels sprouts (*Brassica oleracea*)
cabbage (*Brassica oleracea*)
carrot (*Daucus carota* ssp. *sativus*)
cassava (*Manihot esculenta*)
celery (*Apium graveolens*)
chard and other kinds of beet greens (*Beta vulgaris*)
chicory (*Cichorium intybus*)
chives (*Allium tuberosum*)
cocoa and chocolate products (*Theobroma cocao*)
collard greens (*Brassica oleracea*)
common stitchwort (*Stellaria media*)
curly dock (*Rumex crispus*)
endive (*Cichorium endivia*)
garlic (*Allium sativum*)
goosefoot foliage (*Chenopodium* species)
kiwi (*Actinidia deliciosa*)
parsley (*Petroselinum crispum*)
purslane (*Portulaca oleracea*)
radish (*Raphanus sativus*)
rhubarb (*Rheum rhabarbarum*)
sheep-sorrel (*Rumex acetosella*)
soy protein (*Glycine max*)
spinach (*Spinacia oleracea*)
sweet-potato (*Ipomoea batatas*)
taro (*Colocasia esculenta*)
tofu (*Glycine max*)
turnip (*Brassica rapa* ssp. *rapa*)
two-rowed watercress (*Nasturtium officinale*)
wood sorrel (*Oxalis* species)

There are a great number other plant foods that contain low levels of oxalates. If you consume plants, you cannot avoid oxalates. Many people are quite concerned today and live in fear of (or have actual experience with) stones. Many of these same people will avoid wild plants said to be rich in oxalates, while not avoiding cultivated plants rich in these compounds (a familiar cultural phenomenon of exaggerating the toxicity of wild plants). Such issues were rarely (read "almost never") a problem with hunter-gatherer and traditional groups. One practice that helped to eliminate oxalate content of plant foods was boiling (such as was done for many shoots and greens by indigenous people). While oxalates are heat stable and not appreciably deactivated by cooking, they can precipitate in the water. Through boiling greens and discarding the cooking water, the levels of oxalates can be reduced. Approximately three minutes of this manner of cooking has been shown to reduce oxalates by nearly ⅓, which is a significant reduction for this antinutrient.

The diets of modern people also create several favorable conditions for the deposition of oxalates as stones. Omega-6 fatty acids (FAs) accelerate the deposition of oxalates. Whereas hunter-gatherers consumed a diet with a ratio of ω6 to ω3 FAs of 1:1 to 3:1, most modern diets range from 8:1 to 24:1. Therefore, reversing this and eating a diet more rich in ω3 fatty acids aids in the prevention of oxalate deposition (as stones). Now, most people will read this and assume they need to supplement with a source of ω3 FAs. But that is not what I wrote. Eating a diet richer in ω3 FAs means also that one is eating a diet less rich in ω6 FAs. Moving away from a grain-based diet (which is not to be interpreted as avoiding grains altogether) and eating wild and pastured animals (rather than grain-fed animals) are two very important steps that can be taken. Supplementing with a high quality fish oil (such as fermented cod liver oil) is not a bad practice, but it misses the point that the entire diet must be addressed.

Vitamin B_6 (pyridoxine and other vitamers) is a water-soluble vitamin also effective at preventing deposition of oxalates. There are many possible sources of this vitamin, some of which have been vilified in recent years, including organ meats (like liver, kidney, and heart), unpasteurized milk (cooking does promote loss of this vitamin in most foods), and eggs. Other animal foods that contain this vitamin include poultry, beef, pork, and fish. Plant foods rich in vitamin B_6 include avocado (*Persea americana*), whole grains, sunflower fruits (*Helianthus annuus*), pistachio nuts (*Pistacia vera*), spinach (*Spinacia oleracea*) and bananas (*Musa* species and hybrids).

Another dietary element that helps with oxalates is probiotic food, especially those that are formed with bacterial cultures. Such foods are living foods that contain active bacteria that are capable of producing enzymes that break down oxalates. One of the bacteria with this capacity is *Oxylobacter formegenes*. Almost all children test positive for this bacterium by the age of 6 to 8 years. However, only 60–80% of adults test positive for the bacterium, hypothesized to be a result of antibiotic use (which harms the gut microflora and kills this beneficial bacterium). Fortunately, other bacteria can degrade oxalates, including *Lactobacillus acidophilus*.

In summary, oxalates do not have to be a concern for healthy people who practice eating a varied diet and follow some simple strategies. These include consuming some oxalate-rich foods as cooked foods (after brief boiling and discarding the cooking water). A diet that includes important foods in wild and traditional cultures that supply ample vitamin B_6, a vitamin that inhibits oxalate deposition, is essential. Also, probiotics that degrade oxalates are very important. Frequent use of antibiotics inhibits your ability to break down oxalates, creating a risk of stones that can cause health issues.

omnivorous diet
working together

This section was an introduction to two important antinutrients found in plant foods. The antinutrients discussed here can be reduced or eliminated through relatively simple methods that can be practiced in the home or in the field, or their effects mitigated through other dietary elements (for an extensive list of recipes and step by step protocols for dealing with antinutrients in grains, legumes, nuts, and other seed-like fruits, see Sally Fallon's book "Nourishing Traditions"). These preparation techniques can allow people to incorporate practical concepts into their diet that maximize the nutrition in foods they consume (through reducing or eliminating factors that interfere with nutrient absorption). While Americans are generally lazy about their food, proper preparation becomes second nature with practice (not to mention Americans are some of the unhealthiest people living in an affluent country). In many cases, there is little extra effort needed, only (for example) that a food for the following morning is allowed to soak overnight (note: no extra effort, just the need to think about food ahead of time). Keep in mind that many diets do not account for antinutrients (e.g., Standard American Diet), and avoiding all foods with antinutrients is not a solution. The solution to this dilemma is to recognize that the well-being of indigenous and traditional peoples influenced by diet was generated and maintained through a large number of practices, one of which was proper food preparation. Reinstating these practices allows us to benefit from the dietary wisdom of our ancestors and reclaim health. Personal health is one of the most important factors in individual sovereignty because it allows a person to disconnect from the medical establishment (this connection can act like chains for someone who is attempting to rewild their life).

ARE GRAINS BAD?

While grains (the fruit of a grass) have been eaten in many and diverse cultures around the world, they have been targeted by various dietary factions and described as empty calories and promoters of disease (as alluded to earlier in this chapter). Perhaps most vocal in their stance against grains has been the Paleo Diet and Very Low Carbohydrate Diet crowds (though some authors in the former category are somewhat softening their stance against grains). This section briefly addresses specific criticisms of this kind of food and provides guidance on selecting grains that can be beneficial components of a modern diet.

The first criticism usually waged against grains is that they are a relatively **new food**. In other words, grains are believed to be absent from the paleolithic diet that early humans consumed, suggesting we are not evolved to consume them. This assertion is false and evidence of grain consumption goes back 105,000 years to a relative of sorghum that was consumed by *Homo sapiens* in what is now Mozambique. Stone ovens constructed specifically for baking grains have been discovered dating back approximately 30,000 years ago. There is ample evidence of grain consumption in Paleolithic humans. If one considers the logic of the argument that humans did not eat grain until the development of agriculture (10–12 thousand years ago), it is found to be wanting. The argument could be stated as follows: humans ignore a source of food, and then, in a relatively short period of time, launch into a completely new form of food production never before seen on the planet using a plant they have never consumed. Clearly, it would have taken a considerable amount of time and interaction with these plants to invent a new food production system. The birth of agriculture would have required knowledge of the plant—not just what forms to select and how to grow them, but why this particular food plant would (at least potentially) be a valuable choice. Such knowledge would likely come from consuming grasses for thousands of years.

Some grasses related to modern bread wheat (*Triticum aestivum*) contain a specific protein called **gluten** that provides an elastic character to the dough and allows for certain desired qualities (e.g., texture) in leavened bread. Unfortunately, gluten is an allergenic protein for some that can cause immune system reactions that lead to inflammation in the small intestine and a host of resulting health issues. For this reason, many people prefer to avoid grains, but most of the grains in the world are actually free of gluten. It is members of specific tribe of grasses (the Triticeae), including rye, barley, goat grass, and species of wheat, that contain this protein. Cultivated rice, wild rice, millet, teff, goose grass, and many other species contain no gluten (unless contaminated with gluten-containing dust in factories that process wheat and related grains). The logic of avoiding all grains because some contain gluten is similar to avoiding all foods that comes from the ocean because one is allergic to shellfish. Gluten-containing grains are easily avoided, so this is not a valid reason to cease consumption of all grains.

Grains contain the antinutrient **phytic acid** that, as you now know, binds with minerals and prevents their absorption in the digestive tract. However, phytic acid is not limited to grains, but also found in legumes, achenes, and nuts (the latter of which is not "prohibited" in the Paleo and Very Low Carbohydrate Diets). Using the presence of phytic acid to dismiss one maligned food and then overlooking it in a praised food is highly inconsistent (which weakens the premises of the diets). Further, phytic acid is dealt with through proper processing of the grains, including sprouting, soaking, and fermenting. In other words, this antinutrient is really only an issue in improperly prepared grains (such as those usually sold in American supermarkets). While that may be a reason to avoid most store-purchased grains, it is not a legitimate reason to avoid all grain dishes (or to chastise people who consume properly prepared grains). Stating grains should be avoided due to phytic acid is merely a display of poor understanding of traditional food preparation methods.

Some authors point out that grains also contain **lectins**, biological molecules that bind to carbohydrates and serve a cell recognition function (among others). Lectins are considered to be another antinutrient and can cause health issues when consumed in large amounts. However, lectins are not restricted to grains but are found in almost all foods (including animal foods). Further, many lectins are deactivated with proper processing (which includes sprouting, fermenting, and cooking). Therefore, again, warning people to avoid grains due to lectins fails to recognize that practically all foods contain them and proper processing reduces their concentrations.

Grains are also considered a **nutrient-poor food** by various diet authorities. This assertion is made through comparisons of modern cultivated grains with pastured animal foods. While these comparisons are useful, they are somewhat misleading because they are using grains that do not demonstrate high nutrition profiles. When we examine a species of wild grain, such as annual wild rice, against grass-fed beef, we see a very different story. In fact, annual wild rice exceeds grass-fed beef in several micronutrients (see Table 3.1). The idea that all grains are merely empty calories is a falsehood, as evidenced by the table below. Therefore, nutrient density, while a reason to perhaps avoid some grains, is not a reason to avoid all grains.

nutritional element	100 g of beef	100 g of wild rice
vitamin A	0.0 IU	0.2 mcg RAE
vitamin B1 (thiamin)	0.1 mg	0.1 mg
vitamin B2 (riboflavin)	0.1 mg	0.3 mg
vitamin B3 (niacin)	7.6 mg	7.0 mg
vitamin B6	0.7 mg	0.1 mg
vitamin B9	14.7 mcg	26.0 mcg
vitamin B12	1.4 mcg	0.0 mcg
vitamin C	0.0 mg	0.0 mg
vitamin E	0.4 mg	0.2 mg
calcium	10.2 mg	16.0 mg
iron	2.1 mg	1.9 mg
magnesium	26.1 mg	32.0 mg
manganese	0.01 mg	1.4 mg
potassium	387.0 mg	450.0 mg
zinc	4.1 mg	6.3 mg

Table 3.1. Comparison of nutrition found in 100 g of grass-fed beef (as published by Whole Foods Market) with the same mass of annual wild rice (*Zizania aquatica*) harvested from lake in Minnesota (from Swain et al. 1978).

And the reasons go on for avoiding grains. For example, grains are considered to be rich-sources of **ω6 fatty acids**. Of course, this is not true of all grains (e.g., species of wild rice have ⅓ of their total lipids as ω3 fatty acids) and is only an issue if people consume a very grain-rich diet that is not combined properly with foods high in ω3 fatty acids. For example, a traditional culture from an island in the Outer Hebrides (off the northwest coast of Scotland) consumed grains as a staple, primarily oats (*Avena sativa*). These people experienced health and (more importantly) produced healthy, well-formed children. The grains were combined with ocean fish and shellfish, including cod (and their organs and eggs), lobster, crab, oyster, and clams. These traditional people suffered none of health issues that were found in nearby villages living more civilized lives (such a tuberculosis and frequent dental caries). They stand as evidence that grains used as a staple can be part of a healthy diet.

We can also look to the many hunter-gatherer groups around the world who consumed grains to greater or lesser extents. The Anishinaabe of the Great Lakes region harvested two species of wild rice (*Zizania aquatica* and *Z. palustris*), which they used as a staple in their diets. The Hopi consumed a species of panic grass (*Panicum capillare*), which they ground and used to make bread. The Navajo gathered a species of rice grass (*Acnatherum hymenoides*) and used the grains to make bread and hot cereal. Of course, the consumption of grains by wild people is not limited to North America. African natives consumed goose grass (*Eleusine coracana*) and teff (*Eragrostis teff*), while Australian Aborigines consumed a species of millet (*Panicum decompositum*). All of the indigenous people mentioned here experienced exceptional physical health while on their traditional diets, which included grains. They stand as evidence that grains (at least wild versions) are not harmful foods.

The problem for many people living in affluent countries is that they consume diets that lack diversity. In this case, they consume the majority of their calories as a few species of grain (primarily bread wheat and corn in the United States). Their breakfasts, lunches, and dinners are often centered on grains (e.g., consider the usual breakfast foods, all made from grain: toast, bagels, pancakes, hot cereal, cold cereal, granola, donuts, French toast, waffles, English muffins, Pop-Tarts, and pastry rolls). This abundance of very few foods, which are not combined appropriately, contributes to much of the poor health that Americans experience. The idea that we should avoid all grain might sound like a nice, simple solution to the problem, but this practice would actually avoid some nutrient-dense foods that have been shown to impart health to wild and traditional people. As importantly, avoiding wild foods on your landscape or grown locally in your community is a practice that can only be maintained through long-distance transportation of food (which allows for very unnatural diets). This practice, taken for granted by Americans, has a host of consequences to anyone interested in a more natural, healthier, and secure life. These short comings include (but not limited to): extensive pollution caused by transportation, huge expense of maintaining transportation networks, destabilizing food security by centralizing food production (i.e., it is easier to disrupt), and limiting personal interaction with the local landscape by purchasing foods from distant landscapes. In short, Americans can create very unnatural diets only because they have the wealth to have foods shipped to them from around the world. If they were interested in the health of their bodies and their health of the ecosystems, they would eat more local (and more wild), which would include (on many landscapes) some grain consumption. The real message about grains should not be "avoid them all", but rather this: **choose wild and heirloom grains, restrict or (if necessary) avoid gluten-containing kinds, and eat less grain through diversifying the diet.**

FATS FOR HEALTH

No dietary topic is more contentious and replete with inaccurate information than that of lipids (i.e., fats). As I write these words, I'm also aware that the "Lipid Hypothesis", which states that there is a direct correlation between the amount of saturated fat and cholesterol consumed in the diet and the risk of cardiovascular disease, is so ingrained in American health dogma, that it is unlikely anything I state can overcome this societal bias (at least for some people). That said, I'm going to attempt to describe how baseless this hypothesis is using several different approaches. Anyone truly interested in dietary health should make a strong attempt to clear their head of biases while they read these next paragraphs in order to understand how the usual lipid narrative is flawed in many ways.

First, we must understand that the phrase "artery clogging fats" is a very inaccurate term that demonstrates a poor understanding of human physiology (if your health professional uses this phrase, you might want to consider finding a new one). While it is often used to create a picture of the supposed health effects of consuming fat, it is not a realistic analogy to use—the kitchen sink and the human vascular system are very different things. First, the human body is often 25 or so degrees Fahrenheit warmer than room temperature, which liquefies many fats that would be solid in the kitchen. Second, fats are not water soluble, so they do not travel freely in the blood stream, but must be "carried" by a specialized molecule called a lipoprotein. And, fats do not leap off these lipoproteins and stick to the walls of arteries. If fats truly clogged blood vessels, why wouldn't they clog the narrowest of passages (the capillary beds)? Why is it that they only stick to the walls of larger vessels (such as the arteries)? The point is, fats don't clog arteries. Other factors, such as inflammation and plaques (which we will discuss in this section) can and do clog arteries.

Second, why is it that indigenous people, who not only consumed fats, but relished dietary fats, did not succumb to cardiovascular disease? In fact, examination of indigenous diets by Cordain and colleagues in 2000 showed that 97% of the world's hunter-gatherers exceeded the recommended dietary fat intake (calories from fat less than or equal to 30% of the diet). Even more to the point, northern populations (e.g., Inuit) often exceeded 50% of their calories as fat—yet, none of these groups experienced cardiovascular disease. Historical observations of living people who consumed traditional diets rich in fats showed them to be healthy. Blanket statements that assert all dietary fats are harmful and contribute to a risk of cardiovascular disease are grossly inaccurate because they are contradicted by observations of human beings.

Important to this conversation is the fraudulent origins of the Lipid Hypothesis, where the researchers responsible utilized misleading or deceptive practices in their presentation of data. Ancel Keys was a researcher who published on the Lipid Hypothesis in the 1950s. While there was earlier work, Keys certainly helped to popularize this hypothesis. In his work, Keys published a study that examined six different countries and demonstrated a correlation between dietary fats available and coronary heart disease. First note the word "available"—the data was based on food available rather than food actually eaten. Aside from this obvious issue, the real deception here was that Keys had access to data from 22 countries but analysis of all those data indicated no correlation (as verified by later researchers). He also failed to mention that consumption of fat was correlated with less overall death from other diseases and resulted in a longer life span. Keys cherry-picked the data to find countries that demonstrated a correlation—he selected data to match his personal belief (and left out various benefits). And while the American Heart Association concluded (in 1957) that the data do not support a link between dietary fat and heart disease, they changed their stance in 1960 when a committee—of which Keys was a member—released a report that low-fat diets benefit heart health. As importantly to this discussion was Nikolaj Anitschkow, who fed rabbits high cholesterol diets and was able to induce atherosclerotic plaques on arterial walls. The fact that his work (published in 1913) was able to demonstrate blood vessel injury by feeding cholesterol to an herbivore that does not normally ingest cholesterol is possibly interesting (in the name of science). However, it is irrelevant in regard to an omnivore with a long history of consuming lipid- and cholesterol-rich foods. Interestingly, even Ancel Keys did not believe the cholesterol content of foods had an effect on atherosclerosis (a thickening of the arterial wall due to inflammation) and dismissed the conclusions of Anitschkow's work. However, later health authorities have used it to "prove" dietary fat is harmful. Even the Framingham Heart Study, so widely touted as demonstrating dietary fats are bad for health, actually showed that the higher the intake of saturated fat and cholesterol in a person's diet the lower the serum cholesterol (contrary to what is commonly believed today). The nail on the coffin for dietary fats came in 1988 when the US surgeon general Everett Koop claimed that dietary fat was causing coronary heart disease and that there was a preponderance of data to establish this claim (which was not the case). From that point on, fats became highly demonized.

At this point, some of you may be stating that it is saturated fat, not all fats in general, that is the causative factor in cardiovascular disease. The Mayo Clinic recommends that calories from saturated fat do not exceed more than 10% of the total daily calories and further recommend that to lower your risk of heart disease you should keep saturated fat intake to no more than 7% of your daily calories. These are interesting numbers given that research indicates that most hunter-gatherers consumed 10–15% of their calories as saturated fat (and some were 1–2% higher than this). Therefore, the Mayo Clinic's recommendation to restrict saturated fat intake to no more than 7% of the calories has no basis—humans have consumed more than twice this amount of saturated fat and experienced virtually no cardiovascular disease (compared with the United States with more than half of the people over the age of 45 in some stage of this disease). In fact, a paper published in 2010 by Siri-Tarino and colleagues that analyzed data from over 347,000 people showed no that "there is no significant evidence for concluding that dietary saturated fat is associated with an increased risk of CHD [coronary heart disease] or CVD [cardiovascular disease]". Americans have followed the recommendations of health authorities to reduce saturated fat consumption (e.g., replace butter with margarine), and the result was that the incidence of heart disease markedly increased. Think about this for a moment, which group of people should you emulate the diet of: hunter-gatherers who don't experience cardiovascular disease or Americans who follow various medical establishment's suggestions and experience substantial incidence of this disease? It really makes no sense to follow the dietary recommendations promulgated by US institutions (and, in fact, studies show that following your doctor's suggestions regarding diet lead to shorter overall lifespan).

In order for us to understand dietary lipids and realize that there are differences between kinds of fats (including the processed fats common to the Standard American Diet), we need to present a little background on lipids. While there are many ways that fats are classified, one of the easiest to understand and most useful for the person interested in natural diets is a classification based on available bonding sites (it's not as complex as it might first read).

Saturated fats are those in which all of the available carbon bonds are occupied by hydrogen atoms. As a result, there are no vacant bonding sites (i.e., all of the bonding sites are saturated). These fats form straight molecules, and, as a result, pack together very densely and are solid or semisolid at room temperature. Saturated fats are mostly commonly of animal origin (such as tallow, lard, butter, and ghee), though some also originate from tropical plants (such as coconut oil). Because saturated fats have no vacant bonding sites, they are also more chemically inert than other kinds of fats and are less prone to damage from heat, pressure, and light (hint: these are the best fats to cook with because they are more resistant to oxidation). Saturated fats are necessary for health because they fulfill a number of functions, including providing stiffness to cell membranes, protecting from toxins and pharmaceutical drugs, fueling the heart, functioning as antimicrobials in the digestive system, and assisting with the incorporation of calcium into our bones.

Monounsaturated fats are those that have a single double bond where two atoms are linked together, which means they lack two hydrogen atoms (the remaining carbon atoms have a single bond). These kinds of fats have a bend at the location of the double bond; therefore, they do not pack together as tightly as saturated fats and tend to be liquid at room temperature but become semisolid when chilled slightly. Monounsaturated fats are found in both plant and animal foods. Given these fats have only one double bond, they are relatively stable (from a chemical perspective) and are suitable for cooking (though highly saturated fats are more preferable).

Polyunsaturated fats are those that have two or more double bonds, which means they lack four or more hydrogen atoms. These fatty acids have multiple bends (one each at the location of double bonds), so they do not pack together and remain liquid, even when chilled. Polyunsaturated fats are found in animal and plant foods. Because these fats have multiple double bonds, they are relatively reactionary and can be damaged by heat, pressure, and light (hint: these are the worst fats to cook with and become oxidized unless protected by ample antioxidants). There are two kinds of polyunsaturated fats that are essential because they cannot be manufactured by the body: ω6 and ω3 fatty acids. While both are essential, certain forms of ω3 fatty acids are necessary for eye and brain development. Further, the ratio of these fats in the diet is vitally important (especially considering some of the common forms of these oils in the diet today—industrially extracted and, therefore, often oxidized). Modern diets rely on large amounts of grains, legumes, seed-oils, and grain-fed animals, which collectively supply too much ω6 fatty acids. For example, a truly pasture-raised chicken eating lots of fresh plants and insects lays eggs with a ratio of ω6 fats to ω3 fats at nearly 1:1. A strictly grain-fed chicken lays eggs with these fats in a 19:1 ratio, demonstrating how distorted fatty acid profiles become in foods from primarily or entirely grain-fed animals.

Keep in mind that naturally occurring fats (regardless of their origin) are actually a mixture of these three kinds of fat. Therefore, the overall qualities of a fat are dependent on the relative amount of each kind of fat. For example, coconut oil (derived from *Cocos nucifera*) is approximately 92% saturated fat, making it solid at room temperature. Olive oil (derived from *Olea europaea*) is, on the other hand, only about 15% saturated fat, making it liquid at room temperature. In the middle is butter (derived usually from cow's milk), which is around 63% saturated fat, making it solid at room temperature, but softer than coconut oil.

Fats are a necessity in the diet (all three naturally occurring kinds). Each version of fat has its supportive roles in the health of human beings. Collectively, fats both supply energy and enable energy storage in the body. They also support healthy brain development, reduce inflammation (when consumed in proper ratios), and assist with the absorption and transport of fat-soluble vitamins. Fats also help prevent over-eating. While this might sound impossible, it is the result of the fact that fats are approximately twice as calorie dense as carbohydrates but are four to five times as satiating, which means you fill up faster and remain feeling full longer (i.e., consumption of naturally occurring fats actually helps reduce and maintain weight). However, there are fats that are harmful to human health. These include extracted polyunsaturated fats and hydrogenated fats.

Extracted polyunsaturated fats are lipids that were, in nature, contained inside of a plant or animal and have been removed from its original source through a chemical and/or mechanical process. The most commonly extracted fats are found in nuts, seeds, and fruits, such as corn, cotton, safflower, walnut, canola, soy, and sunflower oils. The usual commercial extraction process for most of these plant-based oils uses immense pressure to squeeze out the lipids, a process that damages the fats due to the heat it generates. Sometimes chemical solvents are also used, which must be boiled off to reduce (but do not eliminate) their presence in the final product. This heat further damages the fats. Remember that polyunsaturated fats are highly reactive, and, as a result of these modern methods, become harmful to humans because they function like free-radicals in the body and cause injury to cell membranes, DNA, and the interior wall of blood vessels, contributing to, of all things, cardiovascular disease. Inside the plant, these lipids are protected from light and co-occur with naturally occurring antioxidants (which include antioxidant vitamins, such as vitamin E). Once extracted, these fats are ripe for damage while they sit on store shelves in clear containers at room temperature. Even worse is the fact that many people use these extracted oils for cooking, subjecting them to additional heat. While there are certain exceptions (such as peanut oil, due to naturally occurring antioxidants), most liquid plant oils are ill-suited for cooking because they become a harmful food (note: olive oil is primarily a monounsaturated fat and is not included here). Further, most plant oils (again, with certain exceptions such as walnut and flax) are very high in ω6 fatty acids, causing severe essential fatty acid imbalances and promoting inflammation in the body.

Hydrogenated fats are those that have been chemically altered to create solid fats from polyunsaturated fats (i.e., fats that would normally be liquid at room temperature). This process begins with inexpensive plant-based oils and subjects them to a high pressure and high temperature environment in the presence of microscopic metal particles. Through several additional steps, including cleaning, bleaching, coloring, and flavoring, these highly oxidized (i.e., rancid) lipids become solid and are sold as food items (often with the declaration that they are more healthful because they contain no saturated fat and less cholesterol). The truth is a very different matter. These lipids have been highly damaged due to multiple exposures to heat and pressure, creating free-radicals that contribute to disease. Not only this, but the hydrogenated fats have an altered configuration from that which occurs in nature. The hydrogen atoms in the fat change from a *cis* configuration to a *trans* configuration, a form much less commonly found in nature. These human-made trans fats become incorporated in your cells and disrupt normal chemical reactions that occur in the body. Research demonstrates that hydrogenated fats are very injurious to humans through several mechanisms, including disrupting immune system function, blocking utilization of essential fatty acids, and increased incidence of atherosclerosis, cancer, diabetes, birth defects, and sterility. Hydrogenation is a new process that creates an unsafe food and such foods should be avoided at all costs.

Extracted polyunsaturated fats and hydrogenated fats are new to humans. In the former case, wild plants rich in polyunsaturated fats were routinely consumed by indigenous people, but they were consumed intact (i.e., within the plant) where they were protected from light, heat, and pressure. These new versions of fats can truly be described as "bad fats" and should not be consumed. They are a perfect example of what happens when humans encounter new, highly processed foods—it usually has disastrous consequences and supports the need to rewild our diets. These human-processed fats are often "lumped in" with naturally occurring fats as evidence that all fats are harmful. This is a poorly supported argument that merely demonstrates a lack of understanding by the persons making such assertions.

As mentioned a couple of paragraphs ago, trans fats are sometimes found in nature. While human-created forms can be very harmful when ingested, the natural forms of trans contribute to the health of people consuming them. These trans fats occur in small amounts in wild and pasture-raised animals, and are even found in human breast milk (the only natural food that can be stated as designed, by evolution, for human consumption). It is important to recognize that simply because a natural food contains some amount of trans fats doesn't imply it should be avoided (i.e., the word "trans" should not immediately throw up red flags). Consider conjugated linoleic acid (CLA). This is a fatty acid with several different forms, of which a trans form is common in grass-fed animal foods (including the dairy produced by grass-fed cows). Research shows that CLA has a host of health benefits, including inhibiting tumor growth and metastases, promoting weight loss, reducing the risk of heart disease, preventing diabetes and improving glucose tolerance, and reducing inflammation. These are very different actions than the industrially produced trans fats. Yet more evidence that modern foods (i.e., foods that have been tampered with) do not have the health promoting qualities of wild and conscientiously raised foods.

So, if saturated fats do not cause cardiovascular disease, what does? In actually, there are a many factors that contribute to this disease (e.g., smoking, obesity). Relevant to this discussion are the extracted polyunsaturated oils and hydrogenated fats that are so frequently consumed by Americans. These free-radical-rich modern foods contribute to the very disease they are meant to prevent. They do so by a suite of mechanisms that ultimately damage the blood vessel walls (through the formation of plaques), promoting calcification of the arteries (resulting in stiffness), and promoting the formation of blood clots. Therefore, consuming plant-based oils rich in polyunsaturated fats and eating lots of deep-fried food (which typically uses polyunsaturated fats that are prone to damage from heat) is a perfect recipe for the development of cardiovascular disease (there is now lots of reliable information on the web about this topic for those interested in more information; see the next section for additional discussion). Add to this a diet rich in refined carbohydrates, foods that further promote inflammation, and it is easy to understand why this disease is so frequent in those practicing the Standard American Diet. None of these foods were consumed by the indigenous who demonstrated excellent cardiovascular health.

Before we leave the topic of fats, let us address one last item: **ketosis**. Ketosis is a metabolic state where the primary fuel is ketone bodies (rather than glucose). Proponents of this diet correctly point to the dismal health of people consuming lots of refined carbohydrates. They also point to the fact that high fat diets can be therapeutic for some diseases, such as epilepsy and type 2 diabetes (in fact, people can reverse diabetes by increasing their intake of natural dietary fats). Using this information, proponents of a Very Low Carbohydrate Diet (VLCD) state that humans should consume a large proportion of fats so that their body is deprived of glucose and must instead burn ketone bodies, made when the body cleaves fats into fatty acids. While ketosis is normal in humans for periods of time (e.g., at night, on fasting, during high-fat consumption periods), proponents of the VLCD assert that humans should exist in a state of chronic ketosis (i.e., continually using ketone bodies for fuel). They often point to far northern cultures, who consumed large amounts of fats and proteins as a result of short growing seasons and limited availability of carbohydrates, as examples of humans who existed in ketosis. There are several issues with this assertion. First, considering people who live in an extreme environment (and do not represent the majority of humans on the planet) to be an example of what everyone should eat is certainly inappropriate. Second, multiple studies have concluded that far northern people (e.g., Inuit) were in fact not in ketosis for extended periods of time. The lack of ketosis in northern indigenous people results from many factors, including enlarged livers found in some populations that is capable of converting more protein to glucose, abundant glycogen (an animal storage form of carbohydrates) found in the tissue of marine mammals they consume, and a genetic anomaly that prevents a state of ketosis in a significant number of some northern populations. The point of this paragraph is that a diet that induces chronic ketosis is a new diet to humans. And while it has been shown to be therapeutic, it has also been shown to have deleterious consequences in some people (including newborns of moms consuming high-fat diets). If we have learned anything in the last decades it is that we should not embark on new diets without careful consideration of all the potential health outcomes for the people consuming them and their yet unborn children.

CHOLESTEROL IS A HEALTHFUL SUBSTANCE

A brief discussion of cholesterol is necessary to help people overcome the nutritional mythology so established in the United States, one that stands in the way of them acquiring a state of vibrant health. Cholesterol is both produced by the body and ingested in the diet. Cholesterol is so important to our health that without it we would not survive. One of its primary purposes is to provide our cell membranes with the necessary strength and integrity for them to function. But this is just the beginning. Cholesterol is a precursor to vitamin D, one of the most important vitamins for immune system function, growth and development, and epigenetic health. Cholesterol is also a precursor for several hormones, including corticosteroids and sex hormones, and for bile salts, necessary for the digestion and assimilation of fats. Cholesterol is an antioxidant and a healing substance. It influences serotonin activity in the brain, protecting against depression and aggressive or suicidal behaviors. In fact, cholesterol is needed by infants for healthy development of the brain (which is why breast milk contains lots of cholesterol and an enzyme to help babies utilize these molecules). Given all these facts, it is interesting that cholesterol is considered a harmful substance by much of the public. They certainly didn't make this up—they learned this from health authorities who provided them with overly simplified and sometimes outright erroneous messages about cholesterol.

Why has cholesterol been so maligned? For several reasons, one of which is an incredible story demonstrating how misinformed we are about the causes of certain diseases. In our blood vessels, when plaques form, they are composed of cholesterol-rich white blood cells (i.e., white blood cells that engulf fat and cholesterol and form a raised lesion). Because these plaques are, at their core, comprised of cholesterol, it became "known" that cholesterol was the cause of these plaques and that it infiltrated arterial vessels and ultimately created constrictions in the vessels. Therefore, it was important to limit dietary cholesterol to prevent cardiovascular disease (even though 75% of the cholesterol in our body is manufactured by the liver). Because polyunsaturated fatty acids contain less cholesterol than saturated fats, it become public policy to promote the use of these fats in the diet. However, the research on this topic was nowhere near concluded, but health authorities jumped and made many premature dietary recommendations. What is convincingly known now (but will take decades to permeate popular health knowledge) is that cholesterol is involved in the formation of the plaques—after it has become damaged by oxidized polyunsaturated fats. The low-density lipoproteins (LDLs, the so called "bad cholesterol") are more easily damaged by oxidized fats (which are common in the Standard American Diet). These damaged (i.e., oxidized) LDL particles initiate a complex set of reactions that ultimately cause white blood cells to penetrate the blood vessel lining and engulf the oxidized LDLs, forming raised plaques. It isn't that LDL is actually bad for health, it is that their membrane is highly subject to injury from modern foods (a very good, though somewhat technical and lengthy discussion of the facts can be found at http://www.cholesterol-and-health.com/Does-Cholesterol-Cause-Heart-Disease-Myth.html). Traditional diets, which do not have the high amounts of oxidized fats, do not injure LDLs and, therefore, are protective of cardiovascular disease.

Given that the problem is not Low Density Lipoproteins, but the foods we eat that damage them, it becomes important for the neoaboriginal, or anyone interested in health, to follow some basic guidelines to avoid the consumption of oxidized polyunsaturated fatty acids. Here is a short list of necessary practices that anyone can employ.

1. Reduce consumption of fried food (or at least use different fats than those that are commonly used). Frying food in vegetable oils (such as soy, canola, and corn) damages the fats, and you consume the damaged fats. If you wish to consume fried foods, one should use lipids that are more chemically inert, such as tallow and lard, fats that have a higher proportion of saturated fat that withstands the heat of cooking much better than polyunsaturated fats.

2. Reduce use of liquid vegetable oils in the diet altogether (this does not apply to olive oil). Liquid vegetable oils, with few exceptions, once removed from the source (i.e., the grain, seed, or fruit) become exposed to air and light, initiating the oxidation of these fats. The only way these lipids should be consumed is within the intact food or shortly after it has been processed.

3. Reduce the consumption of refined foods made of grains. The problem with store-purchased foods made of grains and grain substitutes, is that the grains are not whole (i.e., intact) but have been ground into a fine particle size that provides abundant surface area to expose the polyunsaturated fats to oxygen. This is why grains should never be stored as flour (as most Americans do), but should be ground just prior to use in cooking (after they have been soaked, sprouted, or fermented to deal with antinutrients). Storing grains whole better protects the lipids from exposure to oxygen.

4. Reduce the amount of cold cereal you consume (this includes granola that was not freshly made). Many cereals are made of grains that are first ground (which opens up the grain and exposes the polyunsaturated fats to air), then often extruded at high pressure to make a particular shape (which causes more damage to the lipids), and then exposed to heat and air (yes, further damaging the fats). These "heart-healthy" cereals can be packed with free-radicals that harm cardiovascular health.

5. Reduce the amount of pre-prepared hot cereal you consume. Oatmeal and other hot cereals that are made from rolled and cut grains suffer from the same problem as foods that have been made from flour—the rolling and cutting opens up the grains to more contact with oxygen. Hot cereals should be prepared from properly stored whole (i.e., intact) grains that are rolled or cut just prior to preparation.

6. **Reduce consumption of human-made trans fats.** Margarine and similar spreads are made from highly processed vegetable oils that create trans fats. These spreads are highly oxidized (and must be cleaned, deodorized, colored, and flavored during their processing to make you willing to consume them). These spreads are some of the unhealthiest foods on the planet. Margarine and similar spreads should be replaced with a real food (e.g., butter, nut butter).

I have been polite here and used the word "reduce". This is in recognition that many people are unwilling to make substantive changes in the diet in a relatively short period of time. For some of these guidelines, it would have been appropriate for me to use the words "avoid at all costs", especially number 6. Be aware that all of these foods are only available or available in the form commonly consumed due to the presence of industry. In other words, they are highly unnatural foods that were not part of the human diet until quite recently. A more natural diet (including those enjoyed by hunter-gatherers) is devoid of the number and amounts of cholesterol-harming foods, and produces healthier humans as a result. This is yet another example where we can learn from those who came before us about diets that do not lead to chronic disease. All six of these items can be practiced by anyone living anywhere who is willing to research different menu items from whole foods.

THE FIFTH KINGDOM

Fungi, or mushrooms, are an important kingdom of food that we should seek out from wild and organically grown sources. These are important organisms that are not only responsible, in part, for the breakdown of organic material in the environment but also form symbiotic relationships with plants that help them acquire nutrition. Fungi differ from other kingdoms of life in that they have cell walls that contain a special kind of polysaccharide called chitin (which has important ramifications for natural medicine made from fungi, as discussed in chapter 5). While fungi are a natural and necessary component of healthy ecosystems and can be described as a valuable food-medicine, our society suffers from a deep sense of mycophobia. Domesticated people have become terrified at the thought of poisoning themselves with wild-gathered mushrooms (or wild-gathered anything for that matter). Of course, this fear can only be maintained by not registering the alarming number of food poisonings and severe allergic reactions that are occurring at increasing frequency with store-purchased foods. No different than plants or birds or any other taxonomic group, some fungi are very easy to identify and some are very difficult; therefore, there is no reason for paralyzing fear of all fungi. Fortunately, people who are interested in rewilding their diet need not (initially) be concerned with harvesting wild fungi The nutritional and medicinal benefits of fungi can be, for the most part, enjoyed through purchases made at markets.

Fungi can be a valuable source of certain nutritional elements. Here, we are discussing macroscopic fungi (i.e., not the fungi that we can use to ferment foods). More specifically, we are referring to their "fruiting body", the structure that produces spores, as opposed to the collection of filamentous hyphae imbedded in the substrate (whether that be soil, leaf litter, or wood) that make up the vegetative portion of the fungus. Numerous nutritional assays from around the world demonstrate fungi can be good sources of certain B-complex vitamins and minerals, especially vitamin B_1 (thiamin), vitamin B_3 (niacin), magnesium, phosphorus, and potassium. But much like plants, micronutrient figures vary and the best way to attain sufficient nutrition is through consumption of a diversity of fungi (which is where the knowledge of wild species is a true benefit). Here, we will focus our discussion on four specific topics of fungi nutrition: polysaccharides, mycochemicals, ergosterols and vitamin B_{12}.

The fruiting bodies (called sporocarps) and the sclerotia (sterile masses of hyphae found in certain species) are rich sources of pharmacologically active **polysaccharides**. These long-chain carbohydrates function to provide strength and rigidity to the cell walls of fungi. They are well-researched and are known to bolster the functioning of the immune system. For example, certain fungal polysaccharides (called glucans) have the ability to activate macrophages (which increases scavenging and antimicrobial activity), induce maturation of T-helper cells (which enhances cellular immunity), stimulate B-cell activation (which make antibodies to antigens), increase release of TNF-α (which up-regulates cell death in tumors), and increase production of interferon-α from white blood cells (which increases viral resistance). Studies also show that fungal polysaccharides are able to bolster immune system function for immunocompromised people (e.g., those undergoing chemotherapy). The important item to understand regarding dietary fungal polysaccharides is that they are bound to indigestible cell wall material and are not bioavailable to humans without cooking (heat liberates the polysaccharides and makes them available). Therefore, the benefits of the immune-modulating carbohydrates are not realized when fungi are consumed raw.

Much like plants, fungi are a source of medicinal compounds referred to as **mycochemicals**. These compounds (including the polysaccharides discussed in the previous paragraph) present an array of beneficial actions, including antioxidant, antibacterial, anti-inflammatory, antineoplastic, and antiviral actions. Some fungi are also able to slightly inhibit production of enzymes used to digest carbohydrates, helping to lower blood glucose levels after meals (benefitting people with diabetes). The ability of various mycochemicals to prevent development, growth, and spread of cancerous cells is supported by many scientific papers. In fact, a diversity of fungi in the diet can be a critical part of an anti-cancer diet that keeps the human being free of neoplasties. The antioxidant abilities of certain fungi extend to assisting with certain gastro-intestinal disorders exacerbated by free-radicals (such as irritable bowel syndrome). Equally as important, many fungi are able to bolster or prevent depletion of endogenous antioxidants (e.g., glutathione, superoxide dismutase), thereby assisting with cognitive function (specifically learning and memory) through protecting the brain from chemical and oxidative stresses. The myriad of ways that fungi, along with plants, support the health of humans through exposure to biological compounds gives credence to the idea that humans are, in essence, chemical beings whose health suffers when they experience reduced levels of natural chemistry in their foods.

While mammals have cholesterol, and plants have phytosterols, fungi have **ergosterols**. These molecules perform many of the same functions that cholesterol does in mammals. And, just like in mammals, where cholesterol is a precursor to vitamin D, ergosterols are also a precursor to vitamin D. In the case of fungi, ergosterols can be converted to vitamin D_2 on exposure to sunlight. We have already discussed that vitamin D_2 is not as potent as vitamin D_3, nor does it convert to the active form as quickly, but that is not to say it does not have biological activity (i.e., not to say it doesn't have value). Vitamin D_2 can be used by the human body and can help keep vitamin D levels up during important periods of the year, such as the winter season in northern areas. Freshly harvested mushrooms can be placed in the sun (preferably gills or pores up or sliced up—to increase surface area exposure to ultraviolet radiation) to substantially increase their vitamin D content. One study performed by Stamets and Plotnikoff (published in the International Journal of Medicinal Mushrooms) showed that edible mushrooms can substantially increase their vitamin D levels with exposure to ultraviolet radiation from the sun—as much as 159 times (that is, one species went from 134 IUs of vitamin D_2 per 100 grams of tissue to 21,400 IUs for the same mass). Some species had even substantially higher total amounts of vitamin D_2 (e.g., hen-of-the-woods, *Grifola frondosa*, with 31,900 IUs). Despite the overall lower potency of vitamin D_2, these are significant amounts that can bolster circulating vitamin D levels. Consumptions of sun-dried mushrooms (or placing mushrooms that were dried in a dehydrator in the sun for eight hours) is a strategy that can be used to keep vitamin D levels at adequate levels during the winter season, a practice that can be very important for those without access (or without a willingness to consume) various vitamin-D-rich animal foods.

Vitamin B_{12} is an important B-complex vitamin, called cobalamin, which is used by the body to produce new blood cells and maintain proper functioning of metabolism and the central nervous system. Vitamin B_{12} is not a rare vitamin because it is found in many animal foods. However, certain diets restrict (or avoid) animal foods, a practice with severe ramifications (especially for the infants of those practicing such diets). In this case, deficiency in cobalamin leads to pernicious anemia, an illness that includes such symptoms as fatigue, depression, nausea, gastrointestinal issues, and neuropathic pain. Further complicating this matter is that many non-animal foods stated to possess vitamin B_{12} do not; they actually possess analogs (i.e., pseudovitamin B_{12}) that have structural similarity but not actual vitamin activity (as such, they actually increase the body's need for bioactive vitamin B_{12} through inhibiting certain vitamin B_{12}-dependent enzymes). Fortunately, recent research does demonstrate that a few non-animal foods do contain actual vitamin B_{12} activity, including a few species of wild mushrooms. These include the black trumpet (*Craterellus cornucopioides*) and golden chanterelle (*Cantharellus cybarius*). While the commercially available shiitake mushroom (*Lentinula edodes*) contains some active B_{12}, the amounts varied significantly and analog versions were also sometimes present. Several other mushroom species have been examined, but contained no (or only trace amounts) of cobalamin. It is important to note that the vitamin B_{12} content in these species of mushroom were small relative to many animal foods and could not provide the recommended daily intake without consumption of large amounts of mushrooms on a daily basis. However, knowledge of these species can still be a step toward recovering health for those suffering consequences due to an unnatural diet.

With domestication comes a loss of ancestral knowledge of the wild, other-than-human persons we share our landscapes with. Specifically, knowledge of edible and medicinal fungi appears to be one of the first skillsets that are lost when indigenous and traditional people lose part of their connection to nature. Fortunately, many kinds of mushrooms are often available in supermarkets, providing people with access to these health-promoting organisms. Utilize these species cooked (not raw) to maximize the immune-modulating effects that fungi have. It is important to note that wild mushrooms are species that possess their original mycochemistry as a result of their wild-grown experiences and are preferable when they can be obtained. Fortunately, some species of wild fungi are available in markets today because they cannot be cultivated on a substrate (or are very difficult to cultivate on a commercial scale). Examples include many mycorrhizal fungi, such as boletes, chanterelles, matsutakes, morels, and truffles, species that can impart their vitality to the people who consume them.

OUR SYMBIONTS

Modern humans primarily consider themselves to be discrete organisms that are separate from the rest of the world. However, this could not be further from the truth. In reality, humans are populated with many trillions of microorganisms that perform critical functions (i.e., healthy living would not be possible without these microorganisms). As is often stated, there are ten (or more) times as many bacteria and fungi in our bodies than humans have cells (this is possible because the bacterial and fungal cells are smaller than ours). In fact, most people have a greater weight in symbiotic microorganisms than they do of their brain. Therefore, humans are not a single organism, but rather a symbiotic being composed of hundreds of species of microorganisms living in a cooperative community. These beneficial organisms are called our microflora (or probiotics when ingested in foods or supplements) and they form part of our enteric nervous system (i.e., that associated with our digestive tract). The human microflora has far reaching health consequences that most Americans are oblivious to—a statement that is easily supported by looking at myriad of things people do to harm their gut flora (e.g., antibiotics, chlorinated water, fluoride, agricultural chemicals, unnatural diets). We need to understand that a lack of consideration for our microflora is analogous to willfully ingesting chemicals that harm our livers, our kidneys, or our brains (which humans also do). All of these organs, along with our symbiotic microflora, are necessary for vibrant health and happiness (as we shall see in next paragraphs).

It would be impossible here to explain all of the positives of the beneficial microorganisms that constitute our microbiome—there are literally too many items that could be noted. That said, we need to cover some of the really important features to impress on you how vital this aspect of our being is. Therefore, let's present four essential aspects of probiotics: nutrition, protection, disease, and mood.

The human microflora that dwells in the gastrointestinal (GI) tract plays a substantial role in acquiring **nutrition** for the host partner. These microorganisms both aid in the digestion of foods and increase the surface area of our GI tract, enabling greater absorption of micronutrients. For example, different species produce different enzymes that are capable of breaking down various food molecules, such as the β-galctosidase enzyme produced by fermented dairy bacteria that aid in the digestion of lactose and help to reduce symptoms of lactose maldigestion. The microflora also manufactures certain vitamins, including some B-complex vitamins and small amounts of vitamin K_2 (which are then absorbed by our body). As importantly, our microflora are able to nullify the antinutrient phytic acid in various grains, nuts, legumes, and seed-like fruits through turning phytic acid into inositol, a nutrient that affects mood and insulin sensitivity. Perhaps one of the best examples of the complexity and benefit of our microflora is their effect on our bone health. Through a variety of mechanisms, including increased mineral absorption and expression of calcium-binding proteins (as a result of molecules produced by microorganisms), a healthy gut flora results in stronger bones. All of these facts support the role of our gastrointestinal flora in assisting with our intake of nutrients.

It is estimated that our microflora play a role in 70–80% of our body's immune response; therefore, they are an integral part of the defense that provide **protection** from various insults to health. Research demonstrates that the organisms populating our microbiome are responsible for beneficially stimulating the activity of many kinds of immune molecules, such as T-cells and macrophages. They also activate cytokines, which assist in coordinating the immune response. Our microflora also forms a physical barrier that protects our intestine from pathogens, toxins, and radiation. One of the primary manners they provide protection is through the occupancy of available real estate. For example, pathogenic bacteria and fungi require space to grow, and if the available surface area is populated with beneficial organisms, it is less likely for harmful species to expand and create health issues. Further, our intestinal flora produce natural antibiotic compounds that help reduce populations of pathogenic microorganisms. Studies indicate that a healthy gut flora reduces intestinal absorption of bisphenol A (BPA) and heavy metals. Some strains are even capable of degrading BPA so that it does not exert its endocrine-disrupting activity in the body. Other species have been documented to degrade some notoriously toxic agricultural chemicals (e.g., insecticides). Clearly, our microflora provides a kind of "organic armor" for our bodies.

More than forty **diseases** have been linked to microorganism imbalances in the GI tract. Especially important here are gastroenteritis (and inflammation of the GI tract), irritable bowel syndrome (IBS), and inflammatory bowel disease (IBD), though the role of our microflora also extends to such issues as urinary tract infections, cancer, and autism. An unhealthy microflora leads to an unhealthy GI tract, which promotes inflammation (a characteristic of many chronic diseases). To illustrate how beneficial our microflora is, consider that bacteria in the large intestine produce a short-chain fatty acid called butyrate, which is an anti-inflammatory, up-regulates programmed cell death in colonic cells, and inhibits growth and proliferation of tumors. Studies have demonstrated that autistic children (and others with neurological disorders) have substantial differences in their microflora compared with healthy children, including both the types and abundance of microorganisms. While this might seem coincidental at first, it is important to realize that the GI tract and the brain are intimately connected through a number of mechanisms, including the vagus nerve, neurotransmitter production by microorganisms, and lymphatic vessels in the brain. What happens in one nerve center affects the other.

Even our **mood** is strongly affected by our microflora. Around 90% of the body's serotonin (the "feel good" chemical) and nearly half of the dopamine (associated with feelings of pleasure) produced inside the body are found in the gut. These are just two of the many neurotransmitters, around 30 are known, found in the gut (including the associated enteric nervous system). Nerve signals sent from the gut to brain via the vagus nerve are known to affect temperament, attitude, and even cravings for certain foods. Emerging research is demonstrating the presence of a "gut-brain axis" and poor health in the gut can foster depression and anxiety. This evident connection between the GI tract and the brain is one of the reasons that a natural diet is capable of treating depression (rather than pharmaceutical drugs, which just temporarily mask symptoms).

As is clear from the preceding paragraphs, our symbiotic microorganisms are very important to our well-being. One of the most fundamental ways that we support their health (which in turn benefits our heath) is to realize that our diet is their diet. In other words, foods that support the health of the human being are also foods that support the health of their microbiome. Likewise, poor diets that are rich in refined carbohydrates, synthetic ingredients, and agricultural chemicals, diets that harm human health, also harm the beneficial microflora and exacerbate health issues. One kind of food that is well-represented in many wild diets is called a prebiotic. This is a kind of carbohydrate that escapes digestion in the small intestine and is digested by the microflora of our large intestine. These carbohydrates are called prebiotics because they are a beneficial food for our colonic microorganisms. There are several kinds of prebiotics, including resistant starches and specific kinds of soluble fiber (e.g., inulin). These are primarily found in underground storage organs, legumes, and grains. Not only do resistant starches benefit our microflora, they also decrease the glycemic response after meals, increase insulin sensitivity, and promote improved glycemic health in the next generation (through epigenetic factors). Good sources of prebiotics include inulin-containing roots and tubers (e.g., chicory, dandelion, tuberous sunflower, burdock).

How does all of this mention of our symbionts and foods that benefit them relate to rewilding and nature connection? That's easy to answer—modern humans have substantially different microflora than those of hunter-gatherers as a result of their diets (first and foremost) and their lifestyles, which are rich in exposure to chemicals that are toxic to our beneficial microorganisms. The nature disconnection that we experience has affected so many aspects of our being, including the mood-altering organisms we house in our bodies. Important to this discussion is an understanding that microorganisms do not just inhabit the lower portion of our GI tracts, but also inhabit our mouth, lungs, sinuses, urinary tracts, esophagus, and joints. This means that practices such as use of antimicrobial rinses in the mouth and frequent washing head to toe with soap destroy part of our microbiome (remember: vacancy is the worst thing when it comes to microorganisms, because that vacancy can be repopulated with pathogenic species). Modern humans believe they can simply maintain a poor lifestyle and supplement their way out of everything. However, it turns out that supplemented strains do not remain in the body for extended periods of time (i.e., they are transients). Though they do assist while present, the most important thing we do for our microflora is to rewild our diet. This includes sourcing or (better) making your own traditional fermented foods such as sauerkraut, kimchee, kombucha, kefir, yogurt, miso, and natto. These foods are, in some ways, more advantageous than supplements as they provide benefits outside of the probiotics they supply (which are more numerous and more diverse than supplements). These advantages include making the probiotic foods more digestible (the fermentation is a kind of pre-digestion), providing the microflora with suitable food, and bolstering nutrition through offering vitamins produced by the fermenting organisms. When it comes to supporting the health of the human and their microbiome, diet trumps pills.

WHERE DOES DAIRY FIT IN?

Dairy obtained from other animals is a relatively new food in the human diet. One of things that we have learned (or perhaps more accurately: should have learned by now) is that new foods do not have a track record of safety or promoting intergenerational health, which means they should be avoided by anyone who does not want to make their family a Guinea pig in a dietary experiment. However, dairy has been consumed for at least 9000 years by *Homo sapiens*, providing ample time to identify its effects on people. While many people assert that dairy has a number of harmful effects to the individuals who consume it, several cultures have been observed who relied on dairy as a staple and enjoyed healthy lives free of chronic disease. These include isolated people of the Lötschental Valley of Switzerland and the Maasai of eastern Africa (all carefully photo-documented by Weston Price). These people showed the characteristic broad faces and room for all of their teeth found in populations consuming nutrient-dense diets. Given these observations, blanket statements concerning milk and its role in promoting disease are incorrect (such overly simplified statements have become commonplace today in the nutritional world). The question is not simply "can dairy be a healthy component of a diet"—because this has already been confirmed—but, rather, "what were the qualities of the dairy that was consumed by healthy people who relied on this food". For this, we would need to identify the breed of cows used, the kind of feed they received, the time spent on pasture by the animals, and what processing (if any) the milk received prior to consumption.

First, much like plants, older breeds of cows (i.e., heritage breeds) tend to provide a more healthy milk. Without going into a deep discussion of the specific kinds of dairy produced by different cows, it is important that people realize not all dairy is created equal. Some breeds produce relatively more fat, others relatively more protein. Equally important, some of the proteins found in milk differ among the various breeds. For example, one of the proteins found in milk is called β-casein (read as "beta-casein"). Some modern breeds of cows (e.g., Holsteins) show a high proportion of a specific mutation in one of the amino acids that make up this protein—this mutation is associated with negative health outcomes in some people. This kind of β-casein is called A1. Older breeds (e.g., Jerseys, Guernsey, African and Asian cows) have a lower frequency of this mutation and provide less of the mutated protein. The original protein is called A2. The problem with this mutated form of β-casein is that, when ingested, it releases a protein fragment called β-casomorphin-7 (often shortened to BCM-7) that acts as an opioid in our bodies. This molecule (BCM-7) is associated with a higher prevalence of diabetes, diarrhea, autism, schizophrenia, arthritis, and inflammation. While research is ongoing, it does appear to matter (at least to some people) what breed of cow the milk is obtained from (note: human, goat, sheep, buffalo, yak, and camel milk is entirely or almost entirely A2 milk).

The remaining features of healthy milk are easy to describe: raw, unhomogenized, and from cows that consume a biologically appropriate diet (i.e., grass). Briefly, pasteurization of milk destroys nutrition, deforms milk proteins, reduces its nutritional value, and kills beneficial bacteria. Homogenization strips milk globules of its lipid bilayer, creating a processed food that can be irritating to some people, leading to diarrhea or constipation in people who are otherwise tolerant of lactose (a good discussion of this can be found in Chapter 7 of Deep Nutrition: Why Your Genes Need Traditional Food by Shanahan and Shanahan). Cows who consume large amounts of grain are unhealthy animals with distorted essential fatty acid profiles, little or no conjugated linoleic acid, and with greater amounts of *Escherichia coli* bacteria, a serious food-born pathogen, in their digestive tracts. All of these features of modern milk mean there has been a serious decline in the quality of this food.

While many food and nutrition agencies would state there is no nutritional difference between raw and unhomogenized milk from grass-fed cows and pasteurized and homogenized milk from grain-fed cows, let's actually look at a few differences between these two kinds of dairy. To begin, be aware of that pasteurization kills beneficial bacteria but does not kill putrefying bacteria, which is why pasteurized milk still spoils after a time even though it has not been opened. The heat of pasteurization causes milk proteins to become deformed, reducing its nutritional value. Some authors point to the positive relationship between milk consumption in affluent countries and bone fractures, using this as evidence that milk is not valuable for bone health. This association is very misleading because people in affluent countries are more sedentary and tend to consume more pasteurized dairy (a process that makes calcium less bioavailable). The agencies never mention conjugated linoleic acid (CLA), a nutrient that is found in the fat of ruminant animals (e.g., cows, sheep, goats) that feed on green grass. This fatty acid has been shown to be protective of cancer, lead to the suppression of tumors, support heart health, and assist in the deposition of muscle (rather than fat) in those people who consume the dairy (including butter and cheese) and meat of animals that contains CLA. Grass-fed cows also have milk with higher levels of carotene (i.e., pro-vitamin A) and the active form of vitamin A in their milk. Further, fermenting bacteria in the digestive tract of cows turn vitamin K_1 found in grasses into vitamin K_2, an important fat-soluble vitamin that potentiates the activity of other fat-soluble vitamins (vitamin K_2 in dairy is found at the highest concentrations in butter and certain cheeses). Grains contain very little vitamin K_1; therefore, grain-fed cows produce dairy with very little vitamin K_2. Lastly, grain-feeding of cows shifts the essential fatty acid balance toward omega 6 fatty acids (rather than being nearly equal in grass-fed cows), which contributes to inflammation and depressed function of the immune system. All of these facts illustrate that raw and unhomogenized dairy from pastured animals is superior to the modern, highly refined form of this food. If you choose to consume dairy, this is the form that has promoted health in humans and is the form that should be consumed.

LET THE LIGHT SHINE ON ME

We have already discussed some of the health benefits of allowing sunlight to shine on our skin. Here we will discuss a few strategies that will allow those interested in rewilding to maximize the benefit they receive while participating in this elemental experience. But before we launch into this, we must address the prevailing belief that sunlight causes cancer—a deeply ingrained meme in the United States. People have been taught that the more sun you are exposed to, the more likely you are to develop skin cancer (therefore, it is best to have no sun exposure). But if this were true, why didn't indigenous people, some of who had extensive exposure to sunlight, get skin cancer? This is certainly an important question to ask about the prevailing sunlight hypothesis. Another consideration is the fact that people who today live in areas that receive higher ultraviolet exposure have a lower incidence of many types of other cancers, including bladder, breast, colon, leukemia, lymphoid, pancreatic, prostate, and rectal (all of which suggests that sun exposure helps to protect against many common cancers). And while there is research showing that too much sun exposure is harmful for domesticated humans, there is even more research showing that no sun exposure is even worse, because it not only affects vitamin D levels, but also affects blood pressure and overall vascular health.

When sunlight shines on your skin, your body has the capacity to produce vitamin D (given certain parameters, see next paragraph). Of the many things that vitamin D production supports (such as reducing inflammation and supporting immune system function), vitamin D also up-regulates the production of an antimicrobial peptide on the surface of the skin called cathelicidin. This peptide helps to combat pathogenic bacteria and fungi on our skin and prevent infections. Sunlight also produces cholesterol sulfate (discussed earlier in this chapter) and stimulates production of nitric oxide, a molecule that dilates blood vessels, thereby reducing blood pressure and reducing deaths from heart attack and stroke. Sun exposure also bolsters testosterone production in men, especially naked sun bathing that would expose the scrotum (believe it or not) to sunlight. Given all these benefits, why would be told to protect ourselves from exposure to sunlight? Hold on for just a moment, an explanation is coming.

First, it is important to understand that your body's natural skin secretions are partly responsible for the vitamin D that is produced upon sun exposure. These fats and waxes found on the surface of the skin, called sebum enable the manufacture of vitamin D when they are irradiated with UV light. After exposure to sunlight, the vitamin D is reabsorbed (slowly) by the body where it can be used. Unfortunately, people living in affluent countries tend to bathe (or shower) very frequently and use soap, which washes away the sebum and significantly reduces the amount of vitamin D the body can make. Studies show that even people who receive abundant sun exposure (as much as 11 hours a day) have low levels of circulating vitamin D in their blood due to frequent bathing. Therefore, washing head-to-toe with soap on a daily basis (what is excessive hygiene for most people) is harmful to our health. If you want to make the most out of your sun exposure, avoid soap on most areas of the skin—reserve it for armpits and crotch—unless it is really needed. Be aware that it takes up to 48 hours to absorb the vitamin D produced by our skin; therefore, bathing all over with soap at the end of sunny day reduces most of the value of that day's sun exposure.

Second, it also important to understand that ultraviolet light is made up of different wavelengths, and that only some of these wavelengths produce vitamin D when they shine on our skin. The beneficial wavelengths are called UVB (though these can cause skin burns if allowed to shine on skin too long). Another set of wavelengths are called UVA. These wavelengths actually destroy vitamin D on the skin. This fact is very important to neoaboriginals because UVA passes through windows. Therefore, if you spend a great deal of time indoors or in a car during times when sunlight passes through the windows and contacts you skin, you are causing the vitamin D on your skin to be destroyed prior to its absorption. The take home message here is not to pull shades closed but to offset this destruction of vitamin D by UVA radiation through conscientious exposure to UVB light (i.e., spend more time outdoors near the middle of the day).

To answer the question of why modern humans get skin cancer more frequently than hunter-gatherers is complex and relates to many factors. However, one of the most important details of this story is tied to the kinds of plant foods domesticated humans consume: genetically modified plants that have lower levels of beneficial phytochemicals, including those that protect the skin from damage due to UV light. With the documented declines in polyphenols and antioxidants found in modern produce, our newfangled diet does not shield us from sunlight in the way hunter-gatherer diets did. There is ample research showing that plant-based vitamins and chemicals ingested in the diet are able to offer significant protection from the potential harmful effects of sunlight. While indigenous people did utilize sunscreen made from animal and plant fats, these were very low SPF sunscreens (generally in the single digits). It was, in fact, their diet that afforded them tremendous protection from the sun, while at the same time allowing them to manufacture vitamin D for health. Therefore, the solution to UV radiation is not to completely hide our bodies from it through the use of sunscreen, clothing, and indoor time, because this limits our ability to produce a naturally occurring form of vitamin D, but rather to build our body's innate defenses through a diet rich in wild plants and minimally modified, organically grown plants (including those grown within intact natural communities through polyculture).

THE VEGAN ASSERTION

Veganism, the strict avoidance of animal foods, is a religion. In fact, it has many of the qualities of a fanatical religion, including the intense chastising of people who do not practice the same set of beliefs (in this case, the vehemence is directed toward people who practice other diets). While I don't mean for this to sound impolite to strict vegetarians, and they should be commended for both their passion to stop animal suffering and their willingness to depart from the Standard American Diet. However, there may be no group of people that erect as many dietary myths to support their food choices (some of which even casual self-examination would determine as false) and present as much misinformation to the public as vegans do. Their diet, viewed through the lens of natural human diets, represent perhaps the most extreme departure from hunter-gatherer diets (i.e., it could be considered the most domesticated diet).

Those who practice veganism do so for a number of reasons, among which is generally the well-being of animals and a desire to prevent the subjugation and commodification of animals used to produce food (which are laudable goals). However, there seems to be little concern for the plants that are subjected to factory farm conditions because of the assertion they are not sentient and, therefore, do not need the voice of vegans to protect them. While mammals and birds are avoided as food (and often also clothing), plants are grown in denuded soils, forced to produce food and fiber for their human masters, and then cast aside without much thought. In other words, vegans erect a hierarchy of life, with organisms such as plants, mushrooms, and invertebrates lower down on the ladder and animals, especially those with hair and human-like eyes, higher up. It is important to note that such a hierarchical view of life did not truly occur until the advent of agriculture and the formation of social hierarchy—before that time, all life was sacred. Now, according to vegans, only certain animals are sacred. Such a distorted view of life is only possible within domesticated humans.

Vegans are also interested in a using less resources; therefore, food that could be used to produce animal products can instead be used to feed humans. This goal appears to be a very humane objective because it requires, for example, many pounds of grain to produce one pound of animal food (the ratios vary depending on the type of food we are discussing). The concept goes, if people simply ate exclusively plant foods there would be more than enough food for everyone. Of course, the discussion always centers on grain (an agricultural commodity), rather than an understanding that animals can be pastured in open and forested habitats (depending on the species) and can turn plants that humans can't eat (e.g., certain species of wild plants) into food we can eat (their flesh). This is no different than plants turning sunlight, organic matter, and soil minerals (things we can't eat) into food that we can eat (their roots, shoots, fruits, etc.). More importantly is the idea that if humans all switched to veganism, the food we currently grow could feed all of the humanity (of course, with lots of infrastructure and fossil fuel use to ship foods all over the world). This seems like a very compassionate goal (and it is, it is just a very short sighted one). Feeding all of the existing people on the planet saves everyone from the misery of starvation (something I certainly hope never to experience). However, doing so means one thing: feeding everyone allows for more children to be produced. And feeding all those children means they will have children. Ultimately, the human population will reach levels that no amount of agriculture and no technological innovation can feed. Not even veganism can feed many billions of people. Once we reach those population numbers, the remaining forests will have all been converted to agriculture and every last natural resource that can be eaten will have been eaten. Humans will take the ecosystems down with them, causing massive world-wide ecocide that will not only affect many generations of people but also cause the extinction of many species of animals and plants, reducing the overall biological diversity found on the planet. Extinction is final—the permanent loss of biological uniqueness. I ask you, does this sound humane—protecting all the existing people from starvation now and setting the world up for generations of starving humans who will wander through deserts (that were once forests) created by unsustainable exploitation to supply an insatiable population? I would argue that considering not only the future humans but also the future ecological sanctity (at least that which remains) is a more humane goal than feeding everyone now.

Vegans also practice their diet because it has lots of research showing that it produces better health outcomes. Better than what? It turns out that veganism has demonstrated a reduced risk of hypertension, obesity, heart disease (with exceptions), certain forms of cancer, and type 2 diabetes compared with the general omnivore population (i.e., those that practice the Standard American Diet). However, this isn't a difficult to achieve to goal given that the Standard American Diet is also a radical departure from a natural diet. Keep in mind that hunter-gatherers did not experience heart disease, diabetes, cancer, etc., (and some vegans do). Further, consuming meat (in and of itself) does not cause these issues (as many vegans and researchers with a vegetarian bias would assert). The Standard American Diet happens to have incredibly poor quality meat due to both the diet and living conditions of the animals consumed—but not all omnivorous diets support such poor animal husbandry. For example, conscientious omnivory seeks out wild and free-range animals that are fed biologically appropriate diets, treated with respect, and slayed with humane methods. These diets show similar health outcomes (with regard to the diseases mentioned in this paragraph) as veganism.

But still, there is so much research that asserts that animal foods (especially red meat) cause cancer that this dietary myth must be discussed a bit more (it is a foundation of some vegan arguments). It turns out that omnivory—as commonly practiced in the United States—likely does produce higher rates of cancer, in part through the quality of animal foods ingested (as noted in the previous paragraph) but also through the kinds of animal foods ingested. People in affluent countries tend to focus on lean muscle meats, specific cuts that lack connective tissue (including skin and cartilage). This dietary focus on tender cuts of meat provides an imbalance of certain amino acids, specifically, more methionine and less glycine (glycine is an amino acid well represented in connective tissue, skin, cartilage, and organ meats). High intake of methionine is associated with increased production of insulin-like growth factor-1 (IGF-1), a hormone that promotes cell growth throughout the body, including cancer cells. Therefore, omnivory as commonly practiced by domesticated humans, does appear to increase cancer rates. Restricting dietary methionine has been shown to reverse this trend, but so can increased consumption of glycine-rich foods—both are which balance out the methionine to glycine ratio). In other words, a healthy balance of amino acids, which are consumed when the animals are more fully utilized, does not demonstrate higher incidence of cancer (and explains, in part, why meat consumption in hunter-gatherers did not result in cancer). While many Americans will not want to consume certain cuts of meat that contain connective tissue, the skin of poultry, bone broths, and animal gelatin are easy ways to incorporate glycine in the diet (see "Nourishing Broth" by Morell and Daniel for easy ways to make and cook with bone broths). Emulating hunter-gatherer diets is sometimes as easy as consuming poultry with the skin (which also adds much flavor and nutrition and prevents the meat from drying out). While there is very important information for omnivores in this paragraph, part of the telling of this story is to demonstrate that blanket statements like "red meat cause cancer" should really be refined to read "red meat from unhealthy animals in diets that focus on tender cuts can cause an increased incidence of cancer". In other words, we do not need to turn to veganism to prevent cancer, instead, we can also utilize time-honored methods of consuming animal foods (such as full utilization) to maintain health.

As mentioned above, vegans erect many myths to support their diet and chastise those who do not practice it. I've conversed with numerous vegans and heard many reasons why this diet should be practiced. One vegan told me that humans are not equipped to hunt animals because we lack claws and teeth for capturing animals and tearing their flesh. The fact that we rely on tools to capture and butcher animals (e.g., hunting bows, stone blades) was proof enough we should not eat these organisms. When I pointed out that we also lack powerful digging claws for unearthing tap roots and tubers and must use tools such as shovels and (historically) digging sticks to unearth these plant foods, and we use tools to harvest fruits that grow out of reach in trees did nothing to assuage this person's beliefs. Those tools were deemed as "natural" and hunting tools were not. Even when scientific studies are presented that do not support veganism (studies that are generated by the same process that produces the studies they rely on), they ignore them, claim they are lies, or simply state they represent unenlightened viewpoints. An unbiased examination of these arguments (and many others routinely made by vegans) reveals them as subjective.

The vegan diet is notoriously poor in several vitamins, especially vitamin B_{12} and several fat-soluble vitamins (especially A and D) and docosahexaenoic acid. In fact, a study performed by Louwman and colleagues in 2000 showed that a marginal cobalamin status has measurable effects on fluid intelligence, spatial ability, and short-term memory. In each case they examined,  formerly vegan children scored lower on exams of various cognitive traits than omnivorous children (not exactly the head start I would like to provide my child). This study is corroborated by other studies, including one where Kenyan children who consumed primarily a vegetarian diet were provided various degrees of animal food supplementation. Those who received the most animal foods showed the greatest gains in cognitive function, but also the greatest gains in muscle mass, social interaction skills, and leadership. It should be noted that studies also show that higher IQ scores tend to be associated with vegetarian diets—but these are usually people that were raised on omnivore diets that converted to a vegetarian diet as adults (i.e., they received brain-building foods during developmental years and then switched their diet for various reasons). These studies are often used to imply that vegetarianism promotes a higher IQ score, when in fact the logic here is highly flawed because a vegan diet did not produce the higher IQ score in the adult.

Docosahexaenoic acid (DHA) is a kind of ω3-fatty acid found primarily in animal foods (but also marine algae). Large amounts of DHA are found in ocean fish, especially fat-rich species such as salmon and mackerel (but DHA is also found in non-marine animals). This lipid is required for healthy brain and eye development. It turns out that the body can convert the plant form of ω3-fatty acid (called α-linolenic acid) to DHA through a complex series of steps, but this conversion is very inefficient and worse in males, where only approximately 5–10% of the consumed α-linolenic acid is converted to DHA. This is another example where a nutrient that is found in plants is substantially different than that found in animals. In fact, vegans have been found to have lower levels of DHA in the body (and lower levels in the body means that the breast milk of nursing moms provides lower levels to infants who are breastfeeding). This combined with low levels of iron in many vegan dieters, due to the fact that iron in plant foods is not as bioavailable as it is in animal foods, means that children of vegans tend to score lower on exams of cognition (low iron promotes anemia, which impairs cognitive development). Keep in mind that even reducing the IQ scores of children a few points prevents them from reaching their full potential.

While I don't support strict vegetarian diets in adults because of poor health outcomes that I have witnessed all too frequently (especially a suppressed immune system), adults do choose this diet for themselves (i.e., they give themselves consent to partake in a new and unnatural diet). It is interesting that most vegans are converts—how many vegans do you know that were borne to lifelong vegan parents who themselves were borne to lifelong vegan parents? That's only three generations. But more to the point, developing humans (fetuses, infants, and children) have greater requirements for certain nutrients than can be supplied in a strictly plant-based diet. Vegans actually understand that animal foods are needed by developing humans (without admitting to themselves), as evidenced by the fact that most would prefer their infants to be breast fed for some time rather than consuming a soy-based formula their entire infancy. Human breast milk is an animal food. And while vegans will say this doesn't count as omnivory, ask yourself this question: if a lactating mother pumped her breast milk and fed it to the family dog, would you say that the dog received an animal food or a plant food? The problem is that vegans don't realize that the need for animal foods was present before conception and was needed years after the infant stopped breastfeeding. While some adults can live on a vegan diet (generally with supplementation), that is not proof this diet is appropriate for creating healthy, vital, and well-formed children. In fact, studies show just the opposite.

As I write these paragraphs, I am fully aware that some people may be offended by the words presented here (though no offense was intended). I am also aware that the uncompromising religion of veganism will not be swayed by my words. But they were not written for people with closed minds. They were written for people who are still open to information about natural living. Everyone (including vegans) should realize that much of the research supporting strict vegetarianism is flawed by a factor known as the "healthy user bias". Vegans tend to be health conscious and take part in various health-promoting activities (and avoid harmful ones). The research generally compares vegans with general population omnivores who practice the Standard American Diet and may not participate in other healthy activities (and may even engage in many harmful ones, like smoking, excessive drinking, little or no exercise, etc.). Such comparisons are not valid—they are comparing apples to oranges. If only vegans critically examined so many of the statements they make and the practices that produce their food, they might find that the armor surrounding their beliefs has many chinks. For example, how many vegans are aware that most organic farms they purchase food from use animal wastes (i.e., manure) as fertilizer, and that animal waste was sourced from farms that raise animals for food? If vegans were truly interested in the lowest impact food production, they would participate in conscientious foraging of wild plants, a practice that leaves ecosystems intact (unlike most agriculture systems). But, I have found in my discussions with vegans that this is actually not the over-arching goal—it is an end to animal cruelty (but not plant cruelty). More specifically, it is an end to feathered and furred animal cruelty; however, the hierarchy of life they have established is patently artificial to anyone with a connection to nature. While vegans are to be commended for their compassion (and I genuinely mean that), a diet that leaves children lacking in IQ is not a diet I wish to follow. I will not enroll my young child—who cannot truly provide her consent based on comprehension of all the arguments—in an experimental diet.

THE NEOABORIGINAL DIET

This chapter has been a long one, and it was intentional. Our diet is one of the most fundamental ways we interact with the world. The way a society nourishes itself is a direct reflection of their degree of nature connection (or lack thereof). Societies that are strongly separated from nature will utilize chemical agriculture, unaware (or uncaring) what these chemicals do to the soil and the remainder of life in the area of use and downstream of their use (including other people who are affected by the exposure to the toxic compounds). The humane rearing of domesticated animals becomes too much trouble (it is much easier to raise them in tiny enclosures where they stand in their own feces). Feeding those animals foods they are adapted to consuming is too expensive—the goal is feed animals the least expensive food possible (which sometimes includes newspapers, their own dead, and their own manure). All of this is possible only in a society that is too caught up in its own pursuit of pleasure, happy to stand atop the egocentric classification they have erected—a kind of biologically stratified world. This disconnection from nature is one of the major sources of disease in affluent countries because it allows people to consume other life that is ill or has been prepared in ways that actually maximize its harm (rather than its nutritional value).

Diets should foster health in the people consuming them and in the generations to come. Being sick on a frequent basis or dealing with chronic disease that is nutritionally related (which most chronic disease is) are ways to reduce the quality of life and cause people to have a greater impact on the world through using more resources to care for their failing health. Further, "dis-ease" makes it more difficult to rewild other aspects of your life. Natural diets have a long track record of supporting health and vitality. It is completely possible to emulate hunter-gatherer diets in today's world. The following list presents ten items you can incorporate into your life to rewild your diet. This is not a complete list (much more was discussed in this chapter), but practicing these features will invigorate a connection to nature that will be reflected in your health. While most diets define themselves by what they can't consume (which is an unhealthy way to view the world), this list focuses on positive items that you can commit to. Also, this list is not a rigid set of rules of which foods to consume and in what proportions. We know from examining healthy, wild people around the world that the macronutrient (i.e., carbohydrate, protein, and lipid) ratios were incredibly varied, the amount of raw vs. cooked food differed, and the exact species eaten were not the same (yet, the results of these diets were). Therefore, application of concepts (rather than recipes) allows one to modify dietary planning to best match their lifestyle, their healing needs (if any), and those foods available in their ecosystem.

1. Practice **conscientious omnivory**—the consumption of wild or ethically raised life (including plants, animals, and other kingdoms of life). The conscientious harvest of wildlife leaves ecosystems intact, and organically raised plants and pastured animals produce far less pollution (of all kinds) and far less chemical and antibiotic residues in the environment.

2. Focus each day (or as often as you can) on incorporating foods from all **six food groups**: animals, plants, fungi, bacteria, elements, and experiences. Know that lack of exposure to the elements and lack of positive experiences provides a kind of nutritional deficit that affects your epigenome.

3. Find ways to bring higher levels of **phytochemistry** into your diet. If wild plants are unavailable to you (for whatever reason), focus on minimally modified plants that still possess

much of their chemical potency. Humans are chemical beings and we should support this with natural chemistry in our diets.

4. Consume, to the extent possible, **nutrient-dense, whole foods**. These are foods that have not been overly refined and extracted, nor have they seen the addition of synthetic additives. Humans are supposed to consume the majority of nourishment with intact cells (not acellular foods that are ground into tiny particles and reshaped as modern foodstuffs). Further, supplementation is not the ultimate answer for a diet as it relies on industry and fosters dependence on distantly produced products. Humans have been able to nourish their bodies without supplements for most of their existence (and can continue to do so if they invest in learning about traditional nutrition).

5. Learn to **fully utilize** the animal foods you consume. Organ meats are substantially more nutritious than lean cuts of meat. Learning recipes where stronger flavors can be concealed is relatively easy to do (if you are inspired to do so). Consider bone broths and similar recipes as a way to utilize the bones, cartilage, and/or skin of animals in the diet.

6. Ingest more **raw foods** than is usual in the diets of affluent people. Cooking the vast majority of foods in the diet limits certain heat-unstable nutrients. Raw foods should not only extend to plants, but also animal as well. If safe raw animal foods are unavailable (or represent an obstacle you cannot clear), consider lighter cooking of animal foods that are safe to consume rare.

7. Nourish your **symbiotic organisms** that you share space with. Your diet feeds your body and trillions of microscopic organisms that are vital to your health. Traditional, whole foods from a diversity of sources best support your microflora. Incorporate fermented foods in the diet and find sources of resistant starch and similar carbohydrates that benefit the colon flora.

8. Learn to **properly process** the foods you consume, especially the grains, legumes, nuts, and seed-like fruits in your diet (through soaking, sprouting, fermenting, etc.). Some kinds of shoots and greens are also better cooked than raw (at least for some people who may need time to heal various ailments that antinutrients exacerbate). This allows you to maximize the nutrition from the foods while minimizing the potential deleterious effects.

9. Recognize that **dietary fats** are crucial for health (and brain function). Maximize the consumption of unextracted fats (i.e., limit fats that require industrial methods to separate them from seeds and fruits). Healthful fats are found in many plants and animals (in the latter case, those that are pastured and consume a biologically appropriate diet). Plant-based polyunsaturated fatty acids should be consumed while contained within the seed/fruit to avoid oxidized versions of those fats. As part of rewilding your intake of dietary fats, "normalize" your ratio of ω6 and ω3 fatty acids (the ratio should be between 1:1 and 4:1 of these fats—a task easily accomplished by a rewilded diet).

10. **Offer gratitude** for the life that nourishes your body. This is perhaps best accomplished by abandoning the biological hierarchy that agricultural humans have erected and realizing we are merely one part of the world's biome. The frequent practice of thanksgiving has the capacity to change a person's outlook on life (or, at least, certain aspects of life). Offering gratitude is a fundamental part of generating appreciation and respect for those organisms that become part of our being. Without gratitude, there is only mindless consumption of "food" with little care for its origin and history.

4. Water: life blood and universal solvent

The human body is approximately 70% water (give or take for a number of variables, including age and percent body fat). Certain organs, such as the brain, heart, and lungs, are composed of an even higher proportion of water. Without it, our body could not transport oxygen, nutrients, and antibodies to where they are needed. Water is used to regulate our core temperature, lubricate our joints, keep mucosal membranes moist, and is necessary for the metabolism of the food we ingest. Every single cell in our body requires it to continue functioning. It is clear that this wonderful and enigmatic substance is absolutely crucial for life. While the earth has large volumes of water, most of it we cannot utilize as drinking water without processing it in some way (e.g., ocean water, glaciers). In fact, less than 1% of the earth's water can be used for drinking water. Given the importance of water to humans and the small amount of usable water, one would assume that humans have a very high regard for this water and treat it as sacred. Unfortunately, this has not been the case—domesticated humans have been poor stewards of this vital aspect of our world.

HOW WE SEE WATER

I believe that a case history of a river in the United States will best provide an understanding of how modern humans see water. It will also provide another clear example of nature divorcement. We will discuss what is today called the Androscoggin River of Maine and New Hampshire, a river that has been called by many names. It was called aləssikɑntekʷ, the "river of rock shelters", by one of the indigenous groups of the Maine. This river is one of the major "long persons" in the northeastern United States, flowing nearly 200 miles and draining over 3500 square miles of land. It was of great importance to the hunter-gatherers that lived and traveled along its length, and they have a rich history of experiences upon this river. Some of the earliest human artifacts date back more than 11,000 years. It was a significant source of revered food, including migrating Atlantic salmon, alewife, shad, and Atlantic sturgeon—foods that supplied both meat and roe, which contributed to excellent health and beautiful, wide faces. The river was also an important travel way, by canoe during the ice-free months and by snowshoe during the winter season. The river was not just part of their life, it was an integral, defining feature of who they were. After millennia of occupation by indigenous people, the river was rich with wildlife—though this would change after about two centuries of occupation by domesticated humans.

Around the mid-1700s, things began to change for this river. Parcels of land (formerly occupied by indigenous people) were provided to European settlers and land clearing on a massive scale began. Industries began to spring up on the river, perhaps one of the most impactful early on being the forest industry that used the river to transport felled wooden logs downstream to the mills. The felling of trees was originally accomplished with saws and axes and transported to the river with oxen. New equipment eventually came to the region, such as chainsaws and tractors, increasing both the rate of deforestation and the amount of wood floating down the Androscoggin River. At some points during the ice-free season, so much floating wood moved through the river that the surface of the water could not be seen for long stretches. In fact, one well-known large falls that cascades down over massive cliffs of stone was, at times, completely obscured by enormous mounds of jammed logs. Dams, shoreline modification, and boats were all used to further increase the amount of wood that could move downstream through this river and shorten the transit time. The immense volume of wood eventually harmed the quality of the water. As the bark fell off the logs, it sank to the bottom where it decayed, causing significant reductions in dissolved oxygen. This led to a decrease in adult fish, a decrease in viability of the fish eggs, and a decrease in the aquatic insects that the fish relied on for food. Ultimately, the river's abundant fish inhabitants declined (some downstream stretches of the river could be accurately described as dead zones). Transportation of logs down the river by the logging companies represented monopolization of the river because it made the waterway unusable by others living along it. It wasn't until both state and federal lawsuits were filed that this practice was ultimately stopped (i.e., the companies that benefitted from the log drives were unwilling to modify their practices to protect wildlife and allow others to use the river until they were forced to).

Starting around the early 1800s, mill dams were being constructed on the river and its tributaries, which blocked the movement of migratory fish (including a large dam constructed in 1899 at the head of tide). The abundance of fish prior to industry on the river on the Androscoggin River is well documented in historical accounts, as exemplified by the large numbers of salmon and sturgeon caught in early fishing ventures by settlers. Unfortunately, the dams represented impassable obstacles to the fish that required upriver spawning grounds. Said another way, the hydrological connectivity of the river had been impacted for Atlantic salmon and other prized fish that had once travelled up this river. Salmon, with their rich ω3 fatty acid content, so valuable for developing brains and eyes, became a thing of the past along the river, replaced with crops that were largely rich in ω6 fatty acids (i.e., this transition from wild food to cultivated crops represented a serious decline in nutrition for the inhabitants of the watershed). After thousands of years of movement up and down the river, the migratory fish, a fundamental part of the river, were rather abruptly excluded as the river first came under the dominion of its masters.

Another major insult to the river resulted from public and private discharges of waste into the river. For over 200 years, one of the cities at the head of tide along the Androscoggin River discharged public sewage into the river, with no system of waste containment or processing. This led to epidemics of disease. Later, as paper mills came on line, potent carcinogenic chemicals were directly discharged into the river (and air). This included dioxins, which are a group of highly toxic substances that are produced when chlorine is used to whiten paper. Dioxins are known to contribute to cancer, birth and developmental defects, fertility issues, suppression of the immune system, and learning disabilities. Important to this discussion is that humans are not the only beings affected by dioxins—the wildlife living in and along the river suffers as well. Of note is that chlorine-free paper-making technology exists today, but the paper mills refuse to utilize such technology. The paper mills also released other compounds, including malodorous chemicals like hydrogen sulfide, which would rise off the river and react with freshly painted homes, turning them black (this was documented in the early 1940s). Further degrading the quality of the river were the activities of a former paper mill on an upstream section of the river that resulted in substantial mercury contamination, which continues today as this metal seeps through fractures in the bedrock and into the waterway. Biological surveys show that the wildlife along the river possess elevated levels of mercury downstream of this former paper mill location (now a superfund site), including levels that have prompted the US Environmental Protection Agency to issue warning statements about consuming fish from this river. Mercury exposure results in impaired neurological functioning and negatively affects fetal and infant brain and nervous system development. The discharge of toxins into the air and water has led to elevated rates of certain cancers in some towns along the river (leading to the coining of the name "Cancer Valley"). The health of the river is tied to the health of the people living along it, but those people fail to see the connection.

The Androscoggin River stands as a monumental failure to steward an important natural feature and as a clear example of how domesticated humans see water. Water is merely another resource to be exploited for economic benefit, regardless of the modifications that happen to it and the landscape features that contain it. Rivers, specifically, are seen as convenient ways of moving waste away from the source to another location where it cannot harm those who produce it (though it does harm downstream inhabitants). Our thought process regarding water quality demonstrates the characteristic lack of wisdom that is typical of agricultural and industrial societies—exemplified by the "pollute and move on to clean sources" tact we have taken in this country. The Androscoggin River is no different in this regard. In fact, one of the cities that used to acquire its water from the Androscoggin River decided that rather than cleaning up the river it would be better to switch to another water body (a less expensive solution), allowing Big Polluters to continue the degradation of a river with a rich history of wild human habitation. Now, it has been almost 200 years since Atlantic salmon were seen navigating a set of falls that are positioned upstream of the tidal sections of this river. No restoration efforts are underway because the Maine Atlantic Salmon Commission does not consider the Androscoggin River an appropriate candidate for salmon restoration. Like the indigenous people who formerly lived upon it, the Androscoggin River is also a defining feature of who we, modern people, are. But, in this case, it presents a negative depiction, demonstrating that the river is not sacred to us. Our treatment of this waterway serves to define the degree of harm we are willing to inflict upon the landscape, and how seemingly little we care. Apathy, one of the most important forces of modern society, permeates the hearts of the people who live near this river and clouds their ability to clearly perceive how we see water.

THE REMARKABLE PROPERTIES OF WATER

Water is a truly miraculous substance, and life on earth would not be possible without it. It has a number of chemical properties that influence the physiology and ecology of all living beings. Further, it is a defining force that shapes many landscapes through its abundance (or scarcity) and its movement—either as liquid (streams and rivers) or solid (snow, ice, and glaciers). Gaining an understanding of water's characteristics can certainly foster an appreciation for the value of this unique material, but it can also help us understand how certain forms of water commonly found in agricultural and industrial societies is very damaging (especially over the long run) to our health. It is imperative that we learn to see water differently.

Water can be viewed (from a reductionist standpoint) as a very simple molecule, formed by the union of two hydrogen atoms and one oxygen atom. However, water (the collection of molecules) is very complex and dynamic. For example, water possesses a quality that few other compounds do—it becomes more dense as the temperature decreases until around 4 degrees Celsius (approximately 39 degrees Fahrenheit), at which point it gradually becomes less dense until it freezes. The water molecules become spaced apart and form rigid, four-sided crystals (called tetrahedrons) as they freeze, becoming less dense than water that is near the freezing point. Therefore, ice floats (rather than sinking and freezing at the bottom of the water body). While this may not seem like a remarkable trait, the biological ramifications are manifest. If water were like most molecules on earth, and got denser as they got colder, the ice that formed would sink to the bottom and form layers that would kill much of the aquatic invertebrate life. Without the insulating layer of ice and snow on the surface of water, water bodies in northern areas would be more likely to freeze completely solid (or so much so that only a small area of liquid water would remain on the surface of the frozen water below). Life would be dramatically different on the planet, and in many areas it might not be possible if it were not for this peculiar trait of water.

Equally important is the cohesion (i.e., bonding) of water molecules to each other. In other words, water does not break apart into countless water molecules but, rather, forms a unified body of liquid. This occurs because of the chemistry of the molecule. Water molecules could be described as V-shaped, with an oxygen atom at the bend of the V and one hydrogen atom each at the tips of the V. Because the oxygen atom has a slightly higher negative charge, the water molecule is a polar molecule, which means that one end of the molecule is slightly negatively charged (the bend of the V) and one end of the molecule is slightly positively charged (the tips of the V). Therefore, the water molecules bond to each other through the attraction of different ends of molecules (the positive to negative and negative to positive), creating the cohesive force that holds water together. The bonds, called hydrogen bonds, while not especially strong individually, collectively create the most cohesion of any non-metallic liquid. So what, you might be thinking. These hydrogen bonds are responsible (in part) for the surface tension found at the interface of water and air, a distinct microhabitat that is utilized by countless organisms that can float and travel across the surface. The cohesion of this molecule to others of its kind also forms beads of water on many surfaces, such as plant leaves, causing the water to form droplets and fall off the leaf rather than spreading out over the leaf. If the water did not bead (because of hydrogen bonds), it would remain as a film on the leaf for a longer period of time, keeping it wet, both slowing the absorption of carbon dioxide (which would slow down the rate of photosynthesis) and allowing pathogenic fungi to grow on the leaf surface. Therefore, without hydrogen bonds, plant life on this planet would suffer.

Another very special quality of water is its heat capacity. Simply stated, heat capacity is the capability of a substance to absorb heat without changing its temperature—the greater the amount of heat that can be absorbed, the greater the heat capacity. Water is capable of absorbing lots of energy without changing its temperature very much, in fact, it has the highest heat capacity of any common substance. The best way to understand this is to imagine an empty metal pot placed on a stove burner. If heat is applied to it, it will quickly heat up to the point the metal can become damaged; however, if water is added to the pot, the temperature will rise more slowly and stabilize until all the water is evaporated by the heat (and then the metal pot will heat up relatively quickly to very high temperatures). Water has about ten times the ability to resist a change in temperature than does a pot made of iron. The heat capacity of this liquid is what allows large bodies of water to moderate the local climates that contain them (by acting as massive heat sinks) and to keep relatively stable temperatures for the benefit of the organisms that live within them (such as ocean life). Heat capacity is related to another feature of water (called latent heat) that helps it to cool the human organism (through evaporation). We perspire to help reduce our core temperature when it is over-heated. It requires energy to cause water to change from liquid to gas (which is what happens when our perspiration evaporates from our skin). This energy is supplied by the heat energy we possess in our body—as we give up this heat energy, our surface cools, as does the blood in the capillary beds near the surface of our skin. As this blood returns to our core, it helps to cool our body. Without water's special heat capacity (and the related latent heat), terrestrial and aquatic animals would face very different climatic stresses, and their ability to cope with them would be diminished.

Water is also a phenomenal solvent, meaning there are many other molecules that can dissolve in it; in fact, water can dissolve more items than any other liquid on earth. This occurs because of the polarity (i.e., differently charged poles) of other molecules become attracted to the poles of the water molecules, essentially keeping the dissolved molecules suspended in the liquid (through being surrounded by water molecules). But some materials do not have a charge, such as fats; therefore, they do not become hydrogen bonded to water molecules (so they don't mix, but can be described as being pushed out of the water). But for those things that do have a charge, they can dissolve in water quite well and be carried wherever liquid water goes, such as into plant roots, fungal hyphae, and the mouths of animals. Therefore, water can carry dissolved minerals and salts into other organisms, and it can carry hazardous dissolved solids (e.g., landfill leachate, feedlot waste, sewage) and dissolved molecules (e.g., methyl-mercury, various lead compounds) into other organisms.

These are just some of the truly remarkable properties of the water, the life blood that is found (to some extent) in all regions of the world. More and more is being discovered about water every year. The new frontier, which is not really that new, is exclusion zone water (often shortened to EZ water), a "fourth phase" of water that excludes other molecules and can hold a charge. This is the kind of water found inside our cells and likely has important health ramifications (research is on-going). It is clear that if humans should be thankful for any single substance on the planet, it is water. While all things on this planet are sacred (or should be held as sacred), water requires a certain place in our consciousness. Though the previous section demonstrated that people have not cherished the water resources of the earth, we need to see water in a different way. We need to connect to water, much as we need to connect to all of nature. Connection to this part of our world also requires a basic understanding of its chemistry because, without this knowledge, we will continue to harm our health through the ways we misunderstand and mistreat water.

THE "MIRACLE MATERIAL"

Plastic, the miracle material that "freed us from the confines of the natural word", is now routinely used in almost every aspect of American life. This includes food, medicine, sports, the automotive industry, clothing, and so much more. Americans dove headlong in plastic use, and before its safety and disposal issues were ever really researched or discussed, we became addicted to plastic, unable to imagine a life before this substance. We now belong to a society that is dependent on a substance that was believed to be safe—because it was believed to be inert. By this, I mean that when drinking water (or other liquids) contacted plastic, none of the compounds that make up the polymer would migrate into the liquid. We now confidently know this assumption (of the chemical inactivity of plastic) to be false. As a result, we need to bring awareness of the problems of plastic (bear with me, the following pages appear to deviate from the topic of water, but in fact modern water and plastic are strongly interrelated).

If you have spent any time reading about the potential hazards of plastic, it is likely you have seen the warnings about Bisphenol A (BPA). This is a compound added to create various plastic products. It has been used to make baby bottles, plastic linings of many food cans, some resins, receipt paper, dental fillings, and food packaging wrap (and it is found in recycled toilet paper). Many studies document that BPA disrupts hormone signaling (a property called endocrine disruption)—this should not be a surprise given that BPA was tested as a candidate for synthetic estrogen in the 1930s. Hormones are responsible for directing growth and development, metabolism, immune system and reproductive system function, behavior, and circadian rhythms in humans (among many other physiological processes)—disrupting these natural biochemical messengers is harmful to human health. For example, one study showed that prenatal exposure to BPA adversely affected birth outcomes. Mothers with high exposure to BPA had babies with 20% lower birth weight and 11% smaller heads (i.e., those babies had smaller brains). Even a brief study on the world wide web will reveal a number of studies (which can be observed for free) demonstrating a negative correlation between material BPA levels and fetal growth metrics (i.e., high maternal exposure to BPA is associated with a smaller neonate). Of importance is that BPA acts like a synthetic estrogen, so it is associated with sexual dysfunction in men and reproductive system disorders in both men and women. Further, exposure to BPA is also considered a risk factor for obesity, cancer, neurological issues, asthma, thyroid health, and cardiovascular disease. Of interest (and perhaps predictably) is that industry-funded studies demonstrate that BPA is harmless.

If you have paid attention to the news around BPA, you might be thinking that this compound has been removed from products on the market. That isn't the case; it has simply been removed from a few high profile items, such as plastic baby bottles. It is still found in so many aspects of our life that infants and young children (along with adults) receive constant exposure. Over six billion pounds of this chemical are used each year, and it can be detected (through tests) in 93% of the US population (with children generally showing higher levels than adults). Confusingly, many products labeled as "BPA-free" are actually not free of BPA (due to plastic dust contamination at factories), or have simply been manufactured by substituting other endocrine disrupting compounds, such as BPS and BPAF, which are related compounds that also demonstrate endocrine-disrupting activity. Unfortunately, BPA (and its related bisphenol compounds) is not the only hazard associated with plastic.

Phthalates (pronounced thal–ates) are chemicals used as plasticizers (i.e., they help make plastic products flexible). They are found in a large variety of products, such as electronics, adhesives, waxes, paints, inks, foods, children's toys, detergents, cosmetics, medicines, and many more. Phthalates (similar to BPA) can be leached from their containers into liquids, are released into the environment, and, because they are volatile, are also found in indoor air. Phthalates, like BPA (and other related bisphenol compounds), are also capable of endocrine disruption. Keep in mind that hormones work within our bodies in very tiny doses; therefore, it requires very little of a hormone (or a hormone-like substance) to cause potentially serious issues. Phthalates are linked to social behavior disorders, and a recent study demonstrated that the higher the phthalate (and BPA) concentration in pregnant mothers, the greater the degree of social cognition, communication, and awareness issues displayed by the children years after birth. What's more, some products that contain phthalates (such as drinking water containers) also contain other classes of endocrine-disrupting compounds, like fumarates and maleates, compounds that are not regulated by any health agency. Unfortunately, BPA and phthalates are not the only hazards associated with plastic.

Polyvinyl Chloride (PVC) is one of the most widely used polymers in the world. It is commonly used in piping and home construction and, when made flexible by the addition of phthalates, it is also used in electronics, plumbing, imitation fabrics, and inflatable products. PVC is a material that can be heated again and again and will become hard once cooled. Unfortunately, this heating and cooling process releases a suite of environmental toxins, including chlorine, dioxins, phthalates, lead, cadmium, and BPA, all of which pose health concerns for humans. For example, lead is documented to leach into drinking water from PVC pipes. Another example, when PVC in incinerated, dioxins are released into the environment, which are known carcinogens and negatively affect the thyroid gland, central nervous system, and immune system.

Further, as PVC ages and degrades, it fractures, allowing microscopic pieces of plastic (called microplastics) to be introduced into the environment. These microplastic particles are then ingested (usually unknowingly) by wildlife and become sources of persistent organic pollutants that we then ingest as we consume other animals. Unfortunately, BPA, phthalates, and PVC are not the only hazards associated with plastic. We could continue for many pages listing the different kinds of plastics and the hazards associated with these polymers.

To gain an understanding of the degree to which plastic has infiltrated modern life, it is important to realize how much plastic we are using in the United States. The answer is: more than most people realize. Humans use about 260 million tons of plastic each year, accounting for 8% of the world's oil production. According to The Wall Street Journal, almost 100 billion plastic bags are used here in the US each year. Approximately 8 billion pounds of plastic wraps, bags, and containers enter landfills each year—and at best, about 3% of these bags are recycled each year (note, this is only a fraction of the total plastic going into landfills). Seven billion pounds of PVC is discarded in the US every year, with less than 1% of this being recycled. In the United States alone, over 27 billion plastic baby diapers are used each year (about six oil tankers worth of oil). Plastic diapers represent the 3rd largest filler of landfills (after newspapers and food containers). We have created such a disposal problem that our trash is sometimes shipped to undeveloped countries where it can be incinerated due to lax environmental regulations, emitting dioxins and other contaminants onto those landscapes. There is even a massive area of plastic trash (mostly comprised of tiny particles) floating in the Pacific Ocean that covers over 5000 square kilometers. In fact, ocean water in Maine, a relatively rural state in the US, now has abundant microplastic particles suspended in it (in one study, 100% of the samples showed presence of microplastics).

We eat off plastic, we drink out of plastic, and we dispense medicine through plastic. We even walk and crawl on plastic, though most are probably not aware that vinyl and PVC floors are associated with higher rates of autism. We know that plastic doesn't biodegrade; it just breaks into smaller and smaller pieces that, ultimately, enter the food chain. We are coming to know there is ample evidence demonstrating harm to humans and ecosystems from plastic production, recycling, and use (unless you rely on industry-funded studies, there you will see results that stand in stark contrast with independent studies). And we accept all of this mainly for convenience (no need to do dishes) and expense (plastic is cheaper than glass). We allow convenience and cost to over-ride health considerations. We have to stop and think what we want our legacy to be. Is the fact that something is disposable worth the health risks to you? Is the fact that is costs less money worth risking your child's health? When your grandchildren and great grandchildren look back on this period in time, the point at which we knew plastic products were not safe, what do you want them to say about us? I would hope they will have good things to say. But in order for that to happen, we have to stop being apathetic about plastic. We have to do something that contemporary humans are very poor at: we have to consider our impact on people who aren't even yet born.

ENDOCRINE DISRUPTION

The human endocrine system is a network of glands that secrete substances (hormones) into the blood stream to regulate the function of particular organs. This system controls and adjusts many and diverse aspects of human physiology, including metabolism, insulin levels, growth, stress, behavior, intelligence, sexual development, and reproduction. This is an exquisitely balanced system—anything perturbing this system can lead to serious health problems, including (but not limited to) diabetes, obesity, cancer, reproductive issues, behavioral problems, and stunted intellectual development. There are a number of agents that can disrupt endocrine function, including the various chemicals found in the containers and pipes that modern humans use to store and transport drinking water. As has been alluded to in the previous section, various chemicals in plastics are capable of disrupting endocrine function through their ability to mimic human hormones—specifically estrogen. Keep in mind that plastics are not the only source of xenoestrogens (i.e., estrogen-like compounds originating from outside of the body). Xenoestrogens also include several metals that can activate estrogen receptors (so-called metalloestrogens, including aluminum, chromium, lead, mercury, and others), additional industrial chemicals (e.g., polychlorinated biphenyls, dioxins), and phytoestrogens found in various plant foods like flax, hops, and soy. Therefore, when someone notes that the xenoestrogen content in plastic bottled water is relatively low, remind them that there are many routes of exposure for Americans. Xenoestrogens located in plastic bottled water represents one of the frequent pathways of exposure for Americans—one that is easily avoided.

There are several issues that are important to understand when drinking (and eating) out of plastic on a regular basis. One of the most important is that infants and children are inefficient at removing these chemicals from their body because their detoxification process (which involves the liver) is not as well developed as in adults. Therefore, testing performed in the United States (and other affluent countries) has demonstrated that young people frequently have higher levels of BPA in their body than adults, levels that occasionally exceed the safe limits set by the US Environmental Protection Agency. This age group is also one that is undergoing development (i.e., they are growing into adults) and are much more susceptible to disruptions to their endocrine system. High levels of xenoestrogens in young humans are associated with early onset of puberty and sexual organ malformations, such as cryptorchidism (undescended testicles), hypospadias (urethra opening not at correct location, such as along the bottom of the penis), and male genitalia of smaller size.

Of course, adult humans are also affected by the large number of xenoestrogens that are found in our water, food, homes, and environment. While women are affected, and deal with various issues, including disrupted menses and increased incidence of certain forms of cancer (e.g., breast, endometrial), men are hit especially heavy by the increased incidence of estrogen-like compounds in their bodies. Sexual dysfunction, low libido, reduced motivation, low sperm count, malformed and poorly motile sperm, obesity, and feminization of physical traits (e.g., redistribution of fat, decreased muscle development) are just some of the issues that males experience. While male humans do naturally possess hormones we associate with females (and vice versa), there is a balance to these hormones that produces “maleness”. I’m not writing about modern, pathological male traits like egocentrism, chauvinism, and obsessive pursuit of material wealth and recognition. Healthy male characteristics, which include drive, motivation, physical strength, and sexual energy, can be (and are) negatively impacted by disrupting hormone balances.

Be aware that the other-than-human beings (e.g., animals) exposed to the endocrine-disrupting chemicals we discharge into the environment are also demonstrating signs of impaired reproductive health and distorted gender ratios (this is across many taxonomic groups, including fish, amphibians, and mammals—I have personally worked as a biological consultant on such studies). For example, in a study conducted to identify the impact of waste water discharged into a stream from a water treatment plant in Boulder, Colorado, the researchers found that proportion of male fish immediately downstream of the effluent site were only about half as frequent as they were upstream. The study also reported that nearly 1/5 of the fish downstream were described as "intersex" (as opposed to none of the fish with this classification upstream of the effluent site). Chemical analyses revealed that the waste water from the city contained a complex assortment of chemicals known to disrupt endocrine function. Our actions aren't just harming humans, but all of life within reach of our industry.

At this point, you might be thinking that is all sounding a bit too alarmist. After all, the US government would never allow a substance that is potentially harmful to come into contact with something so important as our drinking water (or our food, our children's mouths, etc.). One of the major problems is that the respective regulatory agencies utilize studies with obvious conflicts of interest to guide their policies. For example, in a study by Saal and Welshons (published in 2006), they found that 100% of industry-funded studies (11 of 11) demonstrated that BPA (for example) was safe, yet 92% of studies without industry funding (109 out of 119) demonstrated measurable health effects due to exposure to BPA. The problem here goes even deeper, given the massive amount of lobbying performed by the American Chemistry Council (11,000,000 dollars in expenses in 2013) and the fact that some governmental reports on BPA safety have largely been written by the plastic industry and those with a financial stake in this chemical (as uncovered by Milwaukee Journal Sentinel and published in 2008). This is a situation very similar to the tobacco industry, where individuals and companies with a financial stake sow doubt (through various media) about the health impacts of a given substance, all the while continuing to earn income for as long as possible (at a tremendous cost to the health of all those touched by this product). I choose not to take part in this experiment with my health or that of my family.

KINDS OF PLASTICS

Plastics are actually a diverse collection of different polymers with different physical and chemical properties. Some kinds of plastics are more harmful to our health than others—this based on which chemicals and/or metals leach into the liquids contained within them. Therefore, it is useful to briefly describe the kinds of plastics most frequently associated with the food and drink industry in order to guide purchases in the marketplace (specifically, to evade the worst kinds of plastic). While it is best to avoid (completely) all beverages found in plastic, this is not always possible for a variety of reasons. Avoiding drinks in plastic containers is best accomplished by avoiding the marketplace (i.e., gathering water from clean sources and storing it in inert containers, such as glass). However, there are times when people find themselves needing to purchase water or other beverages. Therefore, the following brief descriptions are provided to help people understand the specific health hazards of each kind of plastic.

Most plastics contain a number inside of a recycling symbol near (usually) the bottom of the container (a number called the Resin Identification Code). This number identifies the kind of polymer used to manufacture the container. The Resin Identification Code ranges from 1 through 7. The code distinguishes the following polymers.

1. Polyethylene Terephthalate (PET). This polymer is often referred to by the name polyester and is one of the most common plastics used in the beverage industry. It is also frequently used to package condiments. While PET is considered to be one of the safer plastics, studies show that it does leach phthalates and the toxic metal antimony. The longer the storage and the warmer the liquid, the more antimony is found in the beverage. One well known 2006 study revealed that water bottled in PET plastic contained tens to hundreds of times more antimony than what naturally occurred at the bottling source. Chronic antimony exposure can lead to a variety of ailments, including cancer.

2. High Density Polyethylene (HDPE). This is another polymer frequently used for beverages, such as milk, water, some fruit juices, and various bottle caps. This too is considered to be a safer plastic, though studies show that endocrine-disrupting compounds are still released into the beverage.

3. Polyvinyl Chloride (PVC). This polymer is certainly one of the plastics that presents a higher level of hazard to humans. In the food and drink industry, PVC generally is used for packing for deli items (e.g., meats) and sometimes for cooking oil containers. It is also used in plumbing and residential water supply (the latter another route of exposure for home owners and their guests). This polymer should be avoided whenever possible due to the presence of phthalates (especially the flexible forms).

4. Low Density Polyethylene (LDPE). This polymer is used for some plastic wraps and packaging for bread. It is also used to line the inside surface of cardboard and paper containers, containers that would not be able to hold liquids for long without wetting through. Therefore, juice and milk cartons made from paperboard are lined with LDPE to make them waterproof. Some endocrine disrupting compounds are found in this kind of polymer.

5. Polypropylene (PP). This polymer is used for a variety of food containers, including some brands of yogurt, some condiments, certain caps, and packaging for take-out and deli foods. It has been shown that a number of bioactive compounds do leach from this kind of plastic, including chemicals that are added to enhance the durability, performance, and stability, some lubricating agents, and some biocides to prevent bacterial colonization of the plastic surface. While one of the compounds found leaching from polypropylene, called oleamide, is found naturally within the human body, it is a substance that is structurally related to cannabinoids and induces sleep in animals.

6. Polystyrene (PS). This polymer is used solid or foamed containers. It is manufactured into a variety of Styrofoam cups, bowls, plates, food trays, and take-out containers. Styrene has been documented to migrate from this plastic container into the associated food and drink, a compound known to cause mutation in genetic material, produce both acute and chronic nervous system function impairment, and is highly suspected to be carcinogenic (documented as such in animal studies). The rate of leaching increases with temperature, so hot liquids (like coffee) and anything microwaved in these containers will contain more styrene (all things being equal) than cold foods. This polymer is another one to completely avoid.

7. Other. This resin identification code is for all other polymers not listed in the first six designations or for products that contain a mixture of polymers. While the consumer does not always know what kind of plastic, it is important to realize that this number includes the bisphenol class of compounds (e.g., BPA, BPAF, BPS). These chemicals are potent endocrine disruptors and are implicated in obesity and insulin resistance (among other disorders). Because this category of plastics can contain these compounds, products with this resin identification code should be avoided for food and drink containers. Keep in mind that BPA is sometimes used in the polymer linings of foods packed in metal cans and tins.

For those unable to avoid food and drink found in plastic containers or polymer-lined containers, consider drinking beverages (and eating food) only from those with a resin identification code of 1, 2, 4, or 5. Those with the numbers 3, 6, and 7 should be avoided at all cost (these kinds of containers are very harmful to human health). While the former set also are harmful, they are generally considered to be "safer plastics" (which does not imply they are safe, especially when we consider life-long exposure to these substances). As Yang and colleagues identified in their research published in 2011, almost all commercially available plastic products that they tested (95% of them) demonstrated measurable estrogenic activity when leached into liquids. In fact, they found that some "BPA-free" plastics had greater estrogenic activity than those known to contain BPA. These products ranged from baby bottles to rigid and flexible packaging, plastic bags, and food wrap. They included samples of polylactic acid (PLA), the thermoplastic made from renewable sources (such as corn starch), which showed frequent estrogenic activity. The take home message is that when you imbibe liquids (or eat foods that have liquids, especially those that are fatty and/or acidic) from plastic containers, metal cans and tins, most paperboard containers, and Tetra-paks, you are usually consuming leached plastic compounds that mimic the hormone estrogen. This represents a relatively new exposure for humans that has far-reaching health consequences. A rewilding path seeks to avoid or limit (to the extent possible) these new exposures in order to restore well-being.

THE RARELY TOLD STORY OF CHLORINATED WATER

In industrialized countries, chlorine is frequently used as a disinfectant for the public water supply. It is used to make water potable by killing pathogenic organisms that can cause sickness in humans, such as the bacterium *Vibrio cholera* (causing cholera), bacteria of the genus *Shigella* (causing dysentery), the amoeba *Entamoeba hisolytica* (also causing dysentery), and the bacterium *Salmonelli typhi* (causing typhoid). This chemical has been used for over 100 years to disinfect water and prevent acute infections. Unfortunately, as with many technological fixes for modern living, chlorine has a large number of drawbacks that are rarely told to the public who rely on it.

First and foremost, if chlorine in drinking water is able to kill bacteria in the water, then it stands to reason that chlorinated water can kill our probiotic organisms that we rely on for health. There appears to be very little research on this particular topic and there is a big assumption that food in our stomachs and materials normally present in our intestinal tracts quickly neutralize the chlorine. That would be all well and good if drinking water were our only route of exposure to chlorine; however, that is not the case. If you live in a home with chlorinated water, you are also exposed to significant amounts of chlorine in the shower. Chlorine can be absorbed through the skin (in small amounts) and one of chlorine's byproducts, called chloroform, is capable of entering your body via inhalation into the lungs (especially easy during a hot shower where water and other molecules are vaporized). Chloroform has been used as an anesthetic due to its ability to depress central nervous system function and it has been shown to damage kidneys after chronic exposure. It is also an antibiotic. An article that appeared in Science News found that after a ten-minute shower, people absorbed more chloroform than after drinking eight cups of water (64 fluid ounces) from the exact same tap. Another study performed at the University of Pittsburgh also demonstrated that washing clothes in chlorinated water represented another route of exposure to chloroform. While we wait for detailed studies on this topic, I prefer to adhere to the cautionary principle. What research on chlorine that has been completed to date suggests this is a prudent course of action (read on).

When chlorine comes into contact with organic molecules in water (including the pathogens they are meant to destroy), they form byproducts called trihalomethanes (THMs). These are chlorination byproducts (also called disinfection byproducts) that should cause concern for people drinking chlorinated water because they trigger the production of free radicals in the body. They include the aforementioned chloroform (in the previous paragraph), as well as bromoform, bromodichloromethane, and dichlorobromethane. The more organic molecules present in the water, the greater the levels of THMs. The regular consumptions of THMs is linked to certain forms of cancer, especially bladder and rectal cancers. This is documented in numerous studies. In fact, an article published in 1992 in the American Journal of Public Health estimated that 18 percent of rectal cancers and nine percent of bladder cancers are related to long-term consumption of chlorinated water. New studies also suggest that THMs may produce a higher risk of breast cancer given that many women with breast cancer have elevated levels of chlorination byproducts in their bodies. Not only are THMs linked to increased incidence of cancer, but also of miscarriage (as elucidated in a study of over 5000 women in California—those consuming the most chlorinated tap water showed the highest risk). This study is corroborated by a similar one in Europe, which also showed an elevated risk of miscarriage with greater ingestion of chlorinated water. The reality is that the disinfection byproducts of chlorinated water are more toxic than the chlorine itself.

Allergies and asthma are also linked to other chlorinated water sources, such as indoor swimming pools and Jacuzzis. Competitive swimmers have been demonstrated to have elevated levels of β-2-microglobulin, an indicator of damage to the kidneys (as described in a 1994 paper examining swimmers in the Netherlands). This is likely due to the inhalation of chlorine and aspiration of small amounts of chlorinated water during exercise. Another study published in 2000 looking at elite swimmers in Spain showed that a large proportion of the athletes had bronchial hyperresponsiveness (a health condition in which people are easily triggered into bronchospasm, making breathing difficult). A 2006 study published in Canada reached a very simple conclusion: swimmers exposed to THMs in the water and air of indoor swimming pools experience frequent respiratory symptoms. Occupational asthma has even been documented for workers who must work near indoor pools (but don't even enter the water; published in the United Kingdom in 2002). Many of these health conditions appear to be more extreme in younger people exposed to chlorinated water of swimming pools.

The point is hopefully clear: chlorine is not a benign substance to add to water supplies. Essentially, chlorine is used as a pesticide, but instead of being sprayed on fields, it is added to water. While certainly it has a role in preventing acute (and possibly life-threatening infections), to state that it is a necessary evil (as many do) overlooks the fact that we can do something about chlorine in our water after it enters our home or office. The information that has been presented here regarding the health concerns of chlorine is not new information, nor is it hidden information. It is widely available to anyone who searches for research articles on the health effects of chlorine in water. And there is much more, including research suggesting increased incidence of heart attacks, decreases in male fertility, more cases of spina bifida, and depressed immune function with higher intake of chlorinated water. There are abundant data from the United States and Europe on this overall topic. Even the United States Council on Environmental Quality reports that the cancer risk is 93% higher in people who drink chlorinated water than in those who don't. It begs two important questions. One, why do so few people do anything about chlorine in (at least) their drinking water? Two, why don't regulatory agencies alert people (more obviously) to the health hazards of chlorinated water? There are certainly many possible answers to these questions. But there is little doubt that, with regard to the first question, domestication (and a concurrent lack of personal sovereignty) robs people of their desire to learn and critically observe what happens around them (i.e., they simply trust authority). In this case, trusting authority has consequences. Fortunately, there are some solutions for this issue, which will be described shortly.

WHY YOU SHOULD AVOID FLUORIDATED WATER

Fluoride has been added (intentionally) to the United States public drinking water supply starting in 1945. The intent was to increase the strength of the enamel in teeth to help them be more resistant to dental caries. It was noticed in the early 1900s that certain locations in the US with naturally occurring high levels of fluoride in the drinking water appeared to confer protection against tooth decay (though it was also noticed to produce dental fluorosis—a condition of white or, in more extreme cases, brown marks on the teeth that may also be accompanied by pitting). Today, it is estimated that around 67% of the United States population receives fluoride in their water (according to the Center for Disease Control in 2012). It is usually one of three fluoride-containing chemicals that are added to the water: fluorosilicic acid, sodium fluoride, or sodium fluorosilicate. The first chemical in the list is the most frequently used (nearly 2/3 of the fluoride added to water is fluorosilicic acid) and is a by-product in the manufacture of phosphate fertilizer (i.e., it is an industrial waste).

Fluoride is not just added to drinking water, but also to a number of oral hygiene products (e.g., tooth paste, mouth rinses) and is now added to some bottled water. It is a practice that is rarely questioned by most people, though a vocal minority in the past few decades has been raising concerns. Fluoridated water is associated with a suite of health concerns—serious enough that you might want to reconsider this common addition to community water supplies. The first thing to consider about fluoridated water is that when imbibing water, it passes over the teeth quickly and does not provide much opportunity for fluoride to protect against demineralization by forming a veneer over the enamel. Clearly, it would be better to keep the fluoride in the oral cavity for a longer period of time (if one was so inclined to use this chemical). Second, it does not prevent cavities, rather, it merely slows the process down. Cavities are caused by a poor diet, especially one that is rich in refined carbohydrates that feed pathogenic bacteria who produce organic acids that demineralize tooth material. Third, there is no benefit (whatsoever) conferred from consuming fluoride. In fact, in the paragraphs to come, you will see there is much detriment from this practice. Again, if one were so inclined to use this chemical, it would be much better to expel the fluoride-containing material from the mouth after it had been applied to the teeth (i.e., it should be a topical application, not an ingestion). Of course, recent studies actually call into question if fluoride really provides any substantial benefit to dental health at all (e.g., Warren et al. 2009, published in the Journal of Public Health Dentistry).

As we get started looking at the health detriments of fluoride exposure, it is perhaps best to set the stage with a quote from Peckham and Awofeso (The Scientific World Journal, 2014):

"The classification of fluoride as a pollutant rather than as a nutrient or medicine is a useful starting point for analysing [sic] the adverse effect of fluoride."

One of the major problems with fluoridation of water is there is no easy way to control the dose ingested by humans (i.e., there is no way to produce an "optimal dose" because people drink varying amounts of tap water each day). In fact, numerous studies have shown that many people (especially infants and children) are receiving more than the recommended dose, as evidenced by the dental fluorosis they are suffering. Research demonstrates that 8–51% of American teens living in areas of fluoridated water are experiencing dental fluorosis. Unfortunately, even infants are exposed to fluoride in the water, especially those that are fed formula that is mixed with tap water. An important question here is: what is the value of fluoride for infants whose teeth have not yet erupted through the gums? In other words, they get all the risks and none of the purported "benefits" of fluoride. As Warren and colleagues stated in their 2009 paper:

"it is doubtful that parents or clinicians could adequately track children's fluoride intake and compare it with the recommended level, rendering the concept of an "optimal" or target intake relatively moot."

Aside from such issues as ambiguous dosing, fluoride is linked to a number of mental and physical health issues. For example, a study published in 2015 shows a strong correlation between attention deficit and hyperactivity disorder (ADHD) and fluoridated water. In the study by Malin and Till, every one percent increase in a state's prevalence of fluoridation resulted in an additional 67,000 to 131,000 additional ADHD cases (and this was after controlling for socioeconomic status). While a specific mechanism of harm was not suggested, it is clear the fluoride is neurotoxic and affects the development of the brain. A 2012 study that analyzed 27 published papers concluded that children in high-fluoride regions have a small but significant reduction in IQ score from children in low-fluoride regions (a mean difference of seven IQ points). This is corroborated by reductions in learning and memory demonstrated by tests of fluoride exposure on laboratory animals (while this is cruel, and I do not support such tests, the data are there for review). None of this should come as a surprise given that fluoride is an endocrine disruptor and can affect one's bones, blood glucose levels, brain, pineal gland, and thyroid gland.

The fact that fluoride has documented effects on the human brain provides ample justification to avoid fluoridated water. At exposures produced through the consumption of drinking water, fluoride has been linked to depressed function of the thyroid gland (i.e., is believed to produce hypothyroidism). The thyroid is an endocrine gland that produces a variety of hormones that govern the growth of and rate of function of many systems in the body. Depressed thyroid function leads to fatigue and weight gain. More importantly, reduced thyroid function in pregnant women is linked to lower IQ scores in their children. Drinking water that is laced with a chemical for which there is no human need is not a wise practice. Said another way, not one person in the world suffers from fluoride deficiency.

Now, bear with me on this one. Let's consider a potential harm that has received very little formal study (to my knowledge). Fluoride is known to accumulate in hard tissues of the body (such as the enamel of teeth) where it replaces calcium. But it also can accumulate in soft tissues, such as the pineal gland in the brain. This small endocrine gland is positioned between the two hemispheres of the brain and is responsible most notably for the production of melatonin, a hormone that alters sleep patterns in circadian and seasonal rhythms. The pineal gland has been referred to as the third eye, and in fact uses information from light sensitive cells in the retina to establish daily rhythms. The pineal gland is known to become "calcified" in some people (especially in age), this resulting from the accumulation of hydroxyapatite (a calcium compound). Once calcified, the pineal gland can also accumulate fluoride (remember, fluoride replaces calcium in tissues), where it has been suggested to destroy neuronal cells and promote synaptic injury (i.e., harm brain tissue). While most of brain is protected by the blood-brain barrier system, the pineal gland is not (it sits outside of this barrier). Therefore, fluoride is capable of damaging this highly perfused portion of the brain. The fact that pineal gland calcification tends to be high in Alzheimer's patients may be more than just correlation. Of interest here is that the rate of pineal gland calcification is higher in Americans of European descent than of Americans of African descent, and African-Americans show slightly higher rates of calcification than indigenous Africans. This is suggestive, as Daniel Vitalis notes in his article "Atheogens", that the degree of calcification of the pineal gland appears to be correlated with the degree of domestication. Yet another reason to be cautious and reconsider a lifetime of drinking highly processed water.

As the World Health Organization asserts, there is no discernible difference in tooth decay between affluent countries that fluoridate their water and countries that do not. Measurable declines in tooth decay that have occurred in the past decades have also occurred in countries that do not add fluoride to their water. Given this and the aforementioned risks associated with fluoride in community water supplies, one has to wonder why this practice is still continued.

BUT WHAT ABOUT PRIVATE WELLS ...

Many people living in rural parts of country have homes that are not connected to public water supplies. Rather, those homes are supplied with well water from a dug or drilled well that is then pumped (in most cases) into the home via a system of tubing. People who have private wells are usually free of continual chlorine and fluoride exposure, so some of the concerns about municipal water are mitigated. The problem for most homes (especially of recent construction) is the material the tubing is made from. There are several kinds of tubing that are commonly used: acrylonitrile-butadiene-styrene (ABS), polyvinyl chloride (PVC), polyethylene (PE, sometimes called PEX), and styrene rubber (SR). While there are other kinds of tubing used, these are the commonly recommended materials by many state agencies for private wells. Each of these materials has its own set of hazards or potential hazards.

Polyethylene, polyvinyl chloride, and styrene-containing polymers have already been discussed. These are not the best choices for piping water into the home. Homes constructed before 1977 (but after widespread plastic use in home plumbing) are more likely to contain PVC piping, a polymer that should be strictly avoided for liquids. That said, most of these leach endocrine-disrupting and/or carcinogenic compounds into water, which would then be imbibed by the home owners. Acrylonitrile-butadiene-styrene, which has a resin identification code of 7, is used in many applications, including the manufacture of Lego toys. Its construction appears to be more resistant to leaching than many polymers. However, there are two important detriments to this material. It does not appear to be impervious to permeation, the situation of certain compounds (especially hydrocarbons from the petroleum industry) migrating through the plastic into the drinking water. This is also true of other kinds of plastics that are being used in home plumbing (like polyethylene piping). More importantly, research demonstrates that ABS is a suitable substrate for colonization by bacteria. Therefore, this kind of plastic requires disinfection in some settings. The disinfectant most commonly used: chlorine. So, when disinfection is required, the home owners are exposed to chlorine and the resulting disinfection byproducts (i.e., trihalomethanes) for a period of time.

Of course, we haven't discussed the adhesive that connects sections of pipe together. These are also known to leach harmful chemicals into home drinking water. We also will not discuss the exposures that occur during the manufacture of piping used in home water systems, nor we will discuss here the ultimate fate of the tubing (a landfill). The point is hopefully clear that modern materials used in plumbing, while creating unprecedented convenience, are not necessarily safe in the long run. Private wells often do offer some advantages over municipal water, but, because of the materials used, are not ideal.

HOW BEING HEALTHY PROTECTS WATER QUALITY

Many people are unaware that pharmaceutical drugs are routinely detected in public drinking water supplies. The primary source of these drugs is people—specifically, those who use pharmaceutical drugs. When a drug is used (whether it be prescription or over-the-counter) some of the drug passes un-metabolized through the body and is excreted into the septic system. Those drugs then enter the sewer systems (or the ground water, depending on where you live) and ultimately end up in the bodies of wild animals or in the bodies of people (especially those that live in an area with waste water treatment facilities that recycle water for drinking). To be perfectly clear, many people in metropolitan areas (and some folks in rural areas) are being exposed to low, constant doses of antibiotic, antifertility, pain-relieving, and mood-altering medications. These include atenolol (used to treat cardiovascular disease), carbamazepine (used for certain seizures and bipolor disorder), gemfibrozil (lipid-lowering drug for "high cholesterol"), meprobamate (a tranquilizer used in psychiatric treatment), naproxen (an analgesic and anti-inflammatory drug), phenytoin (an anticonvulsant used to treat epilepsy), sulfamethoxazole (an antibiotic), trimethoprim (an antibiotic), and others. Even aquifers have been found to be contaminated by these drugs.

The amount of these drugs in the public water system is low (it would be described as trace). This fact has led many water suppliers to claim there is no harm caused by the presence of these compounds. However, no test has shown that exposure is safe (especially in the long run) and some recent research finds that harm is being caused. Remember that most drugs are to be taken for a short time and then discontinued. But in this case, people are being constantly exposed to small amounts of a myriad of chemicals (that may interact with one another)—in one review, 63 drugs were found during testing in watersheds around cities and 56 of those were in the public water supply (as reported by the Associated Press in 2008). These low dose pharmaceuticals in the water have been shown to slow growth of human embryonic kidney cells, speed cancer cell proliferation, and alter blood cell activity. Further, there is evidence that the addition of chlorine makes the pharmaceutical drugs more toxic. In another review, this one conducted by the United States Geological Survey in 2002, 139 streams were examined in 30 different states. They found that 80% of the streams contained measurable concentrations of prescription and nonprescription drugs, steroids, reproductive hormones, and their by-products. There are now numerous studies showing that water across the United States is contaminated with pharmaceuticals (and personal hygiene products). Equally important, municipal sewage treatment facilities are not equipped to remove pharmaceutical drugs and their metabolites. In some cities and towns, if you drink from the tap, you expose yourself (and your family) to a variety of medications (and possibly also chlorine and its disinfection byproducts, phthalates, and fluoride).

Much of the pharmaceutical contamination of water is preventable. The degree to which our drinking water is polluted with drugs is a direct result of how unhealthy Americans are. A study published in 2013 by the Mayo Clinic found that nearly 70% of Americans are using (or have recently used) a prescription medication, and more than half take two medications. The most common type of medication was antibiotics, which suggests that suppressed immune systems are common enough that many people are frequently succumbing to infections. The second-most common type of medication was anti-depressants, indicating (what many realize in their heart) that this modern, disconnected world lacks real, supportive community that people require in order to feel emotionally healthy. The lack of physical and emotional health is taking its toll on the purity of this continent's water, adding to the already long list of artificial items found in industrial water. Being healthy (or regaining one's health) is an important step that anyone can take to protect the natural resources we rely on. Avoiding fad diets and embarking on time-honored nutrition combined with a lifestyle that supplies movement, community, positive experiences, and other aspects of living that humans require for nourishment helps to stop the pharmaceutical pollution of water (for a list of 18 elements humans require for health, see Chapter 3, Epigenetics).

But, regardless of your diet and lifestyle, most people will become ill and be in need of medicine at some point in their life. While most people in this society turn to pharmaceutical drugs (the majority with a litany of side effects), it is better for the landscape (including the water found on that landscape) for people to use natural medicines. Better still if people who live in rural areas use natural medicines that they gather from the open spaces near the homes. Why? Because the plants and fungi that are used for medicine are already part of those environments (i.e., their chemistry is currently present in the ecosystems they are found in). When they shed their leaves, senesce, decay upon death, etc., they release minerals and natural compounds. And when they are consumed by insects and other herbivorous animals, the plant and fungal metabolites are excreted into the environment in the animal's wastes. These natural compounds are in the soil, in the streams and lakes, and even in the ground water. They are all around us when we are in natural areas and wild organisms are constantly exposed to them. When these medicines are used to heal, they pass through humans (as do pharmaceutical drugs) and become a natural part of the ecosystem (unlike pharmaceutical drugs). They do not add novel or synthetic compounds to the watershed. This process (of plant and fungal compounds being released into the environment) is already occurring—with or without humans. Therefore, while being healthy is one of the important ways we protect the quality of water, using natural medicine is another vital strategy to avoid pharmaceutical pollution. A major obstacle for natural medicine use is the way it is perceived by people living in industrial societies—ineffective, backwards, and potentially harmful (all of these myths will be addressed in the next chapter). Of course, the bigger picture here is that humans need to be more aware of what they do (through their actions) to other living beings.

HEALTHY SOURCES OF WATER

Throughout this chapter we have discussed how humans view water and the ways industrial living has impacted the quality of water. It has certainly been an information heavy chapter—the purpose of which has been to create a clear awareness of the degree to which we have impacted our water quality. Domesticated humans fail to understand that what we do to our environment we do to ourselves. When we pollute our water with industrial chemicals, we ultimately pollute our own bodies with those chemicals. The story of our water is a testament to the ineffectiveness of technological fixes—they almost always create other issues that impact the health of humans and other-than-human beings that then require fixes of their own. The water found in urban and suburban areas can be described as highly processed. The first and most important approach regarding healthy hydration is to start drinking raw, wild water. And it is not as dangerous as that might sound.

In many locations in North America (and around the world), clean, safe, and unprocessed water is available from springs. Springs are the result of surface water infiltrating the ground and becoming part of the groundwater. At some location (often the result of topography or bedrock fractures), the water appears on the surface again in the form (usually) of a small stream or pool. This outflow occurs because the recharge rate exceeds the storage of the groundwater region. Sometimes, spring flow can be forced out of the ground at higher elevation than the source area (a phenomenon called an artesian spring). In both of these cases, the water tends to flow through soil and bedrock (sometimes significant distances in these materials), becoming filtered of many of its impurities. Some of the water found in aquifer systems has been underground for a very long time and may predate the industrialization of this continent, meaning it can be free of the many contaminants found on our landscapes today. Along the way, spring water can dissolve minerals, which can alter its pH and taste. While there are too many springs to describe in this brief section, many springs found in North America can be accurately described as providing the highest quality water available to neoaboriginals. The water is clean, of circumneutral pH (i.e., around neutral, neither acidic nor strongly basic), and lacks many industrial chemicals. Most importantly, this water is raw and has not been processed, refined, or added to.

Spring water should be collected in glass containers (if possible). Using an inert material such as glass has many advantages over plastic containers (as has been described in this chapter). Such containers can be purchased (such as the 3- and 5-gallon glass carboys used in wine and beer making) or they can be picked up for almost nothing at redemption centers (gallon-size wine bottles are easy to locate and very useful for water storage). Store the collected water in a cool, dark place to avoid the growth of unwanted organisms (I store 5-gallon glass carboys in a basement setting and have never had an issue with algae or mold growth). We need to think of raw water in the way we think about groceries—it is a necessity. Plan your trips to water sources around other travel (when possible) and gather as much as possible during the trip to avoid frequent returns (both of which save on fuel costs and the resulting pollution of driving).

For those that are convinced that processed, industrial water is not benefitting them, one of the first obstacles they may face is locating a spring. There are many ways to find the nearest springs: questioning friends and family, post to social media, and use the website Find A Spring (www.findaspring.com). Find A Spring lists wild sources of water from all over the world (literally), though the coverage is best in the United States. Searches can provide directions, description of the facilities, images of the spring, and comments if conditions have changed. I encourage people to be diligent in their research—just because a spring exists doesn't mean it is safe to consume (i.e., if you are new to the spring, consider performing web research, questioning locals who live near and utilize the spring, or having the water tested prior to imbibing it).

Another strategy I utilize is clean surface water. I have drunk from streams in northern New England (especially in western Maine—a hilly and mountainous area) my entire life without issue. In fact, the small stream that passes in front of my home has been a year-round source of water for seven years for my family and hundreds of guests and students (none of which have had an issue with this water). I am continually admonished for this practice and it is apparent that modern people's fear of nature is applied to surface water. The general message is that all surface water is dangerous to consume (likewise, it is also dangerous to consume wild mushrooms, expose your skin to the sun, walk barefoot, and so on). While I can only speak about my region, it is clear that this widely held notion is untrue. I seek out streams for drinking water that begin as small rivulets in the forest (i.e., they are not the outlets of ponds and lakes). This is important as our rainwater is not clean (primarily contaminated by coal-fired power plants in the Midwest). As the rainwater lands on the forest floor, it is filtered by organic materials (the surface duff) and clay particles in the soil, both of which chelate (i.e., bind to) the heavy metals found in rainwater. This filtering process removes many important pollutants as the rainwater moves through the ground to the stream channel. Not only is this water relatively clean (when the head of the stream valley is located away from agricultural and industrial influences), but this water has living organisms present in it. It is hypothesized to bolster the functioning of our immune system and reduce allergic responses in the same way that contact with soil does (both wild surface water and soil helps to counteract the problems with ultra-hygienic living). I am not implying here that water-borne pathogens (such as Giardia) are not real and serious in nature, but only that their prevalence may be exaggerated and clean surface water sources have real benefits to provide humans. Again, it is important to do your research in this area and look to historical use of water bodies, known studies of watersheds, and local knowledge.

If you don't live near a spring or clean surface water source, or have no ability to travel to one, you need to utilize other strategies. While I strongly encourage acquiring raw water, using some kind of filtration system to remove industrial chemicals is a next-best solution. Keep in mind that whatever filtration system you decide on, you will also need one in the bath/shower (if you have one) because this is a major source of water-borne pollution for the body in urban and suburban areas. There are many kinds of filters, some more effective than others, and some much more costly than others. Generally speaking, you want to ask lots of questions about the filter and make sure that the contaminants you are interested in having removed are, in fact, removed by the filter you plan to purchase. Preferably, a filtration system would take care of chlorine and its disinfection byproducts, herbicides and other chemical agriculture pollutants, industrial toxins, neurotoxic metals (e.g., lead, arsenic), biological pathogens, and fluoride (though the latter is difficult for most systems that are not extremely expensive). In many cases, a filtration system that uses multiple kinds of filters is the most effective, including sub-micron filters (very small pores), carbon filtration (bonding or absorbing contaminants), and/or ion-exchange (removes dissolved solids). Note that other systems exist, such as reverse-osmosis and distillation (though both of the systems remove fluoride, they also remove naturally occurring minerals that are a beneficial component of raw water).

If a filtration system will not work (or is too expensive), bottled water is a possibility (but this too is very expensive in the long run). Unfortunately, a large proportion of bottled water is (a) merely filtered tap water and (b) is placed in plastic containers. Healthy bottled water should come from reputable springs with water testing data plainly available and be stored in glass. Bottled water is very expensive on a per unit basis. An inexpensive solution for chlorine is to pour chlorinated tap water from the spout into a large bowl or container and let it sit for several hours (such as overnight). This method does help remove chlorine (this chemical evaporates from the water). Unfortunately, that means the chlorine is in the house, so open windows are needed for ventilation (or the container can sit outside with a screen over it). This strategy, while making a small difference, does not deal with chlorine's disinfection byproducts (i.e., THMs). Though this strategy can work for drinking water, it is difficult to apply on a large scale for bathing and clothes washing. It also does not deal with other chlorine exposure, such as swimming pools and Jacuzzis.

Systems now exist for gathering and filtering rainwater, which can offer several advantages (and potential disadvantages, depending on where you live). Water vapor has been distilled through the process of evaporation, so it is initially very clean. However, clouds and rain droplets pick up whatever is in the atmosphere, which includes natural particulates as well as heavy metals, polycyclic aromatic hydrocarbons, sulfur compounds, and more (these often, in significant part, produced by human activity today). Rainwater that is downwind of industry should be treated (i.e., filtered in some way) before it is imbibed. It should also be mineralized, as drinking distilled water can actually leach minerals from your body (water will become isotonic with the body, if it lacks minerals, it will gain them at the expense of the body's mineral stores). There are several companies offering small-scale ways of adding minerals to distilled water (or rainwater), but solutions that require long-distance transport of products are not good long-term solutions. Because of the lack of minerals, rainwater is often best used for things other than drinking water. There are literally hundreds of ways rainwater can be utilized. This includes use as cooking water (after filtration of pollutants) because vegetables and meats do add minerals. Rainwater collection and storage also create their own set of difficulties due to bacterial contamination (which must be considered if rainwater is not used promptly). Impressive systems exist for using the roofs of buildings to filter rainwater through the use of soil and vegetation (which also adds minerals to water, making it a healthful manner of hydrating). Of course, other filtration systems can be arranged to deal with any potential pollutants and an organic matter/biological organisms that have been picked up in the collection system. Whatever strategy you decide to use for rainwater, be sure the necessary contaminants have been removed. This is one of the reasons I like small streams in wild areas so much is that the soil both filters heavy metals and adds minerals to the water (a natural way of accomplishing both of these necessary items). If you consider rainwater, there are many sources of information today online, including (for example) the Harvesting, Storing, and Treating Rainwater for Domestic, Indoor Use produced by the Texas Commission on Environmental Quality in 2007 (keep in mind that some of their suggestions will not necessarily be in line with material presented here, such as the use of plastic for storage and the use of chlorine for disinfection).

THE NEOABORIGINAL STRATEGY FOR WATER

Water is a very special part of our world. Despite the fact that modern people pollute water, they still consider water to be powerful medicine (even if only at a subconscious level). People will pay (on average) more than twice the amount for a home on a water body than a comparable one not constructed on a waterfront. The proximity to water and the daily view of lakes, rivers, and oceans is worth much to people. Water is considered to be more than just cleansing to the physical body, people treat water as emotionally cleansing (as evidenced by the use of bathing in many victims of various kinds of abuse). The water we drink becomes part of the fluids inside our body, including our blood, our lymph, and even the cerebrospinal fluid. People have to ask themselves what kind of water they want to be made up of. There are many solid reasons why drinking unprocessed (i.e., raw) water is advantageous for our long-term health. Sourcing raw water is worth the effort. It serves as a simple way of eliminating one of the most important (and preventable) exposures to industrial chemicals modern humans experience.

This chapter has been more about the quality of water in the modern world than a series of guidelines for how to remain hydrated. There are many topic areas (regarding pollution) that have not been discussed, including agricultural chemicals and compounds associated with fuel for vehicles that are routinely found in drinking water. To give hydration a brief mention, it is a relatively easy task to accomplish for most persons. While many people focus on a specific amount of water (such as 2.2 or 3 liters of fluid each day for females and males, respectively), this recipe does not work for extended exercise in hot or dry environments (and remember, winter time in many northern areas is, effectively, a dry environment regarding air humidity). It is best that people learn concepts that allow them to be hydrated anywhere they travel. It is easy to do by simply observing the color and odor of urine. A person's urine should be relatively clear (i.e., very light yellow) and not have a pronounced odor when that person is well-hydrated.

Dark and strong-smelling urine are clear indications of dehydration. Good hydration with a high quality water can go a long way in keeping the body functioning well and feeling energetic.

As with other topics found in this book, I encourage people not to run up against the Wall of Grief, where things seem overwhelming and you become paralyzed with inaction. Everything has a solution, and given time, you can solve all the threats to your health and sovereignty (or make great strides in your lifetime and help your children go even further). It is difficult to change everything overnight, so embark on this rewilding path one step at a time (remember, it is a path, and traveling on this path is beneficial). Following are ten strategies you can use to incorporate clean (or, at least, cleaner) water into your life.

1. Prioritize locating a spring that provides a reliable source of **wild, raw water**. Such water has not been processed through the addition of industrial chemicals or the stripping away of naturally occurring minerals (as with distilled water). Such water can serve as a valuable way to detoxify your body (through replacing the industrially sourced water that is currently part of your body's composition).

2. Store collected spring water in **glass containers** that will not leach endocrine-disrupting compounds into the water (this also is best for liquid and/or fatty foods). If this is not possible, utilize plastic containers that have a resin identification code of 1, 2, 4, or 5. While these plastics are not "healthy", they are generally less bad choices.

3. If you are unable to locate springs or clean surface waters, consider using some kind of **filtration system** for your tap water. Generally speaking, filtration systems should use multiple methods to remove different kinds of contaminants in the water. Remember that when bathing and showering there can be tremendous exposure to certain contaminants, so consider a filter in the bathroom that removes chlorine and its disinfection byproducts.

4. A **private well** can be a better option than municipal water and will likely be free of some important chemicals discussed in this chapter, such as chlorine, trihalomethanes, and fluoride (unless frequent disinfection with chlorine is required). However, it still may contain endocrine disrupting and carcinogenic compounds because the piping used to bring the water into the home is constructed of one of several kinds of plastic, some of which are quite detrimental to human health. Further, tanks storing automotive fuel, hydraulic fracturing (i.e., fracking) operations, and chemical agriculture can all cause contamination—so test frequently if you reside near these industries. Consider still sourcing drinking water from springs.

5. Think about bringing **travel water** when you are away from home. While certain forms of travel (e.g., air flight, backpacking) do not lend themselves to carrying large amounts of water, travel by vehicle for one or more days may allow a means of transporting spring water in glass containers. When space in the vehicle allows, bring an appropriate amount of drinking water to ensure you have access to healthful water. Containers can be wrapped in spare clothing, blankets, or even specially made foam containers to keep the water cool.

6. When selecting **bottled water**, seek reputable brands that list the source spring and bottle in glass containers. Bottled water is not a good long-term strategy (making and recycling containers is wasteful of energy and contributes to pollution). However, when travel forces such options, do research on known brands ahead of time so you can select those that actually provide raw water (one survey showed that approximately 40% of bottled water is just tap water).

7. Wash yourself, when possible, by **bathing in streams and lakes** that have clean water. While this is not possible for many people in urban settings, it is available to millions of people who live in or near rural and wilderness areas. Simply bathing in the water without soap or store-purchased hygiene products protects the watershed, reduces exposure to water-borne pollutants, and doesn't wash away your sebum (so vitamin D manufacture can continue). When a cleaning agent of some kind is needed, there are many options to do this without polluting the water, including wild-gathered high-saponin plants that will foam and wash away grime or washing with a mild, lard-and-lye or plant-based soap away from the water and rinsing off before returning to the stream or lake. Using natural waterbodies also conditions a person to a variety of temperatures.

8. Consider the items that you **dispose** of down the drain or into the septic system. Household chemicals, hygiene and beauty products, and pharmaceutical drugs all enter the municipal or groundwater systems, affecting other humans and wild beings. Being healthy and using benign home products (discussed further in chapter 11) is one of many ways we steward our water resources. Clean water free of industrial chemicals (which includes pharmaceutical drugs) benefits the entire ecosystem.

9. Using **rainwater** for some portion of your family's water can be a way to avoid much of the commonly added chemicals to processed water (e.g., chlorine, fluoride). While rainwater in many parts of the world does contain contaminants, there are ways to remove these and make the water clean again. Remember that rainwater commonly lacks the minerals found in groundwater, so its use as drinking water has a serious disadvantage. But, that does not preclude the use of rainwater for bathing, washing clothing, irrigating, and for cooking.

10. Offer **gratitude** for the water that hydrates your body. It is a miraculous substance that is necessary for life and contributes to the beauty of this planet. Treating water as sacred is a necessary step to stop the wide-scale pollution today that threatens surface, ground, and atmospheric water. Demonstrate your gratitude by protecting the earth's waters. One doesn't have to stand on a pulpit and preach to the world about the value of water—simply living a life that protects water from pollution is one of the highest forms of expressing thankfulness. Water is truly life blood and we must acknowledge it as such.

5. Wild medicine: healing the human being

The Ani-Yu^{n}wiya (Cherokee), an indigenous people of the southeastern United States, have a story titled (in English) "The Origin of Disease and Medicine". As told by J.T. Garrett, humans were afflicted with a variety of diseases given to them by the animals. This was done in retaliation for the disrespectful treatment they had received from the local people. Essentially, humans were not expressing thankfulness for the lives they took, even though the animals supplied the humans with food and clothing. As the animals told stories of poor treatment by humans, they created more and more diseases for the people. As the number of diseases mounted, it was the plants who spoke up as friends to the humans. They offered themselves as healers and protectors from the harm that might befall humans. It was decided that harmony and balance would be the striven-for goal; therefore, for each ailment humans could experience, a plant would offer a cure. This healing agent would be called the Medicine. And even though the Medicine is still found on our landscapes, it is rarely (now) sought out by the people. Instead, pharmaceutical drugs are considered as medicine, and the drugs are dispensed by legal drug dealers (doctors and pharmacists), who sell products made by drug manufacturers (pharmaceutical companies), to treat symptoms of disease (note: no cure is achieved in most cases).

WHAT'S IN A NAME (THE TRUE ROLE OF MEDICINE)

To begin this section, let's state what might not be obvious to everyone: doctors specialize in pathology, not health. Said another way, they treat injury and illness, restoring people to the condition they were in prior to the ailment in question. But many people are in poor health to begin with, which is why various issues arise. Unfortunately, doctors are not considering those ailments as symptoms of poor diet and lifestyle, but rather as the issues of focus. Most doctors, despite being genuinely interested in their patient's well-being, do not address underlying causes (in diet and lifestyle), a strategy that prevent ailments from ever re-occurring. You might immediately react by stating that doctors do attempt to deal with obesity and addictive smoking and drinking. However, it can be effectively argued that these too are a result of other diet and lifestyle issues that manifest as damaging behaviors. I believe that sharing one of my experiences with the industry will help illustrate this problem.

I practice Brazilian jiu-jitsu, a form of submission wrestling that involves close contact with other people. Before I studied traditional diet and medicine, I used to frequently succumb to staph infections as a result of this sport (sometimes several a year). I would visit the doctor, who would diagnose the *Staphylococcus aureus* infection and then prescribe me a round of antibiotics to treat the infection. Two or three months later I was back, for another diagnosis and another round of antibiotics. The infections were extremely painful and quite debilitating. I eventually decided to perform research regarding the reasons why people experience recurring infections. It became very clear that my immune system was not functioning at a high enough level to protect me from cellulitis (a painful boil created by the staph bacterium). I also became aware that infections of this kind (and this frequency) did not have to be part of my health story. Through my research, I learned that vitamin D up-regulates an antimicrobial peptide in the skin (called cathelicidin), and that independent research showed adults need nearly 10 times the amount of vitamin D that the USDA recommends. This level of vitamin D is difficult to achieve from diet alone. So sunlight exposure is critical (something I was told to avoid to prevent skin cancer), where a special form of water-soluble vitamin D is manufactured from a precursor made of cholesterol (which I was told was bad for me). I then learned that in order for my body to manufacture vitamin D, it is critical that the oil on my skin (sebum) be present. However, washing head-to-toe with soap (as I had been taught to do) removed the sebum and impaired my ability to create vitamin D. All of these details have been discussed in chapter 3—it was my poor (i.e., domesticated) lifestyle choices that were the underlying cause of the infections.

Additional research showed vitamin A is also critical for enhancing our immune function, and some of the foods that are rich in this vitamin (e.g., butter, eggs) had been demonized by the mainstream health authorities (and well-intentioned doctors). Further, I learned that antibiotics interfere with vitamin A absorption, so the more antibiotics I took, the further my immune system was compromised (this was never mentioned to me by the doctors who prescribed the drugs). Perhaps worst of all, I learned there is a positive correlation between the number of rounds of antibiotic treatment someone receives and the chance of contracting cancer. (And we could go on with additional vitamins, essential fatty acids, etc., that I learned about and had not been told by my doctors). For what it is worth, following a suite of guidelines developed by researching traditional cultures, I've been staph infection free for years even though I practice the same activity and have the same exposure to the pathogen.

So this is the important piece: all the doctors did was treat my infection—which means they returned me to my previous state of health. My previous state of health was one of compromised immune function (hence, the frequent infections). I just showed up a few months later and repeated the whole process over again. They shared none of the information about nutrition and infection prevention I just shared with you, which means they either did not know it, or they knew it and did not share it with me. In either case, the doctors failed to generate health. This is not my lone experience. I've helped many people treat various staph infections (e.g., cellulitis, MRSA, impetigo) using plants that can be gathered wild or grown here in the northeastern United States. In no case did any doctor tell them how to boost the functioning of their immune system so that they could avoid staph infections (or at least reduce their frequency). The doctors knew the treatment (i.e., the correct dose of antibiotic to prescribe) but not how to generate real health. In fact, it can be said in this case, their treatment further compromised everyone's health. By focusing on the real issue (poor immune system), the doctors could have also provided vital defense against a host of bacterial, fungal, and viral pathogens (e.g., colds, influenza, cancer, periodontal infections, tinea). This is very important to understand—focusing on root causes strengthens the body against additional health insults.

Let me provide one more example of how doctors provide treatment for ailments but do not generate health. Cholelithiasis is defined as the presence of one or more gallstones in the gall bladder. The usual treatment: if the gallstones are symptomatic, cholecystectomy (removal of gall bladder) may be performed. For those who can't or won't undergo surgery, bile acids can be administered orally to dissolve the stones. I'm hoping that you are asking how any of this treats the underlying cause. Removing a location for gall stones to accumulate or dissolving the stones are ways of treating a symptom. The doctors should be asking: what caused the stones to form in the first place (and then address that issue). There is good evidence to suggest that gallstone formation is largely a result of poor diet, specifically, a diet high in vegetable oils and trans fatty acids. Again, following the treatments provided by many doctors, the patient has not been given health.

When someone who is suffering a health issue visits a doctor, they are looking for definitive care (i.e., conclusive care that treats all the symptoms AND corrects the underlying causes). No one actually wants to experience a relapse of illness or disease. However, most doctors actually perform symptomatic care, as they are focused on the pathology and not the whole human (this is especially true of cancer treatments, where a tumor-centric approach fails to protect the patient from future occurrences of neoplasms). They are not focused on how to prevent disease. It appears to me (from a perspective of someone looking from the outside) that their education paradigm has led them to believe that if the symptoms are not present, a cure has been effected. This is exacerbated by the fact doctors in this country really do not have the opportunity to witness true health. They don't have a gauge by which to measure well-being, which makes it difficult to understand the goal they should aspire to for their patients.

Unfortunately, most of the public considers doctors to be good purveyors of information and practices that generate health. To the contrary, there are studies showing that in some circumstances, if people follow their doctor's advice regarding nutrition, they die earlier than people with the same ailment who chose not to follow their doctor's advice. Please know that this writing isn't meant to speak poorly of doctors. I believe they genuinely want health for their patients (I personally know doctors whom I would consider to be some of the most caring people I've ever met). However, from discussions I've had with them, I don't think they are always cognizant of what their practice actually does—it treats ailments but does not generate true health. The problem with this approach is that many Americans who are not actively dealing with disease are still overweight, pre-diabetic, possess poor cardiovascular health, and have compromised immune function. Therefore, doctors are part of a system of treatment care, one that unfortunately (and not necessarily intentionally) maintains a constant stream of patients. If all doctors were truly part of a healthcare system, they would rarely see their patients because they would address underlying causes that infringe on their patients' vitality (and through addressing those causes they would correct or prevent future issues). Treatments aren't supposed to be the final answer. No one is supposed to take drugs the rest of their life for heart disease, diabetes, and other chronic diseases. Health is the answer. Health is generated through deep nutrition and a lifestyle that engages in frequent movement and maximizes exposure to a clean environment, caring community, emotional fulfillment, and natural experiences. Changing the system's name to **treatment care** would provide an accurate accounting of what the healthcare profession of today actually does. It would also let discerning people know that their health is currently in their own hands.

Of course, the healthcare profession could also remedy this incongruity through ceasing to view patients as the sum total of their pathologies. Each person is unique, and each person requires a customized approach to dealing with their issues. Equally important, they could serve their clientele better by learning about nutrition (as some doctors have done). And not the politically correct nutrition touted by the industry (e.g., low fat, low cholesterol, pasteurized everything, high cultivated grain and vegetable oil intake). It would need to research healthy populations (especially those that used to exist) and identify the commonalities in their diets and lifestyles (rather than create a novel diet and wait to observe the consequences on the subjects—in this case, the American people). They would need to question so many commonly held dietary "truths", those same "truths" that are creating progressive degeneration in health. They would need to learn the real difference between saturated and polyunsaturated fats (and understand the latter's role in promoting cardiovascular disease). They would need to appreciate the real difference between wild and free-range animal products compared with cage-reared, grain-fed animals. They would need to learn about proper food preparation and the importance of deactivating antinutrients in plant foods. It would be critical that they recognize that cholesterol has no more role in vascular disease than do the white blood cells that also play a part in plaque formation (hint, cholesterol is healing a lesion created by a food recommended by the healthcare profession). In short, the doctors would have much to learn, but they would better serve their patients. They could cure disease without drugs or scalpels. Through this knowledge they could produce health. They would practice definitive care. And then they could refer to themselves properly as the **healthcare** industry.

Before we leave this topic, it is important that readers here understand what the actual role of medicine is. **Medicine's purpose is to abate symptoms (i.e., treat current health insults) so that a person can engage in healthy diet and lifestyle practices—which collectively constitute a lifeway—so that the underlying issue is permanently resolved.** In other words, the goal is to stop taking the medicine at some point. Certainly, some people will deal with a true genetic disease or congenital defect that may preclude a medicine-free life; however, these circumstances represent a minority of current prescription drug use. But for most people, they need to understand that medicine is not the cure, diet and lifestyle are. And yes, heart disease, diabetes, depression, inflammatory bowel disease, and a host of chronic ailments can be cured by diet and lifestyle (unless someone waits so long that too much damage has been done).

SOCIETAL BIAS AGAINST NATURAL MEDICINE

The United States can be described as having a strong bias against natural medicine. This is evident in its title afforded to other forms of healing—alternative. However, if one were to objectively examine this given title, it would be clear that what the United States practices for medicine should be considered the alternative. It is estimated that as much as 80% of the world's people use natural remedies, often in conjunction with food, ceremony, and other healing practices. While the United States treatment care system does have some obvious strengths, such as traumatic injury care, pain management, and diagnosis technology, it also has some very important weaknesses. One of those weaknesses is the failure to recognize that many valuable and potent medicines are not found in a prescription bottle.

Before we confront the bias found in the United States against natural medicine, it will be valuable to discuss some of the serious shortcomings of "western medicine", topic areas that are rarely confronted by people who frequently use this healing modality. Gaining an understanding that all healing methods carry risks and benefits can help to illuminate the fact that our prejudice against natural medicine may not be based on rigorous science but, rather, the widespread (and mostly invisible) societal bias against the wild.

We are a society that uses prescription drugs at astounding frequency. Considering that nearly 70% of Americans use a prescription drug (according to a 2013 Mayo Clinic study), with more than half of the country's residents taking two or more drugs, there is little doubt that we are very unhealthy. But, are the drugs that are prescribed safe? While most in the pharmaceutical field would argue these drugs are safe (and necessary), let's examine the statistics. In the eye-opening publication by Gary Null and colleagues titled "Death by Medicine", they report 106,000 deaths annually from prescription drug use. It is estimated that there are over 450,000 preventable adverse events related to pharmaceutical drugs each year in the United States. Note that this figure does not include all of the adverse events, that number is 2.2 million, but only the ones considered avoidable. Perhaps most telling is that a 2010 American Medical News article reported that medication errors were the second-leading cause of accidental death in the United States (and accidental death was—and is—the fourth leading cause of death in the United States). Further, medication errors were the only cause of accidental death that was on the rise.

To further highlight the potential problems with prescription drugs, let us look more closely at a specific group of pharmaceuticals. Currently, the United States is dealing with a serious epidemic of harm caused by opioid drugs (e.g., codeine, hydrocodone, methadone, oxycodone). Every day in America, 44 people die from prescription painkillers, the vast majority of these an opioid. To put this into perspective, since 1999 over 250,000 people have died from overdoses of opioid drugs. These prescribed painkillers are addictive, similar to other drugs that are chemically related and produce similar effects in the brain, like heroin. As a result, many people who attempt to reduce or stop using these drugs often experience pain and discomfort produced from withdrawal, which is mistakenly assumed to be associated with the initial pain that commenced the use of the drug. Therefore, withdrawal experienced during an attempt to taper off the dose of medication and detoxify the body often results in continued use of the opioid. Unfortunately, the drug is actually treating symptoms of withdrawal at that point and not necessarily the original pain. Further, the body develops tolerance to this class of drugs, meaning that the dosage required over time needs to be increased in order for users to experience the same level of pain reduction, which increases the likelihood of overdose. One study estimates that 80% of users of prescription opioid drugs experience some kind of negative consequence (and yet these drugs remain highly prescribed). Of course, the pharmaceutical industry bears major responsibility here as it introduced these drugs in 1996 (Perdue Pharma and Oxycontin) with the statement that the risk of addiction would be much less than 1%; however, this has resulted in an estimated 2.1 million people in the United States suffering from a substance use disorder due to prescription opioids (these are 2012 numbers, published in the Results from the 2012 National Survey on Drug Use and Health: Summary of National Findings). According to the Center for Disease Control, 1 in 4 people who use these drugs long-term for non-cancer pain struggle with addiction. And due to the chemical similarity of opioid drugs (prescription and illegal kinds), these pharmaceuticals frequently lead to the use of prohibited opioids. A recent study found that ¾ of high school heroin users started with prescription opioids. While certainly many people have experienced a relief from their pain as a result of opioids, many too have been harmed (or died) from these drugs. While pharmaceutical companies regard these drugs with high favor, the statistics (which are available to anyone with access to the internet) suggest Americans should be more critical of medical opioids.

It would take pages for us to properly illuminate all of the potential non-lethal side-effects of pharmaceutical drugs. One of the more important of these, which is seldom presented to the people using them, is cognitive impairment. This has been documented in several group of drugs, but is especially prevalent in a class of drugs called anticholinergics, pharmaceuticals that block the neurotransmitter acetylcholine. These include many commonly used over-the-counter and prescription drugs for hypertension, congestive heart failure, allergies, insomnia, pain relief, and depression (at present there are 136 drugs known to cause cognitive impairment). The drug-induced cognitive decline is most noted in elderly people and the more anticholinergic drugs they take, the more significant the decline is. Symptoms range from mild losses in mental acuity, to delirium and dementia, with losses in language, mental function, and performance of routine activities. In fact, elderly people using anticholinergic drugs have lower survivorship (on average) than those using non-anticholinergic drugs. The use of drugs (or dosages) that diminish one of human's most amazing abilities—intelligence—doesn't seem that ... well, intelligent.

And the medical system, how does it compare? An article in the New England Journal of Medicine in 2010 reported that 18% of the people admitted to hospitals were harmed. In another study, after researchers analyzed over 40 million Medicare patients' records from 2007 to 2009, it was determined that 1 in 9 people developed a hospital-acquired infection. This same study (Thirteenth Annual HealthGrades Hospital Quality in America Study) showed that over 40,000 hospital mistakes occur every day. Long lists of these kinds of statistics can be presented. These are but a few of the powerful (read telling) numbers that suggest the American healthcare industry should not always be considered the first choice for people dealing with ailments, especially if those ailments have safe and effective natural treatments (which is usually the case).

One of the most compelling sets of arguments for the failure of American healthcare follows. First, the total annual cost of healthcare in the United States is 3.8 trillion dollars (in 2014 according to Forbes). Second, the amount of this care that is related to chronic disease—86% (according the US Center for Disease Control (CDC) using 2010 numbers, 2014 numbers are not yet available). This means that 86 cents of every dollars spent on healthcare is the result of chronic disease. Third, seven of the top ten causes of death in the United States are a kind of chronic disease. Fourth, two forms of chronic disease, heart disease and cancer, account for nearly half of all the deaths in the United States. Fifth (and most important), **most chronic disease is completely preventable** (i.e., it does not ever have to happen). You may dispute this fact, but remember that hunter-gatherers displayed essentially no chronic disease, even among the elderly, indicating it is not a “fact of life”. Chronic disease (in most cases) takes time to develop, and is a result of poor diet and lifestyle. Consider, for example, that just slightly less than 1 in 100 infants are borne with a form of congenital heart disease, but heart disease is the leading cause of death in Americans, with 1 in 4 people dying each year of this disease (again, according to the CDC). This means that something has to happen over people’s lifetimes to dramatically change the ratio of people born with a heart condition (nearly 1%) to those dying from a heart condition (approximately 25%). And you cannot state that the reason is simply age (for reasons already discussed). These numbers clearly point to the fact that most people are using the American healthcare system for chronic disease, but this system has a miserable track record of preventing and healing chronic disease. In fact, according to the Center for Managing Chronic Disease, such disease is defined as:

“Chronic Disease is a long-lasting condition that can be controlled but not cured.”

While I do not mean to imply that this belief was created to maintain a steady income stream from sick people, popularizing such a belief certainly does just that (because sick people will not question the fact that they need to take drugs their entire life). However, chronic disease can, in many cases, be cured by altering diets and increasing beneficial lifestyle practices. Even the CDC states that 80% of heart disease, 80% of type 2 diabetes, and 40% of cancer can be prevented by changes to diet and lifestyle (i.e., the contention that chronic disease can be prevented is not solely my opinion). That all stated, the entire intent of this paragraph is this: the US healthcare system should be used for its strengths (e.g., trauma medicine, pain management, diagnostic tools) and should not be relied on for its major weakness—chronic disease. Unfortunately, this is exactly what we are doing (86 cents of every dollar, in fact). For chronic disease, holistic healthcare practices that incorporate medicine with changes in diet and lifestyle based on ancestral lines of evidence will produce the best outcomes.

Unfortunately, it is not only the theory of practice of medicine in the United States that fails to protect the health of many Americans but also some very serious unethical practices. While it is impossible to do this topic justice in a paragraph, let’s highlight a few of the important conflicts of interest that are built into the American medical system. Drugs, generally the treatment of choice of doctors, are considered to be effective and safe by most who use them. However, an

ABC news report showed that when a pharmaceutical company funds the research (which is quite common), the drug will be viewed as effective 90% of the time. This stands in stark contrast to when research on a drug's efficacy is funded by an organization other than a pharmaceutical company—only 50% of the studies provide favorable results. Several pharmaceutical companies have paid massive fines (sometimes exceeding a billion dollars) for marketing drugs for conditions they are not approved for and for payments to doctors. These payments are not technically commissions but still amount to massive amounts of money paid to doctors for various purposes (e.g., lectures, consulting, research, dinners, unsolicited gifts). These monies don't just potentially cloud doctor's judgment; they have been found to actually cloud doctor's judgment (with highly favorable reviews provided to products that were found to be wanting in quality).

The facts that have been presented in the last few paragraphs certainly suggest that we should be, at the very least, open to other forms of healing than those usually employed in the United States. In many other affluent countries (including many European countries), herbal medicine is dispensed by a doctor, and those doctors are aware of formulation, dosage, and (importantly) safety issues (e.g., potential interactions) because they have been published in scientific monographs on plant healing agents. Despite the fact that there are tens of evidence-based, peer-reviewed journals that feature medicinal plants and fungi, use of anything other than drugs and surgery is considered to be "quack science" by many credentialed physicians. As noted by Mark Plotkin in an on-line article in 2014:

> "... our pharmaceutical industry is often dismissive of nature as a source of healing. It seems to overlook the fact that many of the most important classes of prescription drugs like ACE inhibitors for high blood pressure (first developed from Brazilian snake venom), beta blockers (from hallucinogenic Mexican fungi), and cholesterol-lowering statins (from *Penicillium* fungus) came from natural sources."

Why would natural remedies be viewed so poorly by many physicians? There are many potential answers for this. Cleary, and most importantly, is the fact that doctors don't learn about herbal medicine; therefore, they will not use these medicinal plants in their practice. Period. Some doctors are very threatened by any information that allows their patients (actual or potential) to become more self-sufficient in healing. They use their credentials to attack everything outside of western medicine in order to maintain their standing as the only source for evidence-based medicine. I do not mean to imply that all doctors (or even the majority of doctors) are mainly interested in their patients for providing a revenue stream. Some doctors who react poorly may also be dealing with substantial ego issues that cause them to be threatened by patients learning to actually heal underlying issues (something western medicine rarely can effect). For whatever the reason, there is little doubt that many credentialed doctors vehemently attack natural healing (of any kind), using phrases like "natural healthcare is unsafe and a danger to public health". Clearly those making such statements have not looked into their own profession's track record.

Another influential reason that certainly needs to be mentioned is the cost associated with bringing a new drug to the market in the United States. Research and development, clinical trials, insurance, and other factors now bring total expenses to somewhere between 2.5 and 5 billion dollars for some drugs. Given this massive investment, no American drug company is going to commit this money to researching medicinal plants—something that can be gathered for free by those that have a relationship with said plant (i.e., they can identify the plant and understand its ecology and phenology so they know where and when to find the species of interest). This is a major impediment to natural remedies being used widely in the United States.

Any company trying to bring an herbal medicine to market would face overwhelming costs and little chance of recouping those expenses. This is likely one of the major reasons why most research on herbal medicine is performed in countries other than the United States. The American system virtually precludes the general use of botanical medicine.

But is natural medicine effective and safe? The answer is both yes and no (no different than with pharmaceutical drugs)—it depends on what they are used for, how they are used, and what they are used in conjunction with. It also depends on various ethical and practical considerations of those who collect, formulate, and sell herbal medicine. Adulteration of herbal formulas with species (or pharmaceutical drugs or toxic metals and metalloids) not listed on the label, outright replacement of species being sold with cheaper or more easily procured plants, and poor storage conditions (leading to molding of plant material) are all documented to occur. No different than with drugs, the quality of the medicine is dependent on the honesty of those that make it available to the ill (all the more reason to learn to identify, gather, and prepare your own). The fact is, there are cases where a plant-based medicine was found to work equally well or more effectively (in a lab or in a clinical study) than a drug. And in most cases, plants present a greater therapeutic range—there is a greater difference between the minimum amount needed to exert a physiological effect and the maximum amount that can be safely ingested (in most cases) than pharmaceutical drugs, making it much more difficult to ingest toxic amounts. For example, examining 2009 records from the American Association of Poison Control Centers, there were no deaths attributable to herbal medicine, even though nearly ⅓ of Americans use herbs of some kind. The Alliance for Natural Health calculated the odds of dying from drugs and herbs in the United Kingdom (also in 2009) and found that residents of that country were 7750 times more likely to die from adverse reactions to pharmaceuticals than from herbal medicines. If you examine statistics concerning the safety of herbal medicines vs. pharmaceutical drugs in places where both are used, you will find herbal medicines to be orders of magnitude safer.

Americans typically reject herbal medicine, believing it to be both unsafe and ineffective, even though many pharmaceutical drugs are, in fact, derived from plants. Americans recognize that some plants can produce phytochemicals that cause harm, indicating they believe in the potency of plant chemistry, but they appear not to consider it possible that plants can contain a suite of compounds that can be beneficial for humans—even though there are at least 320,000 species of plants worldwide (some estimates go as high as 500,000), numbers that suggest some species would offer benefit simply by chance. These beliefs, perhaps without realization, consider all humans who have used herbal medicine (especially those living in the distant past) to be deluded individuals who willingly ingested plants that did nothing to assuage their ailments and poisoned them in the process. Of course, these beliefs are held by a population of people who consume highly processed foods devoid of nutrition, oxidized lipids that contribute to cardiovascular disease, and synthetic food ingredients that promote allergic reactions. In other words, these people willingly consume items that do not support physical health (are ineffective) and contribute to disease (are unsafe). Perhaps it is understandable to you, the reader, when I write that this opinion, held by people who consume highly unnatural things that are not safe to consume, is not an opinion I would hold in high regard.

The fact is, while past use of natural medicine is not the same as a controlled, clinical trial, the information we gain from this historical context is still of value to modern humans. Long history of use helps determine safety and presents anecdotal evidence for efficacy. When we combine this with contemporary scientific research, which helps validate efficacy and determines mechanisms of action, we can paint a more confident picture of harmlessness and effectiveness—two criteria a given medicine should possess (how many modern drugs do you know that possess both of these criteria?). Viewing medicine through this filter (i.e., the intersection of folk use and modern study) is a much stronger method of determining safety and efficacy (rather than simply modern research alone). Remember, every pharmaceutical drug recalled by the Food and Drug Administration for safety reasons was first approved for use.

Natural medicine has a number of benefits to offer those on a rewilding path when it is used appropriately (i.e., when use is guided by education in the topic). Herbal remedies can support organic agriculture and sustainable wildcrafting (if sourced correctly), rather than chemical and biotech industries. Many plants and fungi that have been used for millennia in herbal medicine actually provide multiple benefits to the human body (aside from the issue the remedy is being used for). For example, while someone is, hypothetically, using Japanese knotweed (*Reynoutria japonica*) for a staph infection, this plant also supplies antioxidant, anticancer, anti-inflammatory, cardiotonic, and immune modulating actions (among others). Medicinal herbs provide another source of nutritional intake due to their vitamin, mineral, and phytochemical content (which can be very high in some plants). Plant-based medicines are often much less expensive than pharmaceutical drugs, and they do not contribute to the pollution of the landscape and our waterways. As important, they contribute to the self-reliance of a family or community, something that is going to become more and more important with increasing interruption of services (due to extreme weather, economic hardship, terrorism, etc.). And these medicines supply connection to a landscape—something that is sorely missing in American society (and one of the reasons we allow ecocide to occur). When we finally realize that potent medicine can be sourced from our open spaces, we may look very differently upon the forests, prairies, and wetlands that surround our homes (or are found beyond our city limits). We can recognize that there is value in a natural area that can be appreciated (and utilized) that does not involve its destruction.

CUT, BURN, AND POISON

Cancer is a prevalent (and misunderstood) disease that warrants special mention in a book such as this. It is very common in the United States with approximate life-time odds of 2 in 5 for contracting this disease. There were 577,190 deaths from this disease alone in 2012. It is one of the leading causes of death in both affluent and non-affluent countries and is now the leading cause of childhood death according to some estimates (it was, until recently, accidents). The frequency of contracting cancer is on the rise. It was 1 in 7 in 1980, 1 in 12 in 1950, and so on (these numbers from the National Cancer Institute). Many authors who are fond of attacking various groups who promote a natural lifestyle are quick to point out that the death rate from cancer is declining. While that is true, it is a very deceptive statement. In the year 2000, cancer was responsible for nearly 1 in 50 deaths here in the United States. In 2011, cancer killed 1 in 54 people. So it has declined (a little). But of course, in 1900, cancer killed only 1 in 156 people—so it is a much more frequent way to die now than then (these numbers compiled from information published by the US Public Health Service and US National Center for Health Statistics). Longer life is frequently touted as the reason why cancer is so prevalent by many credentialed authorities. In other words, you should not concern yourself with rising rates of contracting cancer because it is to be expected with our longer lives. Of course, this does not explain rising rates of childhood cancer. And it does not take into account that cancer was virtually unknown among indigenous of any age (so long as they practiced their traditional lifeway). Certainly, a greater life expectancy does contribute to the rising frequency and tremendous death toll of cancer in some way, but it cannot explain away all that we observe.

Changes in diet and lifestyle (for the worse) with concomitant increasing exposure to carcinogenic and mutagenic factors does explain (in large part) why we have such high rates of cancer here in the US. In other words, the further we move along the spectrum of lifestyles from hunter-gatherer to agriculturalist to industrialist (i.e., the further we become divorced from nature), the more prevalent cancer becomes in the story of humankind.

Cancer is now one of the most costly ailments to manage. How much money does it cost to treat cancer? One estimate placed the spending on cancer in 2012 at 124.6 billion dollars. This does not include the 6 billion dollars in tax-payer monies that are cycled through various research agencies searching for a cure. It is clear that treating cancer is big business. In a 2012 study examining records from 28,530 patients who had cancer in their last six months of life, the average cost of cancer treatment in those last six months was 74,212 dollars (keep in mind, that was just for the last six months of life, most of these people would have also had expenses in the months prior to the study period). With this kind of income being generated, it is perhaps clear why the current (and often ineffective) cancer paradigm is maintained.

What is the paradigm I'm writing about? It is this: massive amounts of money are poured into searching for a cure to cancer and very little research is directed toward preventing cancer. This may not seem like an important distinction, but it is an essential part of the discussion. Would you prefer to avoid having your house catch on fire (prevention) or wait until it is burning and then do something about it (curing)? While certainly you would say that you want both (and I would agree), you clearly would prefer to take steps to prevent a fire from occurring (proactive) rather than placing nearly all your money into putting out a fire once it occurs (reactive). But this is exactly what the cancer industry in the United States does. Worse, they have confused the public, conflating early diagnosis with prevention. If one were to visit almost any cancer charity's website, there are volumes of information on early diagnosis (i.e., finding cancer in the early stages of development), even in the brief sections on how to stay healthy (as if it is a form of prevention). While I do agree that finding a disease early is important for successfully treating it, using our analogy from earlier in this paragraph, that amounts to finding the fire when it is still very small (i.e., it is still not prevention).

Unfortunately, citizens of the United States are primarily reactionary beings, waiting until a problem occurs and then trying to figure out what steps to take in order to mitigate the problem (this strategy often requiring much more effort to effect). This is evident in our massive promotion of cancer charities, some of which have been found to be frauds, others of which have been found to direct a large proportion of the donations to for-profit fund-raising businesses (this is not to write that all cancer charities are disreputable because that is certainly untrue, and, before I go any further, I want to be clear that I think those who donate have the best intentions and are trying to help those in need). One of the activities performed by cancer charities is the donation of money to pharmaceutical companies to identify a cure. However, pharmaceutical companies then turn around and make large profits from the sale of their therapies. Equally important, companies also own the research, meaning they don't have to publish results that are unfavorable for their product (a phenomenon called "publication bias"). This means that the public (including oncologists) may have a skewed opinion of the efficacy of a particular cancer therapy.

Susan G. Komen for the Cure, whose mission statement is "Ending breast cancer forever", actually promotes the use of materials that are known to contribute to cancer. Komen for the Cure denies the link between bisphenol A (BPA) and cancer, despite studies that link BPA to breast cancer. Bisphenol A is a component of the pink-capped polycarbonate water bottle distributed by its partner DS Waters. Komen for the Cure receives donations from 3M, maker of Scotch Tape, who is a member of the American Chemistry Council, a trade group that argues for the safety of BPA. Clearly, Komen for the Cure has ties to industry that creates carcinogenic materials. More to the point, many breast-cancer-related charities still promote the use of mammograms, even though mammograms expose women to ionizing radiation that can increase their chances of developing breast cancer. The more mammograms a women receives, the higher her odds. Each mammogram increases a women's lifetime odds of contracting breast cancer 1 to 2 percent. But, you say, mammograms help detect cancer. Yes, they do, with an over diagnosis (and over treatment) rate of 30% (as revealed in the 2011 meta-analysis by the Cochrane Database of Systemic Reviews). Further, a 2015 study in the Journal of the American Medical Association Internal Medicine examining over 16 million women found no evident correlation between the extent of screening and ten-year breast cancer mortality (i.e., mammography screening does not extend life). Now there is a new three-dimensional mammogram (called 3D tomosynthesis), which exposes women to twice the radiation as a traditional two-dimensional mammogram. Doesn't it seem strange to attempt to detect breast cancer with a device that produces radiation that can promote breast cancer? I think so, especially considering devices such as ultrasound and infrared (i.e., thermography) do exist that are far less invasive and do not expose the breasts to ionizing radiation. A final question for you to consider: how do the funds given to pharmaceutical companies by Susan G. Komen for the Cure (money originating from donations) to develop treatments once you have succumbed to breast cancer, actually promote their goal of "Ending breast cancer forever"?

Our approach to cancer is somewhat barbaric, if one examines it objectively. We primarily use surgery (cut), radiation (burn), and chemotherapy drugs (poison) to attack tumors, often resulting in harm to the remainder of the body and rarely ever realizing that cancer is a symptom of an overwhelmed immune system. The cure for a cancer is not the removal or destruction of the tumor (that is simply a treatment), rather it is an increase in the functioning of the immune system and a reduction in the exposure to carcinogens. Western Medicine's tumor-centric approach often fails (ultimately) to prevent death because without diet and lifestyle changes, cancers can and do return (the rates of recurrence dependent on the cancer and the therapy used). In fact, the cancer therapy is considered a success if the patient survives for five years (even if the cancer returns shortly after). Equally important is that many cancers are considered by oncologists to be genetic diseases, giving people the impression that there is no hope for prevention because it is their fate. As a result, some women prophylactically remove their breasts and uterus, even though there was no guarantee that cancer would appear and there can be tremendous quality of life factors that come into play. Some people who have genes that are considered important risk factors for breast cancer (such as BRCA-related genes) do not develop cancer. Given what we know about epigenetics, this makes perfect sense. The expression (or silencing) of genes is based on our diet and lifestyles (i.e., our lifeway). Poor diets, stressful lives, abundant exposure to endocrine disrupting compounds, and similar features likely promote the occurrence of such "genetically predisposed" cancers. Remember, as previously stated in this book, we inherit a lifeway (with the corresponding genetic expression) from our parents. Lifeways are something that can be changed, and in doing so, we have the ability to make significant positive impacts on our genetic health.

It is a shame that many oncologists fail to see cancer as a symptom of a poor lifeway. Thinking of it as the underlying issue means the focus is placed on removing or shrinking the tumor, regardless of the price the rest of the body pays as a result of the cutting, burning, and poisoning.

Further, few, if any, lifestyle changes are implemented to prevent the recurrence of cancer later in life. I have assisted many people with complementary strategies because their oncologists provided them no guidance on diet, movement, and other lifestyle changes to bolster their overall health. Fortunately, some oncologists do practice more holistic strategies, and I encourage you to find such practitioners should cancer become part of your medical history (and you choose to use conventional therapies). It has been shown, for example, that some adaptogenic herbs have the ability to potentiate western cancer therapies, meaning that lower doses can be used (which also means less harm to the body and decreased severity of side effects). Other natural remedies can help to maintain proper function of the immune system during treatments. And certainly, regardless of what mainstream oncologists may tell you, there are natural remedies that can be used to treat cancer that do not cause extensive injury to the body. It is frustrating to realize that cancer was incredibly rare amongst non-acculturated hunter-gatherers and that this information does not appear to have worked its way into our thinking about this disease (i.e., it does not influence our prevention methods). Said another way, we know that a lifeway that is deeply immersed in nature is highly resistant to cancer. Cancer is a disease of civilization. Its unchecked growth and harm it causes to the host organism is remarkably similar to the modern-day manifestation of humans' interaction with the earth. As I have written previously in this book, we don't need to seek a cure for cancer because prevention is plainly possible.

ANTI-LIFE DRUGS

An antibiotic drug is a drug that is "opposed" (anti-) to "life" (biotic). So antibiotics are substances designed to kill other life. The "other life" is usually a bacterium, but some fungi are also targeted with this class of drugs. Antibiotics are used with increasing frequency in the United States and are having waning efficacy (for several reasons). The antibiotic era, which could be stated to have begun with the discovery of penicillin, was thought to mean the end of ailments caused by pathogenic organisms (bacteria in particular). Modern people focused on excessive hygiene and ample use of anti-life drugs, not realizing that these practices would come back to harm them. While their use in serious and life-threatening infections is not being called into question here, what is being questioned is the overuse, the kind of drug used, and the side effects (which are rarely mentioned by credentialed doctors who prescribe these drugs). To reiterate from writing earlier in this chapter, antibiotics represent symptomatic treatments—they are not addressing the root cause (which is often a susceptibility to infection due to poor immune system function).

There is little controversy regarding the overuse of antibiotics. Doctors, naturopaths, and herbalists alike all agree on this fact. Reuters' pediatricians recently estimated that annually over 10,000,000 unnecessary prescriptions for antibiotics are issued, often for items such as influenza and asthma (ailments that are not caused by bacterial infections). Each use increases the chances that a specific bacterium develops resistance to an antibiotic. Once resistance occurs, the antibiotic will no longer work for that strain of bacteria, meaning it becomes more and more difficult to treat infections (using pharmaceutical drugs). Important to this topic is the fact that antibiotics are routinely added to animal feed because it has been found to increase growth rates of livestock and fish. This practice has been known for decades to lead to the formation of antibiotic-resistant bacteria, bacteria that can, and are documented to, infect humans. Antibiotic-resistant bacteria originating from farms that include antibiotics in the animal feed have been identified in the areas surrounding farm operations and on meat available for purchase in supermarkets. This practice of supplying antibiotics in feed to otherwise healthy animals is a dangerous one. It supplies yet another reason to consume wild and conscientiously raised animals.

One of the real limitations of many pharmaceutical antibiotics is that they are comprised of a single chemical. For example, Erythromycin (a very common antibiotic) is a molecule produced by the bacterium *Streptomyces erythreus* that has the molecular formula of $C_{37}H_{67}NO_{13}$. It also goes by the name (3R,4S,5S,6R,7R,9R,11R,12R,13S,14R)-6-[(2S,3R,4S,6R)-4-(dimethylamino)-3-hydroxy-6-methyloxan-2-yl]oxy-14-ethyl-7,12,13-trihydroxy-4-[(2R,4R,5S,6S)-5-hydroxy-4-methoxy-4,6-dimethyloxan-2-yl]oxy-3,5,7,9,11,13-hexamethyl-oxacyclotetradecane-2,10-dione. It functions as an antibiotic by inhibiting the synthesis of proteins in some species of pathogens. Given that it is a single molecule, operating through a single mechanism, it is more likely for a species of bacterium to become resistant to this antibiotic (through genetic variation or mutation). In fact, this has happened in some pathogenic bacteria in the genus *Streptococcus* for this pharmaceutical antibiotic. Contrasting this are herbal remedies that utilize whole-plant preparations (i.e., medicines are made using relatively crude methods such that the entire suite of phytochemistry is present in the medicine). These medicines often possess suites of antimicrobial compounds, all acting in concert on the pathogenic bacteria. For example, consider cultivated garlic (*Allium sativum*), with over 35 known compounds that work synergistically to treat infections. I have used this plant many times to help people with staph infections, including Methicillin-resistant *Staphylococcus aureus* (MRSA). Whole-plant preparations of this kind offer tremendous advantage for many infections because of their efficacy and inability of bacteria to gain resistance.

Pharmaceutical antibiotics, especially frequent use of these drugs, come with some significant drawbacks. One of those is that our symbionts (specifically, the probiotic organisms that inhabit our digestive tract) can be harmed by the use of such drugs. Loss of our symbionts means several things, including a reduced ability to derive nutrition. While many mainstream doctors are still unaware of the tremendous importance of our symbionts (as evidenced by the fact that they prescribe drugs that kill them), we need to consider different approaches than using pharmaceutical drugs. Vacancy in our digestive tract is a recipe for altering our flora to something less than beneficial because pathogenic species can colonize the free space. This idea, of vacancy in a biological world being potentially detrimental, is perhaps best exemplified by the (attempted) sterility of a hospital. The removal of microbial life from the hospital setting creates an opportunity for other bacteria to invade, which is exactly why one of the most probable locations to contract a staph infection is … a hospital. This is exactly what happens in our intestinal tract with the frequent use of pharmaceutical antibiotics: beneficial organisms are partly replaced by those that can cause pathology (e.g., evidence is growing that this may be one of the contributing factors to the obesity epidemic in the United States because some altered gut microbiomes can derive more energy from the diet and contribute to weight gain).

At this point, you may be thinking this all sounds well and good but the infection must be treated to protect the individual. And I agree with that thought, but here is another reason to use herbal antimicrobials: there is documentation that they do not harm our probiotic flora. We know this through several lines of evidence, including the fact that many food plants consumed by indigenous people are known to possess antibacterial action (as documented in a laboratory setting), but indigenous people did not experience problems created or exacerbated by altered microbiomes in the digestive tract. There are many widely available (in the field or in the store) antimicrobial plants that can be used to treat bacterial, fungal, and viral infections. It simply requires an acceptance that safe and effective treatments can be found outside of a pill bottle.

When we overlay on all of this the fact that the number of antibiotic treatments is correlated with increased rates of cancer (this is documented in several studies), it suggests we should be willing to identify other agents to treat infections. Such agents exist, but it will require people to step outside of their industrial mindset to "see" these medicines.

SELF AS ENEMY

A group of diseases that are on the rise in developed countries are collectively termed autoimmune diseases. Nearly 24 million people are afflicted by these disorders in the United States alone, though that number is likely a significant underestimate because it includes data on only 24 diseases with good epidemiology studies—but there are over 80 autoimmune diseases. The real number is likely closer to 50 million people (according to American Autoimmune Related Diseases Association)—which represents 15% of the US population (or approximately 1 in 6 people). These diseases, which include type 1 diabetes, rheumatoid arthritis, celiac disease, lupus, psoriasis, inflammatory bowel disease, and Grave's disease (among many others), have one important thing in common: the body's immune system cannot distinguish between self and other; therefore, the immune system attacks some portion of the body and, in the process, causes serious health issues. This is in contrast to an allergy, where the body attacks a harmless particle from the environment in an overly vigorous manner. The exact causes of autoimmune diseases are still poorly understood, though there are a number of factors that are known to be associated with a high risk for development of one or more of these diseases. The biggest risk factor of all—civilization. Autoimmune diseases were absent in hunter-gatherer cultures and are rare in non-industrialized countries.

Civilization has a number of insults on our health that predispose modern people to autoimmune disorders. These include excessive hygiene, poor nutrition, exposure to environmental toxins, disturbed microbiome health, diet rich in inflammatory and allergenic foods, underlying infections, and sedentary lifestyles. At the point where our immune systems consider our own bodies (or some portion of our bodies) as an enemy, we can state we have reached a new level of "dis-ease" in our society. Fortunately, some holistic medicine practitioners (this field sometimes called functional medicine) are having success not only treating symptoms of autoimmune diseases but also curing the disease outright by addressing these aforementioned insults.

Our immune systems require challenges to help them function at a high level (keep in mind, a challenge is different from something that overwhelms). Just like our skeletal system, which gets stronger when our bones are stressed, our immune system reaches a higher level of functioning when it receives many small challenges during our developmental years. Excessive hygiene and lifestyle that avoids contact with soil, leaf litter, wild water, and animal life is an existence with reduced contact to the earth. Think about it, people in industrialized countries are actively trying to raise children in a way that reduces interaction with the planet we live on. Is it any wonder that that practice leads to health issues? Autoimmune diseases (and allergies) are, at least in part, a symptom of a nature divorced life. Of course, this aspect of autoimmune disorders is remedied by rearing children with ample free time to connect with the earth and the other-than-human beings that we share this planet with.

There is a growing body of evidence demonstrating that poor nutrition can be responsible for autoimmune diseases, or at least an increased severity of autoimmune disorders. Research shows that vitamins A and D work in concert with each other to protect against factors that lead to autoimmunity. Chris Masterjohn has summarized some of the research in an article titled "New

Evidence of Synergy Between Vitamins A and D: Protection Against Autoimmune Diseases". Given that many people in the United States have low levels of these fat-soluble vitamins, it is not surprising that autoimmune disorders are on the rise. But, environmental toxins play an important role in this story. These chemicals, such as polychlorinated biphenyls, chlorinated herbicides, some synthetic pyrethroids, and organophosphate insecticides (among others), cause even greater harm than simply their chemistry's primary effects on the body. That is because they also have the secondary effect of limiting the body's ability to protect itself by essentially depleting circulating stores of important vitamins. This occurs through the chemicals' ability to prevent activation of vitamin A or reduce the body's ability to circulate this vitamin. Some of these chemicals are routinely used in chemical agriculture—and people are exposed to them not only through consumption of conventional produce but also through living in areas where chemicals are sprayed.

Autoimmune disorders, which will likely become an even greater collective health issue in the coming years, are excellent examples of how human physiology becomes impaired when we move away from natural living. Further, they are yet another group of diseases for which synthetic drugs will never cure the underlying cause (they can, at best, treat symptoms). Most of these diseases are entirely preventable, but prevention needs to start early in the life of the human at risk. Nature connection in all facets of our life is one of the most important ways to avoid autoimmunity because such a life will avoid many of the commonly believed factors for development of these pathologies (including food, environmental, lifestyle, movement, and symbiont factors). Depending on the autoimmune disease, curing can be as straightforward as:

1. removing offending foods and/or substances;
2. replacing allergenic foods with high quality wild and organically raised foods;
3. healing with specific remedies;
4. and focusing on microbiome health.

While these four steps cannot work with all conditions, they do offer significant promise (for an actual cure) with many autoimmune diseases. The specifics of the offending foods, replacement foods, and specific remedies will differ for each condition but a qualified holistic medicine practitioner could design a healing protocol that would produce virtually no side effects and would, in the implementation, support the body in many beneficial ways. The specific remedies will often include herbal medicine to treat chronic inflammation (a symptom present in most autoimmune disorders). While such a system might be considered "quack science" or "wishful thinking" by many doctors, I have personally witnessed this approach succeed for many people who were diligent with diet and lifestyle changes.

SYMPTOMS THAT ARE SOLUTIONS

One of the common features of living in an industrial country is an over-medicated populace. More specifically, residents of such a country often are unable to distinguish symptoms of health insults that should be treated and symptoms that are the body's way of coping with a health insult that will clear on its own (if we trust our bodies). In fact, people sometimes medicate in a way that is working against the body's own mechanisms of dealing with issues, potentially causing the issue to become exacerbated. Part of taking back the sovereignty of our own health is realizing that not all issues we experience require a visit to a doctor or a drug (whether prescription or over-the-counter).

Three excellent examples of symptoms that are not necessarily problems are swelling, diarrhea, and fever. Swelling is the localized edema that occurs as a result of an injury (such as a sprain or laceration). This process increases blood flow and brings white blood cells to the region. The swelling helps to splint the region to enable healing without additional injury due to excessive movement (the pain is a part of this response, helping to "favor" an injury by keeping it from bearing weight). Potent anti-inflammatories can reduce swelling and discomfort, allowing an injury to bear weight prior to healing. Diarrhea, the presence of loose and watery stool, in a healthy individual is often the result of a bacterial, viral, or parasitic infection in the gastrointestinal tract. It is, in this situation, an evolved response to purge the unwanted pathogenic organisms. Stopping this kind of diarrhea can worsen the situation and delay recovery. A fever is an increased body core temperature over the usual 37 degrees Celsius (98.6 degrees Fahrenheit). It can be caused by a number of agents, a common one being an infection by a bacterium or virus. The body enters a state of pyrexia (i.e., increased temperature) to kill pathogens in the body, ultimately clearing the infection and allowing a person to recover. Using drugs to reduce a temporary and minor fever may prolong the sickness.

The previous paragraph has presented a few of the many possible normal body responses to mild injury and infection. These responses are frequently medicated in the US, actually working against the body's natural healing mechanisms. The point of this section is that every minor discomfort we experience should not be attacked with drugs (which themselves carry risks). Modern humans need to learn to listen to their bodies and respond accordingly. A headache that is not the result of a disease can be easily treated with some time laying down in a comfortable location, a minor injury will heal with some days of low activity, and diarrhea often requires no medical attention at all—the body clears the infection and health returns. Of course, prudence must be used on the part of the person experiencing these symptoms. Severe and/or chronic episodes of such symptoms can be caused by serious underlying issues. Even normal reactions by the body, such as diarrhea, can cause dehydration if people are not cared for while the symptoms persist. It is pertinent to note that people frequently do not study human health and physiology. Such a lack of information provides them with no basis to understand the severity of the symptoms they are experiencing and if any medication is required at all. Part of learning to heal ourselves and our families is learning when no medicine is needed. The mild pain and discomfort we experience is a message that we are to "lay low" for a time and allow healing to occur. Natural medicine practices recognize normal physiological reactions and seek to support them (rather than work against them).

PLANT ALLIES

The majority of medicine in the world (past and present) comes from the plant kingdom. Collectively, these beings possess a diverse array of natural compounds that have numerous effects on the body. Depending on the species, those effects can be mild or significant (even serious). Those developed countries that have mostly turned their back on healing with natural remedies (like the United States) all hail from people with strong traditions in herbal medicine. North America, for example, is now populated with numerous plant species from Europe that were brought here by colonists for medicine. Examples include motherwort (*Leonurus cardiaca*), horse yellowhead (*Inula helenium*; often called elecampane), single-veined sweet-flag (*Acorus calamus*), milk-thistle (*Silybum marianum*), colt's-foot (*Tussilago farfara*), and common comfrey (*Symphytum officinale*), species that have escaped the garden setting and can be found naturalized in the Western Hemisphere. These medicines were often incorporated into the pharmacopeias of the indigenous of the continent, who could see how valuable these plants were for healing. Nowadays, when pharmaceutical drugs possess a litany and severity of side effects sometimes more severe than the symptom being treated, it is time for a rebirth in the understanding of how plant allies can assist us. These medicines are effective, often supply a multitude of beneficial actions, and have a frequency of harmful events orders of magnitude lower than drugs.

Hunter-gatherers around the world have used plant remedies for healing. An important question that can be asked is whether or not the purposes for which they used different plant species have any verified merit (i.e., do modern scientific studies validate their use of these plants?). The answer is, for the most part, yes. Hunter-gatherers had a significant knowledge of plants and their pharmacological properties. This has been confirmed in a number of studies. For example, in a study performed by Omar et al. in 2000, they examined the crude extracts of 14 different deciduous tree species found in eastern North America for their antimicrobial ability. These trees were all documented as medicine amongst various Native American tribes. All of the trees that were used for infections by hunter-gatherers possessed significant antimicrobial activity (i.e., the extracts killed bacteria in laboratory tests). Of interest is that the results showed also that all of the trees used for infections possessed activity against Methicillin-resistant *Staphylococcus aureus* (MRSA). The researchers then grouped the trees into three categories (high usage, medium usage, low usage) based on the how many different tribes used the trees as medicine. Those trees that were more widely used (i.e., used by the most tribes) had the highest activity against the bacteria they tested, indicating a kind of cultural understanding of the degree of efficacy of the plants being used. In another study performed by McCutcheon et al. in 1992, 96 different extracts from wild medicinal plants used by native people of British Columbia were examined for their antimicrobial ability. They found that 95% of the plants that could be categorized as antimicrobial plants based on the historical usage demonstrated activity against at least one bacterial strain. Most were active against two or more strains of bacteria (85%), and 75% were active against MRSA. These studies, and others, showed that hunter-gatherers possessed an understanding of plant chemistry, even without the use of laboratory equipment. Numerous similar studies indicate their use of plant medicines was not random, but generally correlated (sometimes highly so) with verified use from contemporary scientific study.

Many people in industrialized countries are simply so unfamiliar with any form of "natural living" that the use of plant medicine is simply too extreme, as they are fearful of wild beings. While cautiousness is prudent, fear is simply unhelpful and, sometimes, outright detrimental. It is easy to locate information in books and on the internet that describes the toxicity and cancer-causing potential of many wild plants that have been used as medicine by wild and traditional peoples. This information is frequently based a reductionist method of study, one that can provide highly misleading results in the field of herbal medicine. The study goes something as follows: isolate a single compound from a plant, feed it or inject it into laboratory animals at high doses (i.e., unrealistic amounts), identify health problems that arise, and then ban all natural or alternative food and medicine that contains said compound. As I wrote in 2015 in Ancestral Plants volume 2 about an eastern North American tree called sassafras (*Sassafras albidum*):

"Safrole, one of the constituents of the root bark (also found in the leaves) is considered to be carcinogenic (producing cancer) and mutagenic (promoting mutation in genetic material) by the Food and Drug Administration (FDA). Understand how the FDA comes to this conclusion: highly refined extracts are delivered at high doses over long periods of time to laboratory animals living on a nutrient-poor diet; when cancer develops in the test subjects, the FDA reports it is carcinogenic and prohibits its sale. There is no reality in their test procedures (in fairness, at least not in this case). No one consumes Sassafras albidum for 72 weeks straight as injections (though rats that developed cancer were subjected to this). The FDA does not mention that the root bark of *Sassafras albidum* contains antimutagenic compounds (β-sitosterol, boldine, eugenol, and tannins) and cancer-preventing compounds and minerals (α-pinene, β-sitosterol, anethole, myristicin, and 14 others) that would temper the effects of safrole in crude extracts (such as those used in home medicine). The problem is that they test in isolation and at ludicrous dosages. Anyone consuming an occasional root bark beverage or using *Sassafras albidum* infrequently as a medicine (for short duration) should not be concerned about the FDA's warning. Further, the FDA seems to avoid mentioning that safrole is also found in *Theobroma cocao* (cocoa) and *Ocimum basilicum* (basil), among many other plants."

There is simply so much dubious information that has influenced our opinions on various herbal medicines. As noted above, scientists often extrapolate from a single chemical constituent to what the outcome will be from consuming the entire plant or a large suite of chemicals from the plant, which is not always reliable. Another confounding issue in the discussion of herbal medicine toxicity is that scientists use large volumes of animal studies, some of which may not be appropriate because of tremendous differences in the physiology, overall diet, or lifestyle of the animals being used as test subjects. A great example of this is the warnings generated from observations of light-colored livestock who develop photosensitivity after consuming common St. John's-wort (*Hypericum perforatum*) in the fields where they are kept. The observations result in warnings that people should avoid this plant because of the potential adverse reaction. The reality is, despite being dispensed by the millions of doses each year, there are very few actual cases of photosensitivity in humans. What is rarely stated by those warning people away from such a remedy is that studies have shown no adverse reactions have been confirmed as a result of this plant with appropriate dosages (up to 1 mg of total hypericin). In fact, one study showed that therapeutic dosages of St. John's-wort are 30–50 times below the phototoxic level. Further, some episodes of photosensitivity that have occurred are based on work with high doses of a synthetic form of hypericin being injected intravenously for experimental anti-viral treatments. This example, and many others that could be written about, indicate our civilized prejudices of wild and cultivated botanical medicines are the result of the way civilization studies the world. In an attempt to control for all variables, we study a single compound (or synthetic version of that compound), eliminating many of the beneficial aspects of a plant's total phytochemistry, including compounds that temper (or even alleviate) potential harm. Such practices generate biases against valuable healing remedies, ultimately continuing the high reliance on pharmaceuticals.

If you are someone who has not previously used herbal medicine and is interested in such practices (or you are someone who has but limited familiarity with this form of healing), I strongly suggest you find experienced herbalists and holistic doctors who use herbs in their practice to learn from. Much like foraging for wild foods, these are skills that require study and time to gain a base level of expertise. That said, you do not have to learn the use and preparation of 100 herbs before you can implement what you know. Treat each herb (and each condition you are interested in treating) as a single skill. You can be learned in dealing with minor cuts, bruises, stings, and similar soft-tissue injuries without necessarily knowing how to treat cancer. Don't simply focus on the plants but learn how to formulate different kinds of medicine and what proper dosages should be. These are important aspects of herbal medicine that contribute to safe practice. Use yourself as a Guinea pig. While many people would immediately raise concern about that statement, I'm not advocating you treat serious cardiac myopathies in your first month of study. Start with relatively benign issues that do not have pressing reasons for timely treatment. Examples could be dandruff, dermatitis from poison-ivy (species of *Toxicodendron*), a wart on your finger, short-term stress from a large project at work that is keeping you awake, or discomfort from menstrual cramps. As your education continues and your experience builds, you can move on to other issues. Given that plants are the most commonly used healing agents in the world, various versions of plant medicine, such as dried material for tea, tinctures, capsules, and salves, are often available in health food stores. These prepared forms of plant medicine can be useful until one learns how to create such medicines for themselves. And please remember two more things. One, you do not need to import "mystical" or "sacred" plant remedies from Asia or South America. That is because every continent is filled with natural healing remedies that can treat a wide variety of issues. Two, keep in mind practices of sustainable harvest if you gather your own medicine. Eradicating plant populations to treat illness ultimately means we will have no plant allies to rely on.

MEDICINAL FUNGI

An important class of natural medicine comes from the fungal kingdom of life. These enigmatic organisms, perhaps even more than some other life we share the planet with, are subject to tremendous bias from modern humans. Because some species are poisonous, people living in industrialized countries often suffer substantial mycophobia (i.e., the fear of fungi). However, this fact alone (that some are poisonous) cannot completely explain the fear possessed by domesticated humans, for many of our food plants have close relatives that are themselves poisonous in sufficient doses (especially members of the celery and nightshade families). It is likely that lack of interaction and virtual absence of education in public schooling creates a societal mythos around mushrooms (one that is not favorable). If you consider the general knowledge held by most residents in developed countries, those people cannot identify any species (or perhaps only a few in a general sense) from this kingdom of life (Fungi). This would be similar to watching a blue jay fly by, a coyote run by, or a brook trout swim by, and the people viewing could only discern the life form as an "animal" (kingdom Animalia). In fact, we see that some of the first food and medicine information lost in indigenous groups is the cultural knowledge of fungi. Their unique role in the ecosystem, combined with unusual morphology (relative to other organisms) may create an atmosphere of mystery or, worse, one that exaggerates common sense precautions to outright fear. In any case, wild fungi are no different from other groups of wild organisms. Some are useful to humans, some are not. Some are edible, some are poisonous. Some are easy to identify, others are very difficult. Learning about medicinal fungi that may occur in your region is especially useful for developing health sovereignty for a family or community.

Edible mushrooms, in general, do contain some important nutrients, such as several B-complex vitamins and minerals (e.g., potassium, magnesium, calcium, and others). They are rich in ergosterol (i.e., pro-vitamin D_2), which is converted to the active form of vitamin D_2 if exposed to sunlight (e.g., such as occurs when they are sun dried for later use). You can even take dried mushrooms from the store and expose them to sunlight to increase their vitamin D concentration many-fold. Mushrooms also contain important functional aspects of nutrition, such as anti-inflammatory, antioxidant, and anticancer compounds.

But perhaps the most important reason to consume them is the immune modulating compounds they possess. Fungi contain a special group of carbohydrates, complex polysaccharides called glucans, which are known to beneficially activate components of the immune system. Glucans are known to stimulate or activate a suite of lymphocytes (i.e., white blood cells) for the benefit of human health. For example, the glucans rouse Natural Killer Cells to destroy malignant cells, increase the scavenging activity of macrophages, induce maturation of T-Cells to enhance cellular immunity, stimulate B-Cells to produce antibodies to tumor antigens, increase release of

Tumor Necrosis Factor-α to induce programmed cell death, up-regulate production of Interferon-α from white blood cells to improve viral resistance in the body, increase the concentration of some Interleukins that are responsible for triggering the maturation of other immune cells and, well, you get the point. Mushrooms improve the functioning of our immune system in a manner that protects us from bacteria, viruses, and cancer. It is important to note that to get the full effects of the glucans in fungi, they must be cooked to liberate these compounds from indigestible cell wall material (called chitin). Without some kind of prolonged heat activation, these polysaccharides are not bioavailable and a major reason for ingestion as medicine cannot be realized.

Recognize that over 300,000 people are hospitalized each year in the US eating "safe food". Knowing this, are you going to avoid store-purchased food? Probably not. We all know some car accident horror story. Does that mean you will avoid riding in cars? Doubtful. It's time to be rational about fears of nature and realize the United States' mycophobia has gotten a little out of control. These species have numerous benefits to our health (see below) and contribute to our self-reliance. Understand that some species of mushrooms are very easily identified and don't have close look-alikes. It simply takes a little time to learn the necessary skills to recognize them.

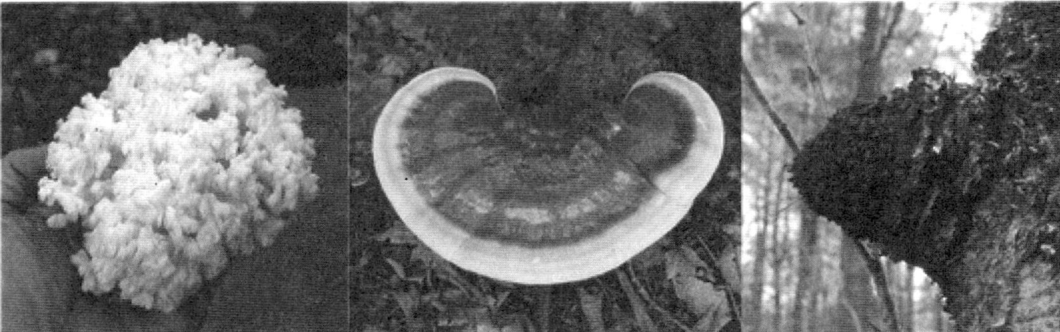

Figure 5.1. Species of medicinal fungi found in the northeastern United States for which there are no poisonous look-alikes and have scientific study supporting their use. Left—coral tooth fungus (*Hericium coralloides*), a species that has use in dementia and Alzheimer's diesease. Middle—hemlock reishi (*Ganoderma tsugae*), a fungus that can help in the treatment of cancer. Right—chaga (*Inonotus obliquus*), a potent antioxidant that has use in diabetic therapy.

Instead of fearing all fungi, learn the distinctive ones by spending time with a skilled mycologist (i.e., one who studies fungi). Bring these special organisms into your life (as food or medicine). Even edible fungi, after thorough cooking, act as a functional medicine through supplying bioavailable glucans that benefit the immune system. Think of how interesting your children would find it to gather and prepare these foods and medicines (it teaches them an actual skill that can help them break free of dependence on pharmaceutical companies). Fungi and other wild healing allies provide us with a means to armor our body against infection and cancer. Avoiding these medicines due to inexperience or hearsay simply means you are missing out on an important aspect of wild medicine. Learning from someone skilled in the identification and preparation of fungi serves to cut through the misinformation and allows neoaboriginals to embrace more of this planet's life.

ENTHEOGENS AND THE DIVINE WITHIN

An entheogen is a substance or a practice that generates the divine within. Though this definition means different things to different people, entheogens are able to produce altered states of consciousness that facilitate expanded awareness, deep self-examination, healing of physical and psychological issues, and generate a greater sense of awe and connection to existence. Entheogens are primarily plants, though fungi, animals, and various practices (e.g., syncopated beat, fasting) are also capable of generating an entheogenic experience. Most affluent societies consider entheogens to be substances that produce intoxication without benefit; hence, the names provided to these medicines generally carry a negative connotation: psychoactive, hallucinogen, psychedelic, dissociative, and deliriant. Given that most people in these societies have not truly experienced a sacred ceremony involving entheogens, these names are based more on ignorance and fear, rather than first-hand witnessing and understanding.

Entheogens have been used virtually around the world by indigenous people. The people of the Andean highlands of Peru used a species of column-like cactus now called San Pedro cactus (*Echinopsis pachanoi*) in their ceremonies. Documented use of this cactus goes back to a stone carving over 3300 years old. In Mexico, the indigenous people used peyote (*Lophophora williamsii)* to attain realms beyond the material one. Some groups considered peyote to protect the people so that they need not fear hunger, thirst, or all dangers. Through a large area of South America, including parts of Bolivia, Chile, Columbia, and Peru, the blood-red angel's trumpet (*Brugmansia sanguinea*) is used as a teacher plant to diagnose disease and divine the future. On portions of the African continent, the dogbane relative iboga (*Tabernanthe iboga*) is used to speak with the ancestors. The fly agaric mushroom (*Amanita muscaria*) was used in northeastern Asia among herder-gatherer shamans. There (and elsewhere), this fungus was used to attain an altered state during divination ceremonies. And the listing of species and indigenous people who used them could continue to great length. Throughout most of the world, indigenous and traditional people employed one or more entheogens. It was a common feature of life.

Now, we enter the Neolithic (or perhaps better called the polymer-lithic), where traditional dietary, medicinal, and ceremonial practices have been interrupted or completely lost. In a world now filled with people afflicted by disease, depression, addiction, greed, and dissension, who simultaneously lack awareness, empathy, healing power, and spirituality free of bureaucracy, it may be time to admit that the loss of traditional lifeways, which included entheogens, may be having major impacts on the quality of our existence. In fact, modern studies are finally beginning to reveal the value of entheogens to contemporary (i.e., domesticated) humans.

Studies have demonstrated the value of iboga (*Tabernanthe iboga*), a west-central African shrub, in treating opiate addiction. The roots contain an indole alkaloid called ibogaine, which produces dream-like visions followed by deep introspection. Characteristics of addicts, such as a desire or intention to use a drug, have seen substantial improvements in human studies. Some cocaine and heroin addicts have experienced tremendous value from this entheogen, reducing or eliminating their need for these drugs in the span of days (rather than months), without the discomfort associated with substance abuse treatment. Studies have also shown that mood is generally improved with less depression experienced by those utilizing this healing strategy. While the alkaloid ibogaine is metabolized relatively quickly in the body (by action of liver enzymes), it is transformed into noribogaine, a metabolite that is cleared very slowly and continues to exert its beneficial pharmacological effects on the central nervous system. Studies have also shown iboga may assist with other types of addiction, including nicotine and alcohol.

A study conducted at Johns Hopkins School of Medicine interviewed volunteers who ingested psylocybin, an indole alkaloid produced by some 200 species of mushrooms (including members of the genus *Psylocybe*). The participants were questioned 14 months after ingestion of the mycochemical, and 94% stated they had had one of the top five most meaningful experiences in their life; 34% stated it was the most meaningful experience in their life. Friends and family members were also questioned about the study participants, and they stated the participants were kinder, happier, and calmer after the experiment. Other studies demonstrated that psylocybin could help treat depression through its ability to stimulate the formation of new neuronal connections, without any of the side effects caused by pharmaceutical anti-depressants. In this arena, psylocybin has shown marked reduction in anxiety experienced by advanced-stage cancer patients, helping them cope with dying and ease psychological trauma. In these studies, no clinically significant adverse effects were observed (i.e., no negative side effects).

Ayahuasca (*Banisteriopsis caapi*) is a forest liana of northwestern South America. Its name derives from a Quechua term meaning "vine of the soul". This entheogen has been used to treat several different kinds of cancers. One gentleman was diagnosed with liver cancer (after treatment of colon cancer) and given a 15% chance of survival by one physician and a 20–25% chance by another. He participated in two ayahuasca ceremonies and found his carcinoembryonic antigen count was lower than normal (this test measures the abundance of a protein associated with certain cancers, a lower score is better). There are also published accounts of positive treatment outcomes with breast cancer, ovarian cancer (including advanced ovarian cancer with metastasis), and uterine cancer. People that have used ayahuasca as part of a cancer therapy have reported that this teacher plant had profound effects, usually described as life-changing, and contributed to their sense of well-being. Ayahuasca contains several alkaloids in its bark, including the β-carbolines, harmine, and harmaline. These compounds inhibit destruction of other phytochemicals found in species of plants combined with this liana during preparation of the medicine. Though many species are combined with ayahuasca, the two most common are chacruna (*Psychotria viridis*) and chagropanga (*Diplopterys cabrerana*), both of which are dimethyltryptamine-containing plants. The pharmacological effects of these chemicals are still being studied but preliminary work suggests that collectively they block tumor angiogenesis (i.e., the formation of new blood vessels), up-regulate apoptosis (i.e., programed cell death), and positively affect cell metabolism.

With all the positive outcomes described in the previous three paragraphs, it is difficult to understand why these entheogens are not being employed more widely in the world. It is important to realize there are many factors at work promoting a fear of (and even disdain for) these sacred species. Efforts by European colonists to eradicate the use of the teacher plants and fungi began when they first arrived on the North and South American continents. The ceremonies involving these species were considered by early colonists to be highly inappropriate, and they went to great lengths to suppress the knowledge and practice of entheogens. For example, Spanish priests considered the use of the peyote cactus to possibly lead to people sucking blood, eating the flesh of other humans, and conversing with demons. This stance has continued today, though it is much easier now because the populace is trained to respect a credentialed authority (in this case, someone with a degree in medicine or psychology) who prefers the use of synthetic drugs over naturally occurring substances that humans have been exposed to for long periods of time.

Entheogens produce what can be described as mystical experiences. They have been demonstrated to promote enhanced cooperation among the different brain centers, producing an enlightened awareness and an ability to perform non-linear thinking. Entheogens are responsible for the birth of some religions (possibly more than just "some"). While many domesticated people doubt the therapeutic effects of entheogens, most of them do not realize how subjective their experience of reality is. The altered state of consciousness achieved through ingestion of entheogens has dramatic effects on the ego and how information is translated by the brain. It can be said that the normal separation of the world and the individual ego we experience in everyday life is reduced or even removed. This allows the ability to perceive the world in different ways and on different levels. Given that these teaching tools have been used by indigenous people around the world, their ceremonial use is certainly part of the rewilding path. However, we should not forget that of the approximately 320,000 species of plants in the world, it is a mere 1000 species known to possess potent levels of psychoactive constituents. The great value of these species to humanity makes them vulnerable to extinction. The loss of teacher plants from the world would have a profound effect on our ability to perceive, understand, and heal.

The words presented in this section are not meant to imply that entheogenic substances are right for all people in all situations. These plants, fungi, and animals need to be approached with awareness, openness, and respect. The purpose of the words here is to explore the deep societal bias against entheogenic medicine, a bias based largely on a significant misunderstanding of these species and how they are properly used. For me, teacher plants are not to be used as a means of escapism but, rather, are to be used with ceremony, which includes an expression of intent and gratitude. Many people have heard of someone having a "bad trip" and, as a result, have written off any possible interaction with teacher plants. Such experiences are often the result of ingestion of too much medicine, combining medicine with other drugs, and failure to establish sacred space through ceremony. Of course, it is appropriate to ask how many people have had severe side effects to pharmaceutical drugs and continue to use them—a clear indication of our prejudice for the industrial world (or worse, a decline in an ability to apply logic equally to different facets of the world). Entheogens are widely known to produce a deep connection to the earth, something that is apparently (and unfortunately) threatening to some modern religions, which consider these medicines synonymous with addictive drugs (for the record, entheogens are not addictive). I am not suggesting that everyone should begin "experimenting" with mind-altering substances, though I do hope that people realize that the bias shown by many affluent societies only serves to prevent communication with valuable members of our wild landscapes. Those interested in rewilding may wish to find people who can help provide a safe and meaningful experience.

NEOABORIGINAL STRATEGY FOR WILD MEDICINE

Before summarizing the chapter and presenting concluding concepts, I want to share a brief version of another of my interactions with wild medicine (for whatever help it may be in your journey on the rewilding path). A number of years ago, I was experiencing frequent cardiac arrhythmias. These manifested as a brief period a rapid, uncoordinated heartbeats in which no blood was moved through my heart because the valves were not operating in a coordinated manner. These would sometimes occur multiple times each minute. I had several doctor's visits and even some monitoring performed to identify what was occurring (but they were not successful in identifying the cause). I decided to accept this health insult as something I needed to solve. After some research and reading about various anti-arrhythmic herbs, I decided to use hawthorn (species in the genus *Crataegus*) to attempt to restore a proper heartbeat. These woody plants (related to apples) have a long history of use in various instances of cardiac myopathies. Examining various evidence-based sources, I could find no mention of serious side effects (even after continuous use for years). Starting with store-purchased tinctures from a local company with a good reputation, I was able to completely avoid these arrhythmias. Eventually, I started making my own alcohol-based preparations using wild-collected medicine from the forest edges near my home. Being a scientist, I had to know for sure that it was the herbal medicine acting on my heart and not some other factor I wasn't considering. Therefore, I started and stopped the routine of medicine five times. Each time I was using the hawthorn medicine, the arrhythmias would cease (after about a week or two of doses), and I would remain asymptomatic until about a week or two after stopping the medicine. This happened consistently all five times. Eventually, I realized that I needed to continue this medicine (at a frequency of a dose every second or third day) to maintain a proper heart rhythm. Skip ahead a few years, and I was in the Sonoran Desert of the southwestern United States and participated in a ceremony using an entheogen with three close friends. It was a powerful experience (my first ever interacting with a teacher plant). There were many lessons presented during the altered state of conscientiousness. The next day, I had an awareness that I would not need to use hawthorn anymore. And I haven't now for many years.

Rewilding our lives is much about relearning how to do things for ourselves—things that human communities have always been responsible for. This includes medicine. The realization that much of what we suffer can be treated by plants and fungi collected from our landscapes (or purchased from organic farms) builds self-reliance—which is to say an independence from industry. This realization also forms connections to our landscapes. Real (and healthy) communities exist in an "indirect reciprocal gift economy". Briefly, this means that everyone gives, but not necessarily back and forth to each other. So, in this system, person A gives to person B. Now, person B has an obligation to give to someone else in the community. It may not be person A, it may be person C. But, ultimately, person A will receive gifts from some member of the community (possibly person B, but maybe person D). In a web of reciprocal gifts, all members of the community are provided for. This is exactly what wild medicine promotes. One gathers black elderberry (*Sambucus nigra*) fruits in the late summer for use as an antiviral and immune system modulator during winter cold season. They remember this gift, and find ways to repay other wild beings for this generosity.

Rewilding our medicine isn't about ignoring doctors, but it is about recognizing that their credentials don't supersede your personal sovereignty to find real solutions to your health issues. Those solutions shouldn't cause you additional harm and put you in financial hardship. If you want to step away from this paradigm, it is going to require some study on your part. Learning about healing has always been part of being a human (at least until quite recently). To learn about healing, wild people needed to learn much about the ecology of the plants they used in healing. They developed deep relationships with these species and stewarded the populations they collected from to insure their continued existence. Through healing with wild plants, they actually learned more about the world they lived in. To those who don't want to make the effort, I would ask: when did learning about our world become a chore?

While conventional medicine (typically a pathology-centered system) addresses symptoms with drugs that do not remedy underlying causes, holistic medicine uses drugs (or herbal remedies) to get a person "back on their feet" and then identifies the root issues that are leading to the appearance of disease symptoms. One way of describing the differences to these approaches is to imagine a person standing on a nail that is piercing the bottom of their foot. Most practitioners of western medicine address the primary complaint (pain) with a powerful analgesic, as the pain grows, so too does the dose of pain-relieving drug. A holistic medicine practitioner would utilize an analgesic to provide relief from the pain, but would then remove the nail from the bottom of the person's foot so that the condition could heal and drugs would no longer be needed. It will behoove you to find a holistic medicine practitioner who has knowledge of more than just drugs. The following table (4.1), which summarizes the characteristics of two medical systems in the United States, may further clarify the differences between these two approaches to healing.

From the Delta Institute of Natural History	Pathology-centered Approaches	Holistic Health-centered Approaches
Ultimate Goal	Abatement of Symptoms	Restore and Maintain Health
Underlying Philosophy	Reactive	Proactive
Action Prompted By	Appearance of Symptoms	Ongoing Desire for Health
Focus	Pathology	Health of Whole Being
Symptoms Represent	Treatment Target	Underlying Health Issue
First Line of Tools	Pharmaceuticals, Surgery	Diet, Movement, Community
What is Actually Practiced	Treatment-care	Health-care

Table 5.1. Characteristics of medical two medical systems that are practiced in the United States (and elsewhere). Some people and professionals practice a mix of aspects of each system. The more one practices from holistic health-centered approaches, the less likely one is to require pathology-centered treatment for chronic disease and other preventable issues.

While it may seem to some readers that this chapter has been about attacking western medicine, this has not been my intent. The discussions have centered on demonstrating the strong bias for this form of treatment despite the documentation of important shortcomings in some areas. I would advocate for a merging of the two forms of medicine, utilizing the strengths of each system. Unfortunately, contemporary humans often view things in an "all in or all out" approach, frequently unable to find a positive middle road. Regardless of this, I hope to inspire some to consider the value of natural medicine (in all its forms) for their curative needs. Following are ten positive actions you can take to improve your understanding of the concept of medicine and heal your person. In doing so, you will better yourself and impose less impact to the world in which you live. Further, you may find holistic healing to be a way you can contribute to your community.

1. Remember what the **purpose of medicine is**. Medicine helps speed the recovery from illness and injury—it is not something we are supposed to ingest our entire lives (with the obvious exception of rare congenital and genetic disorders that cannot be cured). Medicine is not the cure, it is a way of treating, managing, or preventing the appearance of symptoms.

2. **Diet and lifestyle are the cures**. While medicine helps with the symptoms, diet and lifestyle ameliorate the underlying causes that contributed to the appearance of illness. With few

exceptions, a lifetime of taking medicine is an obvious message that your diet and lifestyle are promoting disease. The way to stop the appearance of symptoms is to improve these aspects of your lifeway.

3. **Get yourself off drugs**. By this I refer to both addictive and medical drugs. While pharmaceutical drugs can have a place in healing, most can be substituted with natural remedies that incorporate beneficial lifestyle practices. Drugs anchor you to civilization by eroding your self-reliance. Freedom from pharmacies is an important step in the rewilding of our lives.

4. **Use rest and downtime for treating some transient discomforts** (when possible). We need to stop medicating every discomfort we experience as it is building a populace who cannot tolerate any physical discomfort. It is important to realize that every time we ingest drugs for something that will pass on its own, we experience a risk of side effects or worse (e.g., poisoning due to illicit tampering with drugs).

5. **Explore the true causes of fear that influence your perception of wild medicine**. It takes a very aware and honest person to look closely at biases they hold. If those biases are based simply due to ignorance of the topic, this is easily remedied through identifying plant knowledgeable persons and authors. If those fears center on efficacy and/or safety issues, then go back and read this chapter again.

6. Depending on your level of skill, **use herbal remedies for the ailments you face**. If you are new to herbal medicine, you might begin by purchasing prepared medicine from reputable companies that offer sustainably wild-gathered and organically grown plants. If you have some expertise and live in an area with open space, gather your own and learn to preserve it (through drying, tincturing, infusing in oil, etc.). Continue expanding your knowledge by interacting with new plants each growing season.

7. **Learn the identity and ecology of medicinal plants** so that you can potentially use them when illness and injury occur. Identification of some plants is very straightforward, others are complicated by close look-alike species that require careful observation and understanding of plant morphology to differentiate. A broad knowledge of wild medicine requires an understanding of natural history so that rewilders can find the species we use for medicine. Plant ecology incorporates an understanding of the habitats they grow in, the other plant species they are frequently found with, and the development of the plants through the growing season (i.e., the timing). Without these skills, one will be confined to store-purchased or garden grown remedies.

8. **Develop skill in formulating natural remedies**. Preparing valuable remedies can only be effected only through an understanding of how the medicine will be delivered to the body. There are a number of traditional and modern ways this is done. Formulating medicine is primarily performed by using an extractive medium (e.g., water, alcohol, oil) to draw out plant compounds and then deliver them to the body. Each medium has its advantages and disadvantages that can be learned from elders and authors. None of this information is beyond your capacity to learn, it simply requires some education and practice.

9. If you consider **ceremony incorporating entheogens**, do not treat these plants, fungi, and animals as a means of escape. These are important teachers, and interaction with this medicine should be preceded by entering a proper mindset and voicing a statement of intent. Ceremony should be followed by introspection and expression of appreciation. Find a skilled person (or

even a shaman, curandero, or motewolòn) who can guide you through this process—it can increase the benefit of this practice immensely.

10. Offer **gratitude** for the medicine that heals your body. Practice reciprocity, both direct and indirect, to show the gratitude you have for natural remedies. Express thankfulness not only to the life you have used as medicine but also to the persons and authors who have helped you learn to heal naturally. Remember, you are part of a super-organism (called Gaia), and when you are healthy, the earth is ultimately healthier.

6. Native awareness: learning to see again

Awareness is the ability to use our senses to perceive our environment. It is not solely a capacity to recognize the biotic and abiotic elements of our landscape but also the capability to understand interactions, relationships, and dynamic interdependencies (i.e., ecology). It also helps us determine cause and effect (if we are attentive to our surroundings) that is not influenced by political affiliation. Native awareness was an observational skillset that took generations of living in a location (such as a valley, a watershed, a mountain range) to develop. It went far deeper than simply labeling the life that lived in the region—it was a state of cognizance that allowed an understanding of the web of life and helped to diminish the frequency of short-term-benefit decision making. Awareness shapes consciousness and worldview. If you do not see relationships, you will act as if they don't exist. This chapter is about rekindling our multisensory awareness so that we might recognize how domestication has shaped not just our ability to perceive the world around us but even our willingness to receive the information that tells a crucial story that we must listen to.

MUTED AWARENESS

Indigenous people relied on their awareness for everyday survival. They needed to open up their senses—all of them, and there are more than five—extending them as far out into their environment as they could in order to find resources they needed and keep distance between those elements of the landscape that could harm them (e.g., large animals, poisonous plants, venomous reptiles). Today, as domesticated people, our urban existence tends to narrow our perception of the world, down to about the size of a computer, tablet, or smart phone screen. And we don't use all our collection of senses to their full capabilities (i.e., our existence is becoming more and more confined to the visual and auditory senses). We even sometimes decide to intentionally limit our senses to block out the features of everyday life, including sounds (e.g., honking horns, people yelling, construction equipment), smells (e.g., factory discharge, truck exhaust), and so on. This strategy, of purposely blocking the sensory information coming to our person, is a strategy that would have probably meant the death of a wild person and has severely impacted our ability to perceive the modern world for what it is.

But this is exactly how many of us pass through our lives. We are so bombarded with sensory input from non-natural environments that we have learned to shut down (as a preservation mechanism). And we apply this strategy to many facets of our life. For example, we get so fatigued with all the warnings about this and that being harmful to our health that we just shut down and stop paying attention. We have lost the motivation that drives the art of questioning, a mindset that is exemplified by a young person's curiosity of their world. When we stop trying to perceive the world, problems will ensue. This occurs because we are now unaware of the hazards of our landscape, whether that be human predators lurking in the shadows, industrial predators that rely on people avoiding researching the products they purchase, or poisonous plants that can cause dermatitis (which we blindly walk into).

Most modern humans possess a muted awareness of their surroundings. The process of domestication, with humans spending more time in constructed environments, has been one of the primary drivers of this decline in perceptual abilities. Humans are accustomed to projecting their senses only to the nearest walls, limiting their awareness to the confines of a single geometrically simple room. Even more restricted, their time in the cabin of automobiles has limited their senses to a relatively small bubble, their world perceived by windows strategically oriented for vision in certain directions. Their time on floors, patios, sidewalks, and roads—all level surfaces—means they must look down continuously as they walk in natural locations to avoid tripping or falling. Staring at the ground and using sight to make up for our overly protected feet that cannot sense the environment means people fail to witness the life around them. Unaccustomed to truly using their full sensory capabilities (these commonly over-stimulated in urban landscapes), they are more like children than sensory-competent adults. Fortunately, all of this can be undone. Humans can rekindle their wild senses and learn (again) how to perceive their world in a more natural way.

SENSING OUR WORLD

Rekindling a powerful ability to perceive our world requires two important things. We must both open up our senses again AND rekindle a desire to learn about our world (i.e., ask questions). It is going to create some hassle (and grief) at first—you will be amazed to learn how much our landscapes have been altered and how many products are detrimental to your longevity (for examples). But these are crucial items we must learn and pass on to our children so they have the facts to make informed choices (uninformed choice making is one contributing item that has led us to this point in history).

In order to develop a deep awareness of our surroundings, we must first understand that there are more than just five senses. We have been told repeatedly in our education that we perceive the world through sight, hearing, feeling, tasting, and smelling. However, this is patently false. Do you sense the passage of time? Can you not sense gravity? Do you sense your balance and your position relative to other things? Do you not sense the temperature and its change through time? Can you sense hunger or the need to breathe? What about a sense of belonging? There are many more senses than the five we have learned about during our childhoods. Some authors consider us to have a total of 53 senses, though some of the senses they list may be a composite sense. For example, the ability to sense the mood of someone may be facilitated by seeing their facial expressions and posture, listening to their voice, and perceiving their body positioning relative to ours (and possibly more). But, nonetheless, there are more senses that we can use to understand our world. And limiting our understanding of human senses through stating (and believing) there are merely five may have, to some extent, created a weakened ability to perceive in domesticated humans. (See Reconnecting with Nature by Michael Cohen for a more complete list of senses.)

Questioning is just as vital to awareness as using all our senses. Through a desire to question, we continue to look for information upon which we can build a more complete understanding of the topic of interest, whether that be an unidentified track in the snow or the curious statements made by a politician. Questioning, while used extensively by young children, is documented to decline (extensively) in most adults. Keep in mind, questioning is not just the literal asking of someone for an answer to something but also our own questioning (i.e., study) of various topics. Questioning is a direct reflection of our curiosity to learn. Learning does not (or, at least, should never) stop in our lifetimes. The quenching of curiosity so often seen in modern people is a direct reflection of the quality of life they have experienced (why ask, it is just going to be more bad news). Time in nature and the intentional seeking of a more natural lifestyle are important items that can help rekindle the innate curiosity we were born with. Without a deep desire to question, we simply move passively through this industrial life, our health (and that of the world) under the control of other people and corporations. The book you are now reading is the result of a desire to question.

NATURE OBSERVATION

Observing can be described as more than just seeing. It is seeing (or hearing, smelling, etc.) and comprehending the significance of what is being witnessed by our senses. In that regard, modern humans rarely observe things outside of their fields of expertise. In fact, there are many things, especially natural features, they don't even see at all. There are many contributing factors that have fostered a loss of awareness, a broad topic that could be a book unto itself. One of the most important of these contributing factors is familiarity.

There is a frequently cited phenomenon that states when people look at natural scenes filled with plants and animals, it is the animals that are seen and the plants merely form a background in the image. This aspect of perception has been called "plant blindness" and is blamed on a number of issues by the researchers who have studied this. Familiarity is one of the primary issues at work here. The education received by young people in most affluent countries has a definite zoocentric bias, which unfortunately leads to people not only failing to see plants but also considering animals to be more worthy than plants. However, I would argue that people are not actually plant blind. If you fill an image with familiar plants, such as apple trees loaded with ripe fruits, people will see both the animals in the scene and the plants. In fact, if you send people into a supermarket, where they can find plants that they are accustomed to seeing (i.e., cultivated produce), they will not only see the plants but also be able to make subtle distinctions between cultivars of the same species (i.e., demonstrate they are capable of making fine, taxonomic distinctions, even in the absence of labels). The idea that humans intrinsically see a "wall of green" when they look upon a forest is not true. Unseen items (inattention objects) are more likely to be seen items (attention objects) when the items are part of the person's collective experience. In other words, if they are familiar with the forest trees, they will see the individual species that make up the forest landscape. In essence, there is no background when you have a deep familiarity with your landscape.

Of course, lacking familiarity with wild plants has contributed to a broad spectrum of issues that modern humans face. The fear it generates, unfortunately, causes people to be hesitant about interacting with wild plants at all. Given that plants are, in many ecosystems, an extremely significant portion of the life that occurs there and, in some cases, even define various ecosystems (due to their abundance and essential roles), it is perhaps understandable why I am emphasizing plants in this section. The absence of familiarity creates some very inaccurate ideas about plants (or fungi or lichens or algae, etc.). Consider, for example, wild carrot (*Daucus carota*), an edible plant that is native to Europe and Asia that is naturalized on the North American continent. Whenever this plant is discussed, especially on social media sites that feature discussion of wild edible plants, there is a frequent warning about confusing it with water-hemlock (*Cicuta maculata*). Water-hemlock is a native plant of wetlands that is toxic if a sufficient amount of the foliage is consumed. Aside from the fact that wild carrot occurs in uplands and water-hemlock occurs in wetlands (i.e., they have very different ecologies), there is really no way these two plants should be confused given the tremendous dissimilarity in their foliage (see figure 6.1). If these two species of plants truly look similar to people, it is evidence that those people are unable to discern basic differences in the shapes of leaves. This is an important skill considering leaves are a very common feature on most landscapes and are used extensively in the identification of plants.

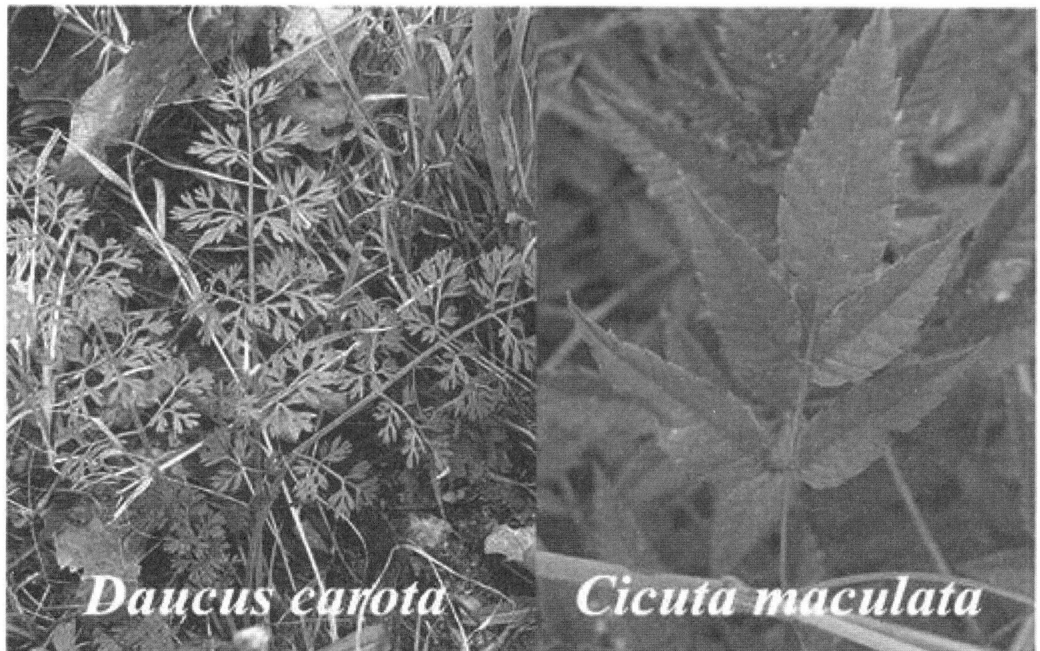

Figure 6.1. Leaves of wild carrot (*Daucus carota*) on left and water-hemlock (*Cicuta maculata*) on right, two species of wild plants that are said to look similar enough to one another that they can be confused. Photos by Arthur Haines.

Nature observation is a necessary skill for those interested in rewilding. It is a talent that must be developed once we step away from the market-oriented world—a realm where each item on the shelf is identified through information found on its associated shopping tag or barcode. Only in the virtual market place do we enter a search term and matching goods are presented on the screen. Creation cannot be automatically sorted by filters that group items by price or color or relevance. Neoaboriginals, like the wild people that came before them, need to use their own senses and mental faculties to discern the interconnected elements of the landscape. This process begins with recognizing the life we share the planet with but, ultimately, goes much further. Once the question of "who" is answered, information gathered from observation can allow the other kinds of questions to be answered (e.g., what, why, where, when, how). It is not simply enough to know, for example, the name of a plant. We must also know what the plant looks like, where it can be found, and when it is to be observed or gathered. As our observational skills improve, we can delve into additional questions—why does it occur here (and not there), what is its role in this region, and how can we cooperate with one another. Of course, to accept these questions as valuable inquiries (as opposed to esoteric or even useless information), we must also tear down the constructs of our modern living. Rewilding requires this to happen on a large scale. We need a full and accurate view of civilization to understand the need to rekindle our native awareness.

THE GROUND IS A MANUSCRIPT

Awareness provides the opportunity to learn that we are not alone in this world; that we share our landscapes with an array of other-than-human persons. Some of these organisms are mobile and some are sedentary. Some communicate by sounds and behaviors, others by pollen and complex chemistry. But regardless of their life histories, all of the world's life leaves behind a record of its existence—though this record may be fleeting in some species. Tracking is one of the skillsets that humans use to read the evidence left behind of an organism's passage. It is a talent that was learned by ancient hominids and passed down through our ancestral lineage to those alive today. It is more than merely an ability to identify the organism who left the track. It is also the ability to create a story from a collection of marks and other signs left upon the ground (or in the snow, on vegetation, etc.). As Mark Elbroch describes it, it is the union of science and storytelling. It is a uniquely human trait. While wolves, for example, can bring the scent of an animal back to the pack by rolling on its carcass or in its feces, this behavior cannot describe the scene, detail the events, and interpret the meaning of actions carried out by the wildlife (or domesticated life) in question. Truly, when humans relearn the art of tracking (i.e., when they recover tracking literacy), the ground is a manuscript with detailed stories that will come alive for anyone with skill and creativity.

Tracking, once a universal skill of wild humans, is a faculty that most alive today only develop to a superficial level. Aside from a few distinctive or commonly encountered tracks, such as species of deer, domesticated dogs, house cats, or car tires, most tracks either go unnoticed or go un-interpreted. There was a time in our history when tracking provided critical information about our landscape, such as the movements of various animals that may have been important sources of nourishment. It was developed to such a high level that hunters could track while running and continue to follow a specific animal when its tracks crossed others of the same herd. As Elizabeth Thomas described of the Ju/wasi (also known as the !Kung) of southern Africa in her book "The Old Way", hunters would need to recognize the tracks of a wounded kudo who is travelling with six or seven other kudu. Given that all the animals were of approximately the same size, it was a significant feat of tracking. This is especially true given that the tracks were just dents in the sand among others dents made by animals of the same herd. The Ju/wasi were expert interpreters of the tracks, as even miniscule signs, such as the tracks of a specific beetle, were useful to them because they understood that that specific insect moved about once the daytime temperature had reached a certain point (for example), and the beetle tracks could be used to age other tracks the beetles had walked over. This is but one example demonstrating the tremendous knowledge and experience that went into following and interpreting the tracks of an animal.

The degree of sophistication in track interpretation even allowed trackers to determine incredible amounts of information from tiny variations in the track created by the animal's size, gender, speed, change of direction, and so on. Even today, where most people derive their nutrition from agricultural or industrial sources, a rekindling of tracking talent opens up many possibilities, including biological inventory work, finding a lost child, security (i.e., tracks left by unwanted persons near a home), recreation and photography, and hunting. Given that many mammals live fairly secretive lives, especially predatory species, tracking allows us to identify their presence and (potentially) consider them in our decision making. But more than this, tracking opens up our awareness to read information from our forests, prairies, and wetlands. It reconnects us with the earth and the life we sometimes forget also inhabits the world.

While a section here in this book cannot do tracking justice, I will take the time to open up this subject a bit more to help readers understand the power of this observational skill. When tracks are encountered, probably the first question most humans ask is **who**? We want to know who left these marks behind. To accomplish this, we do more than simply glance at the track. We study the details of each print, noting such features as the dimensions of the track, the number of toes that register (which can be different on the front and hind feet), if claw marks are visible, and the shapes of the metacarpal pads. Our examination then broadens to examine the gait pattern of the animal, including the width of the trail and distance between steps or bounds, any hairs that may have been removed from the animal when it passed through vegetation or under a fence, and details of its scat or droppings. The "who" question is certainly one of the most fundamentally important questions we ask in tracking, a question that might not be able to be answered until we have gathered enough information by following the trail for a distance.

As we gather more information from the collection of tracks and signs present, we can ask additional questions, queries that lead us from identification to interpretation. Another important question is **what**. With this, we are attempting to identify what the animal was doing at the time the tracks were made. To determine the "what", we use a great deal of information, including the location of the tracks (is food or shelter nearby?). The speed of the tracks can tell us if the animal was walking, bounding, or galloping, which can indicate whether the animal was calm or fleeing from a threat. Are there signs on vegetation, such as browsing, scraping, or scratching? Is there an abundance of feathers, hair, or bones, indicating a kill or a cached food source? The more familiar one becomes with their landscape, the greater the detail that is possible with determining what has happened.

The identification of tracks and interpreting what has happened is even more valuable if one can determine **when**. Without "when", we cannot determine how long ago the tracks were made or if the animal routinely uses a trail in the morning or during the night (for examples). In other words, we simply have a set of observations that are not grounded to any time reference. When is identified through a large set of criteria, ranging from microscopic details of the drying and crumbling of ridges within the track to the identification of more macroscopic events, such as the effects of weather on the track (e.g., is the track filled with debris from a windy night two days ago, is the track obscured by rain from earlier in the day). When provides us with an important frame of reference, ultimately helping us determine the "what" with even more accuracy.

The ability to follow a set of tracks across various kinds of substrate (if necessary) allows us to determine **where**. With this information, we are able to determine where the animal is going and where it has come from. Trailing allows us to compile more and more information about the animal we are following, ultimately giving us greater insight into his or her life. While snow and sand are easy substrates for following tracks, gravel and leaf litter can make it much more difficult to determine the "where" of the animal. Shape shifting into the animal (in a figurative sense), is perhaps the highest ability of the tracker. By "becoming the animal", we follow our wild instincts to identify the direction of travel where the ground is too firm to register obvious details, all with the intent of picking up a lost trail. Trailing is a necessary skill to develop for hunters who may need to locate prey that has travelled some distance before death. It is also a valuable skill for those who assist with the search for missing persons.

Finally, we come to the **why**. The "why" is actually a large set of questions that begins to develop a real relationship with the animal being tracked that answer questions about its biology and personality. Why does the animal come here? Why does it pass this area only near dusk? Why does it bed in that area of the forest? Why do these set of tracks indicate travel in extreme haste? Why do these tracks follow the gravel road and those seem to avoid the road (or vice versa)? These questions begin to enter the realm of ecological tracking, where we start to unravel the mystery of wild animals and become intimately familiar with them. An ability to answer "why" is an important step in realizing a connection to the world, made possible through an understanding of the ecology, which is another way of writing "the sum total of connections", each form of life has to another.

An ability to locate and interpret the meaning of tracks on the ground is a significant advance in the awareness of any contemporary person. Many spend so much of their life on relatively impervious surfaces (e.g., pavement, concrete, flooring) that they are simply unaccustomed to even looking for these temporary chronicles of life. But that can change. There are good manuscripts that register signs of animals in most parts of the world (even in urban areas). We need only look for them, or perhaps begin our journey as trackers by rekindling a curiosity for learning about life. Said another way, we must reawaken the desire to question we had early in our lives. Tracking is the quintessential questioning activity. It involves all the major queries we use to gather information—who, what, when, where, and why. Trackers are seekers of information. They move from track to track (or fact to fact), reconstructing the movements of the animal (or the events leading to an outcome), building a story to share with others. Those stories are sometimes curious or magical, and they are sometimes tragic and sorrowing. Regardless, being aware of our environment (whether it be urban, rural, or wilderness) is not a luxury, it is a necessity (even an obligation for the trackers of the world).

THE LANGUAGE OF BIRDS

When a stone is cast into a pond, concentric rings of small waves flow outward from the point of impact. These waves can be seen by an observer, who can use the waves to surmise something has disturbed the surface of the water and identify the general direction of the disturbance (by tracing backward the path of the waves). This is a good analogy for what happens when a domesticated human (or their domesticated dog) steps into a wild area. Generally, the human is making noise and plainly visible to the wild animals that may live in the area. Many secretive animals and birds that are routinely found on or near the ground will rapidly flee the area to maintain a level of safety afforded by the distance. The rapid retreat of these animals may be accompanied by alarm calls of various kinds, especially among the avian residents of the area. Birds that typically feed high in the canopy may not respond at all to the rapid approach of a human because they are safely located high in the trees and are accustomed to certain animals walking below them. This pattern of behavior—the rapid retreat of a certain group of animals at the advance of a potential predator—can be used by observant people to identify and locate a disturbance in the forest. The fleeing animals are similar to the waves on the pond. All people need to do is tap into what Jon Young refers to as "bird language" to become more aware of the happenings in wild (and not so wild) places.

Bird language works by understanding the patterns of vocalizations and behaviors of birds. Each kind of sound they make, for example, is indicative of their mood, activity, and perceived threats. It can be simplified to two categories (which is a gross simplification that omits much information): baseline and alarm. When birds are in baseline, they are relatively relaxed. Males will sing their particular songs, companions of a flock will call back and forth using specific vocalizations to keep track of one another, juvenile birds will present begging calls to adults for food. Likewise, there will be baseline behaviors, such as feeding, preening, and other maintenance behaviors (e.g., dust and water baths). In alarm, birds stop performing maintenance behaviors and exhibit varying degrees of anxiety. This could be ceasing singing to agitated movements to outright fleeing from a threat and vocalizing specific alarm calls. Birds even flee from different predators in different ways. For example, a terrestrial predator, such as a house cat or a red fox, causes ground-feeding birds to fly to perches in tall shrubs and trees (using height above the ground as a safety). In contrast, an avian predator, such as a species of accipiter or falcon, can cause birds that feed in the canopy to rapidly descend into denser understory vegetation. Ultimately, each bird has a suite of vocalizations and behaviors that can be learned that offer anyone who is tapped into this form of natural communication a greater ability to understand the happenings on the landscape about them, including the approach of other persons.

While it would require many years to learn the significance of all the nuanced vocalizations of birds in a given region (as wild people did over their lifetimes), this topic is often best approached by taking a few common species that are tolerant, at least to an extent, of human-modified landscapes. In this way, people living in suburban areas (or parks within cities) can observe birds and learn to use bird language. It also helps to find birds species that are frequently observed, have small territories, and (when possible) are year-round residents of the area. Species such as the American robin, dark-eyed junco, and song sparrow are birds that are common near my home in northeastern North America that work very well for bird language (though all of these migrate due to our cold winters). In other parts of the world, species of sparrow, wrens, and towhees also are excellent choices to learn with. Simply spending time watching this species respond to approaching people and house pets can be very informative.

It is of interest that bird language is something that people living in less developed countries may learn as part of their upbringing—it was certainly part of the education of hunter-gatherer youth. It has real world application to them, such as locating large (i.e., dangerous) predators and venomous snakes (all of which birds will respond to). People living in highly developed landscapes typically have not learned bird language. In those areas, their settings have been expunged of apex predators by years of concerted effort to make the world safe, and they rely on the police forces to keep them safe from human killers. Therefore, the obvious alarms of birds responding to some threat, which could be a threat to the human as well, are often overlooked as background noise.

Birds can certainly be thought of as the alarm system of different ecosystems (e.g., forests, wetlands, prairies). However, they are not the only group of organisms an alert observer can utilize to understand the current state of the landscape (in terms of baseline, concern, alarm, etc.). For example, many small mammals, such as chipmunks and squirrels, will also vocalize various kinds of whistles, chatter, and barks when disturbed by the approach of a human or another potential predator. Amphibians also produce a chorus of sounds in many regions of the world and, in this case, the absence of sounds can be thought as a potential alarm (when the chorusing amphibians abruptly stop). In eastern North America, the white-tailed deer will create a loud exhaled snort or blow when it alarms. Even insects alter behavior and produce or stop producing sounds as a result of being disturbed. Birds are simply one of the easier groups to tap into and utilize as a kind of awareness of the landscape. While this been called bird language, it is really better described as animal language. But, even then, this name falls short, because it is more than merely vocalizations; it is also the observed behaviors that indicate events that are occurring in the forest or other open spaces. Therefore, bird language can be thought of as simply paying attention to the wild and interpreting its meaning. It is a form of tracking, but rather than tracking prints or signs (made in the past), we are tracking the flow of life very close to the present. We are following the response of one or more organisms to another organism (or organisms). In this way, we are tracking wild relationships and learning more about the ecology of the world we live in.

CIVILIZATION IS ANYTHING BUT CIVILIZED

Anyone reading this book is likely to be a citizen of a civilization. Further, most citizens (especially those in affluent countries) would likely consider civilization to be a magnificent product of human ingenuity. The structures, the art, the music, the sciences, and the collective drive of a society for progress are frequently used as evidence for the beneficial nature of society. People rarely examine civilization in a critical fashion—for if they did, they would see that civilizations carry out actions that would be considered quite barbarous to the objective observer. In any chapter (or book) that is attempting to create an awareness of the detriments of modern living, some discussion of civilization must be presented. While this section is not a call for the dismantling of industrial society, it is intended to generate a better understanding of the outcomes of civilization; which is to write about another product of humans when they become divorced from nature. If we are ever to have any chance at all of building a truly ethical civilization, we must recognize and publicly acknowledge the injurious features of all civilizations—past and present. Without this acknowledgment and action on this information, there will be no wild land left upon which people can rewild. This may read as very pessimistic and gloomy but it is an unfortunate truth that we need to embrace. Ultimately, we need more people living in communities, and the "civilizations" of the future need to evolve (in specific ways) from those of today.

First, we must briefly define civilization so that we are all on the same page. While I am not attempting to establish Wikipedia as the ideal source for all accurate information, the definition used on that web resource does provide a place to begin discussion.

"A civilization (US) or civilisation (UK) is any complex society characterized by urban development, social stratification, symbolic communication forms (typically, writing systems), and a perceived separation from and domination over the natural environment. Civilizations are intimately associated with and often further defined by other socio-politico-economic characteristics, including centralization, the domestication of both humans and other organisms, specialization of labor, culturally ingrained ideologies of progress and supremacism, monumental architecture, taxation, societal dependence upon agriculture, and expansionism."

There are a lot of points that could be discussed in this definition, with many notable departures from the cultural systems of wild humans. Important to our awareness are the ideas of progress and supremacy, two features of civilization that lead to some very poor outcomes for the environment and people (and not just the people from outside the civilization, but also the people within it).

The writing here has suggested that civilization is not all good. So, what is so bad about it (aside from the physical and emotional health effects that we have already discussed)? First, and perhaps foremost, civilization is based on violence. Without this, essentially no civilization that has existed could have occurred. This is because civilizations (which are comprised of agriculturalists) have taken land from hunter-gatherers, people who did not voluntarily allow the land they lived upon to be usurped and damaged for resource extraction. In fact, history has clearly demonstrated that traditional peoples (including hunter-gatherer cultures) were often a thorn in the side of large companies and nations who wished to obtain timber, precious metals, and petroleum from land occupied by these people. Such traditional communities were destroyed in the past through murder and displacement. Today, civilization acculturates hunter-gatherers, bringing them into the modern world under the guise of improving the quality of their life (though in reality doing exactly the opposite). Such actions amount to ethnocide, essentially destroying the culture (without killing the people outright) so that resource extraction can continue.

Civilizations are well known for their expansionist ideology, increasing their territory through various means, most often with military activity. As a result, these expansions are rarely without violent conflict. Each civilization arrives at the conclusion that its hostile taking of land from other people is acceptable for one or more reasons (e.g., its contribution to the world is more beneficial than that of other civilizations, its creation story is more accurate and this story must be shared with more people). The people within each civilization are usually accepting of the expansion because they have been raised with an ideology of patriotism (the social conditioning for the acceptance of a country's decisions and actions). And it is not simply the establishment of a nation that involves violence but also the maintenance of a nation (through competition for resources, defending of borders, forcing religious or political systems on other nations, etc.). If you don't believe civilizations are violent, you should spend time examining the history (and current events) of civilizations. Taking a look at the United States, it was founded on a violent taking of land from the indigenous inhabitants and has not even gone a full decade without being involved in some military action since the American Revolutionary War. The longest stretch of relative peace I'm aware of is 5 years, which happened between the Banana Wars and World War 2 (note: police actions and occupations that involved the deployment of military troops and use of lethal force are here considered to be what they actually were—wars). According to Washington's Blog (which updated Danios' original article from 2011), the United States has been at war 93% of the years since its independence in 1776. While the United States did not initiate all of these conflicts, it nonetheless demonstrates how aggressive civilizations are. The primary issue is that civilizations' borders, their ability to take resources from distant lands, and their ability to "govern" the member inhabitants would all breakdown without violence or at least the threat of hostility. While we are fond of noting the humanitarian aid that affluent countries provide, it pales in comparison with the money spent on their militaries. While violence certainly existed in hunter-gatherer cultures, those cultures were not based on violence (i.e., if all violence disappeared, the cultures themselves would not also disappear).

There are several notable authors that would argue we currently live in the most peaceful time for humanity and that violence is actually declining in the world. I politely but strongly disagree with such a statement and would note that it requires both an overlooking of certain kinds of violence and a twisting of data to allow Steven Pinker and others to come to their conclusions of this age being a peaceful one. To begin, they must use a very strict definition of violence—human on human violence. Any other violent acts, such as human on environment (i.e., ecocide), are not considered in the equations. It requires a fundamental lack of awareness to consider our industrial efforts as peaceful while they cause another mass extinction event. If anyone were to stand in the middle of a northern forest and witness the devastation that comes with oil sands extraction (for example), they might better understand how this is a form of violence. And as we deplete natural resources and pollute the air, water, and soil we require for living, it is clear that we are also committing violence on unborn people—human on future human violence. This is also not considered in Pinker's work. But even if we stick to the present-day arguments and limit our discussion to people vs. people, there are still many problems with the idea we live in peaceful times. War time figures are distorted, considering only those that die directly in battle, and not necessarily those that die years later from starvation, sickness, and disease in the aftermath that follows armed conflicts. Are the deaths from upheaval and turmoil that result from planned assassinations and remote drone strikes included in these figures? What about torture (which affluent countries still use, though more covertly), rape, work camps, child labor, sex trafficking, and so on? These are all prevalent forms of violence that exist today, most of which were not found or rarely found in egalitarian cultures. Of course, it must be mentioned that the reason many affluent countries don't engage each other today in direct armed conflict is for fear of nuclear war. This does not make us peaceful, it makes us fearful of the most destructive weapons ever created. I hope that I am not alone in realizing that fear and peace are different things. There is little doubt that we currently live in a violent period.

It is interesting to note human civilizations function very differently from ecological systems. In the latter, diversity and complexity are traits that provide stability. In regions with limited numbers of species, such as arctic landscapes, the ecology of the region is less stable and populations are more subject to boom and bust cycles. Essentially, the more species that exist in an area (which is another way of writing that more interactions exist), the more stable an ecosystem is against perturbations. However, this is exactly the opposite seen in civilization. The more complex a society becomes (i.e., more classes of people, more laws and regulations), the more fragile it is and more likely to experience collapse. The most enduring human cultures have been those that are simpler, with fewer categories of people (both professionally and hierarchically). However, it is completely possible that this observation is only valid because of the way we define complexity. It may well be that egalitarian communities, where work is performed without supervisors to direct efforts, are actually more complicated than they appear on the surface. The coordination of hunting and gathering, seasonal tribe migration, communal ceremony, and similar features of life in a culture where everyone is autonomous and contributes to decision making may actually demonstrate a greater degree of social complexity (especially in cooperation), given that consensus is reached among the members of the culture. This stands in stark contrast to civilizations, where one or few people (often elected or appointed) make decisions on behalf of others. Therefore, the opening statements of this paragraph may require modification—the kind of social complexity that emerges in civilizations (e.g., political, religious, bureaucratic) contributes to a fragility of those societies.

It should be very telling that no human civilization that relies on agriculture and/or industry has ever been "sustainable". They always damage their landbase and ultimately collapse for one or more reasons (sometimes, this collapse is precipitated by the invasion of another civilization). Instead of covering the reasons for societal collapse, we could, instead, examine what frequently happens after a society collapses. The qualities possessed by those post-collapse civilizations could be seen as features that exist in more stable versions of human society—and can be used as guiding principles of rewilded communities. Certainly, civilizations that are overthrown or completely obliterated will not necessarily display the characteristics discussed in the following paragraph.

The collection of ruling power into the hands of relatively few people (sometimes even concentrated within a particular region of a civilization) is undone when a civilization falls. During **decentralization** of power, people become more self-governed and the inhabitants of individual communities will experience more personal freedom. Decentralization of the population also occurs because cities are not fertile ground for the gathering or cultivating of food. Therefore, people migrate away from the centers of empires to the less developed countryside. As they migrate to relatively more rural settings, people must commit to **despecialization**. Urban centers are populated with people who have a high level of job specialization. Rural living requires that people be able to perform a larger proportion of the daily tasks for living. In fact, many highly specialized guilds (such as religious and political elites) are forced into self-sufficiency because the base of people who worked on their behalf is largely eradicated. However, this reality will also be experienced by various professionals who focus on extremely limited and complex topic areas. As a society falls, there is a **destratification** that occurs. Hierarchy is often based on features such as wealth, ethnicity, and religion, all of which may become less important or completely irrelevant after a collapse. For example, the amount of paper currency you own doesn't imply you will be better fed during resource scarcity when knowledge of edible plants (for example) is a better indicator of your ability to survive. The civilization becomes more horizontally structured as features that perpetuated social hierarchy, such as a warrior class (i.e., the military) or ruling religious institution, become dismantled. A degree of **destructualization** is often found post-collapse, given that immense structures and large public works require people and resources in abundance (two items that may not be present post-collapse). Therefore, constructed structures tend to be smaller and of more imminent importance. And, of course, essentially all collapses involve some degree of **depopulation**. Most often, the population declines are substantial.

These commonly observed features of civilization post-collapse are especially useful in examining why collapse occurs. Cleary, if decentralization, despecialization, destratification, destructuralization, and depopulation are observed as societies stabilize after a fall, then it stands to reason that their antonyms—centralization of power, an extraordinary degree of professional specialization, a highly stratified populace, extremely structured landscapes, and large populations, in some form or another, are features that create or exacerbate instability within civilizations. In fact, observations of hunter-gatherer cultures demonstrated that their people were relatively autonomous, were highly self-sufficient, were egalitarian, did not erect large structures, and consisted of small, dispersed populations. If these are, in fact, characteristics of people who lived for countless generations without infringing on people's sovereignty and destroying the landbase, then we need to ultimately rethink our perception of civilization. Perhaps most importantly, we need to recognize that our present version of civilization will not permit either wild or rewilded people to exist in large numbers. Neither of these groups would willingly hand over their sovereignty to people who make decisions in favor of a minority of the population (people who are wealthy or otherwise politically powerful).

While you might dispute the statement that our elected politicians make decisions that largely favor those with political power, a recent example will illustrate this idea well. In several polls taken, the American public overwhelmingly demonstrated that they wanted foods that contained genetically modified organisms (GMOs) to be labeled. Several polls taken by various agencies demonstrated between 93 and 96 percent support for the labeling of GMOs. However, the US House of Representatives voted in a manner that would prevent this from occurring (through legislation misleadingly titled "The Safe and Accurate Food Labeling Act of 2015"). This occurred due to the lobbying power of various organizations, and the legal bribery we refer to as "campaign contributions" made by companies that profit from GMOs. Here is a clear example of elected officials making decisions that benefit a small proportion of the country's population (who are coincidentally wealthy) and making decisions that stand in contradiction to the people's long-term health.

Civilization becomes a force unto itself. Its leaders and its people become accustomed to the idea of progress, a growth and development of the civilization that, unfortunately, occurs at the expense of other life. The idea that things are not well enough now, and that we must advance toward a utopian future with humans enjoying even more comfort, privilege, and longevity is flawed from the outset (because such a progression is not perpetually sustainable). The large governmental bureaucracy that a civilization creates becomes convinced that it must continue to exist, even when it is clearly acting against the interests of and harming the long-term survival of its citizens (e.g., destroying the landbase that the population requires for continued survival, entering conflicts that do not involve the protection of its boundaries). It is extremely poignant that exposing illegal governmental actions is itself illegal (such as Edward Snowden's exposing of unlawful collection of cellular phone metadata by the National Security Agency). Rewilding will require neoaboriginals to take a fresh look at civilization. One could go so far as to write that we need to initiate an evolution of this feature of human domestication. To re-examine civilization, we must also consider why we (its citizens) allow it to continue causing harm.

THE OUTCOMES OF DOMESTICATION

We have discussed in chapters one and two various outcomes of human domestication. Here, we must continue to develop awareness and identify what are now intrinsic characteristics of modern humans. While this section (and the previous) may seem as radical departures from the awareness topics of this chapter, it must be understood that nature awareness and urban cognizance are different aspects of the same topic—a greater ability to perceive aspects of our world. As contemporary humans shifted from an ecocentric lifeway to an egocentric one, various features have become part of modern living. I refer to these as the **seven truths of domestication**. These are features that define substantive changes in form, worldview, and lifeway from wild to domesticated humans. These are also features that promote a continued separation from nature.

1. **Humanist ideology**. A fundamental shift in the way humans perceived themselves occurred in the last 10 to 12 thousand years. This transition can be described as a philosophy espousing the great value of human beings and the products of their industry (including landscape modifications). Despite abundant evidence to the contrary, the belief in human superiority is easily accepted in a population with an egocentric worldview (read "pathological ego"). In fact, a faith in human superiority is a common feature of the occupants of civilization. This quickly evolves into some occupants believing they are more valuable than others, and decision making leads to biased outcomes, benefitting certain people far more than others. A humanist ideology requires, at its core, a conviction that humans are separate from the rest of the world.

2. **Spatial framework changes**. Humans have switched from a focus-oriented spatial framework to a boundary-oriented spatial framework. Wild humans utilized sites of importance (i.e., of focus), sites that were scattered about a landscape and connected by travel routes. Their environment was not fractured by human-made objects, and the lack of architectural structures maintained a worldview with less delimitation and categorization. With the advent of sedentism, architecture became an important aspect of life. Buildings, rooms, and walls were commonly encountered features of modern society. As such, there were (and are) ample restrictions to travel (even if only through laws and private ownership that created virtual fences). Space became more important than place. This was especially true as some urban centers become extremely populous (i.e., space was need for expansion). The ideas of restrictions and compartmentalization of the landscape then becomes entrenched in the worldview of the humans living in such a boundary-oriented framework. It falsely creates discrete categories that ultimately affect other aspects of living, leading to thinking in terms of black and white, right and wrong, good and evil, etc.

3. **Disconnection from natural systems**. When humans transitioned to a new worldview, they became gradually more disengaged from the processes occurring around them. Said another way, they spent progressively less time as participants on their landscape and more time attempting to control the landscape through modification. Modern humans engage in destructive practices that harm the very elements they require for survival. Nature divorcement is accepted by domesticated humans because of the erroneous interpretation that the environment is not part of the divine cosmos but, rather, a source of raw materials upon which to build human civilization. Nature is now regarded as something that must be conquered in the push for continued progress.

4. **Altered characteristics**. Domesticated humans possess a suite of characteristics that identify them as a separate form from wild humans. These include a number of morphological traits (e.g., cranio-facial changes, crowded teeth, weaker bones, less robust musculature, increased fat deposition), as well as many behavioral traits (e.g., larger litter size, social stratification, almost complete reliance on delayed-return food systems). These altered characteristics ultimately have shaped humans in such a way that they are no longer supremely adapted for living on their unmodified landscapes. Outside of cities, cyberspace, and agricultural landscapes, most modern humans are incapable of long-term survival.

5. **Reduction in information acquisition systems**. Wild humans living on pristine landscapes required awareness. They perceived and analyzed information from nature to navigate hazards (immediate and upcoming), acquire nutrition and other materials for living, plan activities, and better understand their place. They used a variety of senses and tools for perceiving their world (e.g., tracking, bird language, sky watching). Modern humans, by and large, are not well suited for observing their landscapes—which includes both natural and industrial versions. Information is now gathered about their world primarily from a speaker and/or a screen (i.e., domesticated humans do not gather and analyze the information themselves, rather they receive information about their world from various news and reporting agencies). The deterioration of observation skills has led to a reduced environmental responsiveness, in which facets of the environment are not perceived as dynamically interrelated and ongoing insults to it do not lead to a change in action.

6. **Decline of experience**. Modern humans experience less of creation than wild humans because they have become content with second-hand experience. Sports, reality TV, fictional stories, and similar items are now a mainstay of modern, sedentary recreation. Such activities can be described as a small group of people performing or acting out motions and sounds based on a script or set of rules while others watch and listen. While film, music, books, video games, and other such media can store valuable cultural information, most of these are used to escape the very reality that domesticated humans have created for themselves. As they interact less and less with their outdoor world (and more and more with a virtual, cyber-world), they become more and more removed from real, first-hand experiences. This means they are no longer participating in the present and can feel disconnected from reality.

7. **Increased docility**. A characteristic feature of domesticated animals is tameness. This important change in temperament means the populace is willing to accept decisions (and the resulting conditions from those decisions) made on their behalf by an elected group of representatives who do not often act for the common good. With more dependence on a built environment, modern humans require more comforts, leading to even more acceptance of harmful social trends for fear of losing those comforts. Therefore, despite an accumulation of

knowledge by society, the more docile nature of the populace means that obvious issues may not be addressed in a timely fashion. In other words, there is a social inertia surrounding some important topics (e.g., ecological crises, human rights violations) that would require changing the way they interact with the world. The increase in submissiveness means there is more time engaged in activity that results in no change (e.g., complaining) and less real activism, even when activism is plainly needed. Docility should not to be confused with nonaggression. A docile populace follows decisions made on their behalf, even if those decisions lead to senseless violence.

Rewilding provides us with a way of recovering from domestication and ultimately undoing these seven features of modern humans. "Wildness" is not simply defined as a human living in the wild. It is a human that has a deep understanding of his or her place, which produces an ability to live sustainably in that place (and by sustainable, we are not referring to the "greenwashing" version of this word used by some members of industry). Therefore, wildness is not merely a program of skills and other techniques for obtaining food and medicine (or whatever) from a place but an awareness that develops a characteristic worldview—one that promotes connection to and sustainable living in that place. Using this definition of rewilding, anyone living anywhere can move along this path through learning about the outcomes of civilization and domestication. This learning promotes awareness, and awareness is needed to understand the deep need for a new path.

RECOVERING NATIVE AWARENESS

Awareness is by far the most important aspect of rewilding that must be developed. Without it, we are unable to critically examine the paradigms of civilization and ultimately arrive at informed conclusions (vs. the collective opinions of a given society, which may not align with sound logic or healthy emotion). The recovery of native awareness is much more than abandoning a blind faith in civilization (which is not to write that all aspects of civilization must be abandoned, but that some of its assumptions must be questioned). Many people are willing to question society so long as they have a trusted guru to lead them through difficult decision making. However, blindly following a single person is still failing to grasp the idea that awareness can generate self-reliance. And self-reliance is based on the development of skills that allow a person to exercise their sovereignty. Without awareness, we are all simply automatons of society, whether we follow its political leaders or its health and wellness gurus.

Awareness is not merely the cultivation of philosophical ideas that are more in line with sustainable, traditional communities but also the actual practice of becoming more adept at perceiving our environment. Recognizing the life we share the planet with and understanding its significance (i.e., its role) to the landscape it inhabits requires us to do more than just look—we must also be able to interpret what we see. There are many tools (i.e., strategies) for developing heightened perception, and those tools may vary based on the environment where each person resides. One set of exercises is called the **Seven Points of Awareness**, a teaching tool used by Mike Douglas of the Maine Primitive Skills School that I find very useful for awareness development and recovery. These seven exercises are by no means comprehensive, and they should not be seen as something you practice and then cease to perform (i.e., these can be used throughout your waking hours). They are also highly adaptable to different situations and environments.

1. **Sacred silence**. An organism's ability to perceive its environment is based on its ability to be in a state of mind to receive information. With demanding and frantic lives comes a mind that is filled with thoughts regarding happenings and obligations. Clearly, a busy mind is busy minding and not busy perceiving. Slowing down, letting go of troubling thoughts (temporarily), and being in the present help us to enter a state of heightened perception. This state of being can literally be measured using sensitive medical equipment (such as an electroencephalograph). The brain uses bioelectrical energy as part of its communication, which occurs in rhythmic or repetitive fashion that is described as neural oscillation (i.e., brain waves). Most people spend their waking day in a state that produces beta waves, a neural oscillation at a particular frequency. While normal, too much time in a beta state can be associated with anxiety, an inability to relax, and stress. Neural oscillations at a slightly slower frequency (alpha waves) are observed when people enter deep relaxation, but are possible during waking times (including through meditation). These waves are a bridge between the conscious and unconscious states (i.e., even lower frequency brain waves). During an alpha state, people are primed for learning, imagination, and creativity. This state of being is extremely useful for entering states of heightened awareness. Sacred silence may, at first, be attainable only through sedentary activity, such as meditation. Ultimately, this state of being needs to be attainable in dynamic settings while on the move. The sacred silence can enable prolonged states of engaging all of your senses while interacting with the environment. Without this point of awareness, the remaining six are difficult to achieve to a high proficiency.

2. **Fox walking**. The ability to move quietly and unseen is fundamentally important to observing. If we are to observe other life in its natural state, to learn what we can about its habits, its lifestyle, and how it responds to its world (i.e., its biology), we cannot intrude in such a way as to alter the behavior of the individual or individuals we are observing. In other words, stealth and concealment are aspects of observation. While this is a large topic, it is perhaps best approached by teaching people to walk more quietly so that they do not cause the level of disturbance usually observed at the approach of domesticated humans. Fox walking is a method of moving that uses the feet as sensory appendages and enables the user to move much more quietly in a variety of settings. While it does not require a change in posture, it does require those using it to keep their heads up so that their eyes can continue to scan forward. Each step is done in greater balance than the usual walking step seen on urban sidewalks, with an ability to stop and prevent the footfall from occurring if necessary. It also involves lifting the foot slightly higher in order to avoid objects that could cause a trip (this is in contrast to the usual shuffle practiced by most humans, where the foot hardly leaves the ground). The outside of the foot touches first, sensing the ground for objects (including sticks and other brittle objects). The foot gently rolls toward the inside, gradually transitioning weight to that leg. Fox walking is typically done at slower speeds than the usually observed walk, and it is a transitional technique to stalking (where a crouched form and even hands braced on the thighs is used). Moving in the fox walk keeps noise down and the head up for better sensory awareness.

3. **Wide-angle vision**. This skill allows the use of the entire eye for surveying scenes and quickly detecting movement. It is effected by relaxing focus on a single item and allowing the vision to spread out so that even the peripheral portions of the eye can be involved in viewing (i.e., utilizing a soft stare). This technique is also called splatter vision by some authors. Once the broad, soft stare is achieved, any movement is quickly detected and then focus on that object can help determine the specific "who" or "what" that is responsible for the movement. Wide-angle vision is the opposite of focusing on a specific object, and it represents a broadening of the visual sense to counter the frequently used "tunnel vision" when an object of interest is spotted

(and in which time all things on the periphery are overlooked). Those who use their visual sense to a high degree rapidly transition between wide-angle vision and focused vision as they move through natural landscapes, allowing not just movement, but colors, contours, and textures to become more noticeable to the observer.

4. **Deer ears**. Humans don't have an ability to move their ears or change their shape to help discern distant or weak sounds. However, we can use our hands to do just that. By cupping our hands behind our ears, we can adjust the exterior portion of our ears to direct them both forward. The cupped hands help to gather sounds. This practice, called "deer ears" is an excellent way to amplify and locate sounds that may to too soft to distinguish well with our ears in their natural position. While we don't have the "native equipment" to practice what deer do, we have extremely dexterous hands that allow us to perceive and trace the origin of sound. We can even extend this practice to using the landscape (including boulders and trees) that can help gather distant sounds and intensify them.

5. **Total sensory awareness**. Human eyesight is an amazing gift and often also a serious constraint in that we rely on it too much. Our eyesight can become a limiting factor when other senses are ignored (or not developed over our lifetimes), especially in settings where the eyes cannot function well (e.g., in darkness, in extremely busy settings). Compounding this issue is the fact that many people live in settings, such as urban centers, where information must be intentionally ignored to maintain sanity. Total sensory awareness is opening up and using all of our senses to perceive our environment. It is extending our senses outward as far as they can reach in all directions. And it is also allowing the senses to combine for a composite view of our reality. When in total sensory awareness, people are using those senses they often neglect, including our largest sensory organ (our skin). We often think of about skin as connected to the sense of touch (which is true), but it can do so much more. Our skin can detect wind and its direction, the presence of the sun and shade (based on temperature differences), and all the items we usually associate with touch, including textures beneath our feet. While urban settings are clearly rife with an overload of movement, sounds, and smells, this can be quite true of rural and wild settings when people learn to use total sensory awareness. This point of awareness cannot be developed until the sacred silence can be achieved.

6. **Focal points and dead spaces**. Focal points are those features on our landscape that we tend to center on. These might be mountains, buildings, or gardens. The dead spaces are those places in between (possibly even in the shadows) that we tend to ignore because there is nothing there drawing our focus. Concentrating on focal points means we perceive only part of our environment and potentially miss important items (predators are especially adept at concealing themselves in dead spaces). This point of awareness is about de-focusing on the obvious and observing the dead spaces that we routinely ignore. For example, rather than seeing only the trees, we need to also see the empty spaces between the trees (and between the branches and leaves). Focal points and dead spaces is not solely about our eyesight—this awareness strategy pertains to all of our senses. Therefore, when you vary your vision, try also to vary your other senses.

7. **Avoiding the rut of routine**. This point of awareness is very much related to focal points and dead spaces but it is a strategy we apply even more broadly. Many domesticated people move through life on autopilot, following a similar daily routine. Seeing the same thing day after day has conditioned us to stop looking, even though there may be important things to see. After years of living within a deeply entrenched pattern, it becomes difficult to perceive our

environment, let alone consider another way of living. Certainly, the rut of routine can be so deep as to obscure our ability to be open to new information. Therefore, breaking routine is vital to building awareness. Varying our daily activity (even if just the usual commute to work) forces us to perceive new features on our landscape. As Tom Brown Jr. writes, breaking our habits and looking at the unfamiliar in the places we frequent and looking at the familiar with a fresh perspective help us break free from this tendency. He calls these strategies "the same new thing" and "a new viewpoint", respectively. Both of these are valuable skills for avoiding the rut of routine.

NEOABORIGINAL STRATEGY FOR AWARENESS

Awareness changes a human, and those changes present visible signs that can be seen by others who know what to look for. The changes can be thought of as developmental stages that people go through as they generate a deeper understanding of the world. Anyone who is aware of these changes, these indicators, can even use them as goals to track the development of personal awareness that leads to growth of the individual. These indicators of awareness are sometimes presented using the model of the eight directions. They include such signs as common sense, aliveness, focus, caring, service beyond self, and reverence. I encourage those interested in this topic to pursue the work of John Young (and the schools that follow this model), as these indicators of awareness provide excellent benchmarks on which to assess the extent to which experiential and nature-based education is promoting the development of a healthy human, best exemplified through their increase in awareness.

In this chapter, we have focused on not only awareness as it pertains to our senses but also on awareness as it relates to an understanding of humanity. Cultivating native awareness requires us to focus on both kinds of awareness (i.e., what we sense and what we understand). It requires both child-like curiosity and adult-like focus to grasp how much awareness in modern humans has been muted by domesticated living. Civilization, in its current form, can exist only because of this suppression of our desire and ability to perceive our landscape and the events occurring (this manifests as a general apathy about personal and environmental health). In many ways, this chapter should have gone first in this book. However, it was important that a number of key topics were discussed so that you, the reader, could begin to understand that those things we have learned about diet and water and medicine (and so on) are often very inaccurate (or important aspects of those topics are rarely discussed). At this point, it is hoped you understand the need to reawaken our perceptive abilities. Following are ten strategies you can follow to rewild your awareness.

1. **Rekindle a curiosity for life**. Awareness requires inquisitiveness. If there is no desire to see, very little will be seen. If you are having a difficult time envisioning how to bolster your curiosity, simply follow young children around and emulate their behavior. Explore your world, including your natural landscapes, as if you were a young child.

2. Learn to **quiet your mind**, which is another way of writing "live in the present". This ability to avoid clouding our mind with stressful things (past, present, and future) helps us enter the sacred silence, a state of being that allow us to receive information from our environment most efficiently. While we cannot forget our obligations (e.g., bills, upcoming work, necessary tasks), these do not have to be constantly present.

3. Find a location where you can practice **total sensory awareness**, a place where you feel comfortable sitting and allowing all the information from your environment to be perceived and analyzed by your amazing sensory system. By not blocking information, we can rebuild our body's capability to detect light, sound, odor, touch, and the many other wonderful sensations humans are able to perceive.

4. **Question everything**. We have been led to believe that our present situation is one of technological achievement and social evolution. These beliefs stand on shaky ground when truthful answers are obtained for the right questions.

5. Learn to **move more quietly** so that you can encounter more wildlife when in natural and human-modified areas. Fox walking is an excellent way to move across the landscape without scattering the more secretive (i.e., wary) animal life. Stealth and concealment are important aspects of observation, the more talent you develop in these areas, the more you will see. Consider extending fox walking to be a metaphor for how you move through life.

6. Develop your ability to **track**. This was a universal human talent and you need only find the right mentor to awaken your ability—it is already there in your genes. Tracking is where the science of reading small indentations on the ground and interpreting other signs comes alive with storytelling. Trackers help the world see how much life surrounds us at each moment. Authors such as Mark Elbroch have excellent tracking resources for animals, and Tom Brown Jr. has pioneered (for modern people) the ability to interpret the meaning within a given track.

7. Focus some of your attention on the interaction of wildlife with people and other wild animals. Notice how **bird language** can give you clues to the presence of other animals who may not visible. This language, which includes the vocalizations and noises made by rodents, beaver, deer, frogs, and other species, is a very valuable tool for situational awareness in many kinds of environments. John Young has a number of resources to help people learn this skill.

8. Understand the **seven truths of domestication** and how your life has been influenced by these changes. The very way you perceive your environment and what is beneficial or detrimental is based on these features (and modified by your specific social upbringing). The only way to transcend these detrimental changes is to be aware of them and the factors that produced them. Domestication produces an organism that is adapted to a version of living that is anything but sovereign.

9. Ultimately, awareness is not about seeing a thing, but **seeing the interactions between things**. Awareness at this level helps us understand the roles that each life form plays in the maintenance of life on this planet. It helps humans understand there is no hierarchy of life. When we can perceive and interpret ecology, we can also understand how wild humans have a positive role to play on this earth, one that celebrates life and does not need to rule over it.

10. **Have gratitude for your senses**. Humans have the capability for highly developed awareness and can use these senses for remarkable purposes. Such capability was possessed by wild humans and can be recovered by those on a rewilding path. Thankfulness is a state of mind that assists with the sacred silence.

7. Being wild: unlearning domestication and reconnecting with nature

Humans have been immersed in natural settings for most of their existence. Only relatively recently have people lived in largely constructed environments. These settings lack the complexity and ever-changing patterns that are found in nature (i.e., seasonal decorations in urban centers are poor replacements for the earth's seasonal changes). People can now spend the entire waking portion of the day without making contact with ground or even seeing the sun for those working certain professions. Research is beginning to uncover that disconnection from nature is not healthy for *Homo sapiens*. Considering that we are the descendants of hominids whose form, emotions, and spirits were all influenced by (in fact, developed in concordance with) a deep immersion in nature, to remove us from the natural setting has consequences—just as to remove us from a natural diet has consequences. And while these outcomes may not, in and of themselves, generate disease, they certainly can exacerbate existing conditions, slow healing, and promote depression. Modern humans will ultimately need to recognize that their created landscapes are poor substitutes for the wild reality they are designed to live within.

THE BENEFITS OF NATURE IMMERSION

Natural areas are those places where human architecture, media, and technology are largely (or completely) absent. Such areas include places like forests, rivers, lakes, prairies, deserts, mountains, valleys, glaciers, beaches, wetlands, and barrens. These natural areas need not always be vast regions of wilderness. Humans (and other-than-human persons) derive benefit even from small forest fragments, an undeveloped portion of a lake shore, or a stretch of beach without homes. This is not to write that intact wilderness isn't crucial as well, only that our immersion in nature does not always require us to be extremely distant from civilization. Nor does it mean that the landscapes need to be completely free from human modification (something that is, in fact, difficult to locate except in extreme environments too cold, too dry, or too high to live in). While lawns, mowed fields, and manicured parks are all an improvement over pavement, concrete, and brick, areas without obvious marks of human habitat modification will be more valuable to people who are trying to reconnect with nature (in the long run) because the imagery, sounds, smells, and other features will be more wild.

While it seems we should not require studies to demonstrate a benefit of wilderness (or areas that emulate some qualities of wilderness) to people, the fact is domesticated humans have reached an unfortunate point in history where such a requirement does exist. Human worldview today is shaped by various societal factors (including politics and religion) that promote disconnection from wild areas and even aversion to the very idea of wildness. The modern concept of the world, one where technology is the savior, allows continued loss of time in nature and the natural areas themselves. Of course, it should be apparent that depriving people of wild areas, the very environment that humans evolved within, would be detrimental in some way. But, here we are, living in a time where such arguments need to be supplied. The following paragraphs present some of the results of emerging research that demonstrates a variety of benefits resulting from nature immersion—for all age classes of humans.

Atchley et al. (2012) tested the cognitive ability of hikers backpacking in remote areas of the United States (Alaska, Colorado, Maine, and Washington). The research compared the creative thinking and insight problem solving of two groups: those at the beginning of the hike (i.e., without prolonged exposure to nature) and those who spent four days in a wilderness setting without access to technological media. The research was prompted by several observations of outdoor recreation time that they discussed in the introduction. For example, collected data from other research suggested that children today spend only 15–25 minutes in outdoor play (a figure that is apparently declining). National park visitation (in per capita visits) is declining, as is outdoor recreation in general. Concurrent with less time in nature is the fact that more time is spent on various kinds of media, so much so that the children and young adults ages 8–18 years spend, on average, over 7.5 hours each day on computers, televisions, cell phones, and other such devices. They noted that the modern environment is filled with events that distract attention and deplete attentional resources. Participants of the study designed by Atchley and colleagues who were tested after time in wilderness areas showed marked increase in higher-order cognitive skills (based on the testing they employed). They suggested that:

"natural environments, like the environment we evolved in, are associated with exposure to stimuli that elicit a kind of gentle, soft fascination, and are both emotionally positive and low-arousing."

Time in nature, away from technological media, appears to bolster creativity and allow people to access a broad array of cognitive resources when tasks demand complex problem solving. This is hypothesized to be the result of restful introspection that can occur in natural settings, a practice that may be necessary for peak psychosocial health. More recent studies also corroborate these results that exposure to nature improves certain aspects of cognitive function (such as those by Bratman and colleagues published in 2015).

Proximity to and time in nature has been shown to be correlated with improved moods and overall happiness. In fact, people living within one kilometer (0.6 miles) of nature experience less anxiety and depression based on a Dutch study. Natural environments appear to exert a positive influence on mood. The study examined 24 parameters of health, including cardiovascular, respiratory, and neurological conditions. People living in urban areas experienced increased incidence in 15 of the 24 health parameters. The strongest correlations were for anxiety disorder and depression, with those living in cities experiencing lower emotional health. The research also showed that people living on low incomes and children suffer disproportionately from limited access to nature (including green space in urban areas). Related to this study is research showing that health inequalities between rich and poor people are fewer for those living in areas with access to nature. While there are likely many interrelated reasons for the improvement in health metrics, access to nature is correlated with more movement, exposure to sunlight (i.e., greater vitamin D levels), fresh air, and time in low-stress environments.

Increased happiness has not been reported from only one study—there are additional ones that demonstrate improved cheerfulness and greater well-being when people spend time away from media and in natural settings. Another study worthy of mention was performed in Canada by the David Suzuki Foundation, which examined the effects of time spent in nature on various metrics of well-being. The study asked test subjects to spend 30 minutes in nature for 30 days. Participants were scored at the beginning and at the end of the study on a 21-question exam called the Nature Relatedness Scale developed by Nisbet and colleagues. This exam looks at three dimensions of nature relatedness: (1) internalized identification with nature; (2) nature-related perspective and its influence on worldview; and (3) familiarity with the natural world. In all these dimensions, participants at the end of the study reported greater nature relatedness. Likewise, at the beginning and end of the study, participants were asked to answer questions related to well-being. Again, all metrics showed a positive increase in value, including contentment, energy, enthusiasm, feeling less stressed, lack of negativity, mental calm, peacefulness, sleep quality, and vitality. Participants also reported increases in productivity at work and their ability to work cooperatively with colleagues. The more time the participants spent in nature, the greater the well-being they reported. In other words, a change in the amount of time in contact with nature promoted a change in feelings of nature relatedness, which in turn promoted improvements in well-being.

Evidence showing time in nature has substantial emotional health benefits continues to grow. A 2009 report from the University of Essex in England demonstrated the need for what some authors refer to as vitamin N ("N" for nature). The researchers in this study examined two groups of people: those who went for an outdoor walk in a greenspace and those who went for an indoor walk in a shopping center. Of those who participated in an outdoor walk, 80% of the people experienced a reduction in fatigue, 92% experienced less depression, 70% experienced less confusion, and 56% had more vigor at the end of the time outdoors. For those who spent time indoors, 22% reported more depression and 33% reported no change. Other research indicates that benefits can be experienced after as little as five minutes in nature and that even when the weather is uncooperative benefits are still experienced. Feelings of anxiety, depression, and anger can be subdued (to an extent) by simply spending time in natural settings.

Shinrin-yoku (i.e., taking in the forest atmosphere or "forest bathing") is a term coined in recent years for the practice of spending time in a forested environment. This involves visiting a forest for relaxation or recreation. Several studies now support this practice for its positive effects on the health of people who participate in Shinrin-yoku. Park et al. in 2010 studied the physiological effects of time in forests by having study participants alternate between forested and urban environments on different days. Those spending time in forests showed lower concentrations of cortisol (a stress hormone), lower blood pressure, lower pulse rate, lower sympathetic nerve activity, and greater parasympathetic nerve activity than those who spent time in cities. While some research links these benefits to forest trees (see next paragraph), they are, without a doubt, to be experienced (to some degree) by people spending time in any natural environment.

One of the really interesting areas of nature immersion concerns the effects of phytoncides on human health. Phytoncides are aromatic, volatile compounds that are released by plants into the environment. These compounds exert antimicrobial and/or repellant effects and prevent the plants from rotting or being eaten by various small animals (e.g., insects). In fact, the word breaks down as "phyton" for plant related and "cide" for exterminate. Examples of phytoncides include the α-pinene, carene, and myrcene of pines (genus *Pinus*). Phytoncides are, in part, responsible for the characteristic smells of various kinds of forests. These allelochemicals are documented to enhance the immune function of people who are exposed to them. For example, Li et al. have shown that forest environments enhance the number and activity of natural killer cells, one of the critical white blood cells of the innate immune system that release special proteins that attack tumors. The forest environment also enhanced intracellular anti-cancer proteins in white blood cells. They replicated these immune system enhancements through vaporizing volatile oils derived from an evergreen species (*Chamaecyparis obtusa*) within an indoor setting—while people slept in hotel rooms. The volatile oils, rich in various phytoncides, produced many of the same effects (regarding specific white blood cell activity) as time spent in forested areas (but people spending time indoors without exposure to phytoncides did not see increases in immune system activity). Those exposed to phytoncides also showed decreased levels of stress hormones (adrenaline and noradrenaline) in their urine. As well, increases in memory function and concentration have been observed with exposure to phytoncides. This research suggests another mechanism of benefit for time spent in natural settings.

Before we leave this topic of the benefits of nature immersion, let us direct our attention to the younger humans who are also trying to cope with a deficit in nature connection. Research shows that cognitive development and creativity are stimulated by childhoods that are rich in outdoor time. In fact, educational programs that use (at least in part) outdoor classrooms and various forms of nature-based education report gains in various school topics, including language, math, science, and social studies. Such children also demonstrate greater creativity—a result of outdoor time where they are more likely to create their own games (compared with those who play primarily on flat, open playgrounds). But time in nature isn't just about academic gains and improved creativeness. A 2004 study in the American Journal of Public Health also suggested that children with Attention Deficit Hyperactivity Disorder (ADHD) demonstrated improvement in symptoms after being allowed to play in outdoor environments. Later, a 2009 study by the University of Illinois showed that children with ADHD did better after a walk in nature (such as a park) compared with children with ADHD who instead walked in downtown or residential areas. Additional studies not mentioned here also demonstrate measurable improvements in ADHD symptoms with time in nature.

Time spent in natural settings is clearly important for human well-being. With more than ¾ of the US population living in cities, it makes sense why Americans experience such high rates of depression and other emotional problems. We are supposed to be immersed in highly complex landscapes with ever-changing shapes, patterns, and textures. We need exposure to the sounds, smells, and feels of wild places. Studies demonstrate improvements in health, immune system function, cognitive ability, creativity, cooperation, emotional well-being, and even the level of caring people feel for others. At some point, humans need to stop creating new homes in urban sprawls and recognize that the wild was our original home—a home we need to return to. The more we allow urbanization to claim wild areas, the smaller the extent of natural environments left on the planet. At the very least, they need to rethink their constructed habitats and realize that open green spaces within or adjacent to them are vital to the health of all people living there. Remember, multiple studies demonstrate increased happiness with time in nature. Therefore, it can be stated that the rewilding path is a route to greater joy.

SLEEPING SOUNDLY

Sleep is a necessary and somewhat mysterious part of human life. It is, unfortunately, subject to losses in quality as humans separate themselves from nature (like so many aspects of life that have been discussed already in this book). While there are many myths about sleep, we now have the advantage of research that has studied wild humans for their sleep habits and sleep positions. Of importance is that in those hunter-gatherer groups that have been observed, insomnia is almost non-existent (in fact, it was noted that there was no word for insomnia in the native language of some of the groups studied). Therefore, in many ways, recovering sleep quality is much about recovering our wild dreamtime habits.

The quality of sleep a person receives is understood by most to be important (on some level), yet it is one of the most often neglected aspects of healthy living. Sleep quality affects many facets of human vitality, including immune system function, blood pressure, ability to heal, stress, cardiac and renal health, gastrointestinal function, behavioral issues, and epigenetic expression.

In the United States, more than ⅓ of adults report experiencing symptoms of insomnia in a given year (this number is very close to that reported by Roth in 2007 who found approximately 30% of adults from various countries reported one or more symptoms of insomnia). As a result, four percent of American adults aged 20 and older have used prescription sleep aids in the last month (as reported by the Center for Disease Control and Prevention in 2013). While medicine (or drugs) may have a place for assisting sleep in some people, many would improve sleep quality simply by rewilding their sleep.

What do we know about the sleep of pre-industrial people? Well, there are a few studies to draw from, including one titled "Natural Sleep and Its Seasonal Variations in Three Pre-industrial Societies" by Yetish et al. and published in 2015. While it did not examine a large number of groups, one of the strengths of this study is that it observed hunter-gatherer groups who were very distant from one another. Therefore, any commonalities that were identified are likely to be real, ancestral human traits. And there were some similarities. First, indigenous hunter-gatherers (and hunter-farmers) generally lay down for sleep two to three hours after sunset. Second, they lay for a continuous block of about 6.9–8.5 hours (though this can be substantially longer in northern cultures during the winter season when daylight is limited), and this block was not interrupted by extended periods of waking. Three, they sleep longer in the winter when the period of darkness is greater for each day. Four, they sleep nearly continuously during the time. Five, they slept in relative darkness. Six, they woke before sunrise (while it was still dark). Seven, they woke at nearly the same time each morning. And Eight, their sleep cycles were correlated with temperature, with sleep initiating after the temperature had dropped and waking occurring near the coldest part of the day (which would be early morning before sunrise). Keeping in mind that most of the research on hunter-gatherer sleep has occurred on people closer to the equator than the poles, we can nevertheless create several guidelines for helping people sleep more soundly based on our ancestral patterns (which are "hardwired" into our beings).

The BBC World Service published an article in 2012 called "The Myth of the Eight-Hour Sleep". In that article, the researchers made a case that the ancestral sleep condition was that of two sleep blocks, in between which these people would wake and be active (doing such activities as talking, smoking, sex, and bathroom visits). This pattern seemed intuitively correct for many people who wake in the early morning hours and have difficulty returning to sleep. However, while that research was well done, it turns out the biphasic sleep pattern discussed in that research is not our ancestral condition—it arose long after agriculture had become the usual lifeway. In other words, we slept a single block of time, at some point certain groups shifted to two periods of sleep, and then (in more recent years) we have largely transitioned back to a single block of sleep.

How then can we reconnect with our natural patterns of sleep to improve the quality of rest we receive? First, and perhaps most important, we need to sleep in darkness. This fact is attested to both in our history and in modern scientific research. Our body responds to light and dark cycles. During darkness, our body undergoes a number of physiological shifts, including a lowering of body temperature, slowing of metabolism, and (critically) a rise in the production of melatonin. Melatonin (in animals) is a hormone produced by the pineal gland that is responsible for the synchronization of our circadian rhythm, an approximately 24-hour cycle that is entrainable to local patterns of light and dark. Melatonin anticipates the onset of darkness and helps initiate sleepiness. Facets of modern life that disrupt production of melatonin also degrade sleep quality. These include exposure to bright lights in the evening, shift work, and lack of exposure to outdoor lighting in the day.

With the advent of seemingly inexpensive lighting (inexpensive only if you do not include the environmental costs of energy production), people often remain awake late into the evening in well-lit interiors. In urban and suburban areas, humans also light up the outdoors with street lights, outdoor house lights, various electronic advertising, and continually illuminated businesses. All of these create light that can enter homes through windows and sky lights to brighten the interiors. In fact, research suggests that electric lights have shortened the amount of sleep we receive (as documented by Iglesia and colleagues in their study of indigenous groups in Argentina with and without electricity). Today, there is also abundant use of computers, smart phones, and tablets in the evening hours, all of which produce light rich in blue wavelengths. Blue wavelengths of light (along with other wavelengths) are also produced by the sun, and our body uses these wavelengths, along with the intensity of the light, to signal it is daytime. Therefore, media devices and artificial lighting (including compact fluorescent lights) that produce blue wavelengths interrupt the physiological transition to "night time" and inhibit production of melatonin. This light essentially tells the body that it is still daytime (even when it isn't).

There has been a lot of emphasis in recent years on the need for darkness for producing quality sleep (which is useful information for people to have). However, this focus on darkness has failed to account for the fact that humans need strongly contrasting light and dark periods for the resetting of the circadian clocks (note that is plural—we will get to this shortly). Therefore, people spending their entire day in an indoor setting are not receiving certain qualities of natural light. One of these is light intensity (i.e., the brightness experienced). While indoor spaces are illuminated, the light is usually substantially dimmer. Measurements I'm aware of put outdoor lux units (a measure of the amount of light per unit area) at 100,000 or greater around solar noon, in contrast to values of 100–2000 lux units in a typical indoor setting. Spending time outdoors during the bright portions of the day help to improve the functioning of our circadian clocks, which ultimately improves sleep quality. Instead of bright light in the day and darkness at night, modern humans have dimmed the day (by spending it indoors) and brightened the night (by artificially illuminating it)—the exact opposite pattern of our natural world.

Another feature of modern life that is extremely disruptive to the production of melatonin in shift work. People who work at night (and then in artificially lit environments) and sleep during the day (often with a partially illuminated room because of daylight coming through windows) or those with erratic work schedules (and, hence, erratic sleep schedules) demonstrate many of the problems associated with low melatonin production. Aside from sleep quality, low melatonin is associated with increased risk of diabetes and increased rates of obesity. Further, shift workers have a significant increase in cancer rates compared with the average population. For example, shift nurses demonstrate a 36% increase in breast cancer rates (as noted by Schernhammer in research published in 2001; more recent work has demonstrated an even higher risk). This increased risk of cancer is likely the result of several important aspects of melatonin. One, it is an antioxidant and can quench free-radicals, thereby combatting inflammation and helping prevent cancer. Two, it helps to trigger apoptosis (programmed cell death) in cancer cells. Three, it possessed anti-angiogenesis action, meaning it helps prevent the formation of blood vessels in tumors (which feed the growth of the tumor). And four, melatonin helps to stop the proliferation of cancer cells. It does this through its ability to slow cell division as melatonin travels through the body during the night. Cells in the body, even cancer cells, have melatonin receptors. When melatonin attaches to these receptors, it slows growth and can counteract the effects of other hormones and hormone-like substances that can speed growth (e.g., estrogen and its effect on breast cancer cells). The production of melatonin by the body is a valuable strategy to reduce the risk of cancer. Said another way, losing some of the body's ability to produce melatonin is impacting the body's ability to fight cancer. All of this clearly demonstrates that humans are supposed to be awake during the day and asleep at night. This has been the schedule for nearly all of our existence on this planet. Shift work (again) illustrates the problems of diverging from long-practiced natural patterns.

While the simple answer to the issue of optimized melatonin production is to get lots of bright light during the day and experience darkness at night, this is simply not possible for everyone all the time. There are times when schedule constraints and other issues force work or social events into the dark hours, including extremely long periods of darkness in north-temperate regions and those areas even closer to the poles. There are ways to mitigate the effects of light on our melatonin production. Keeping light intensity lower in the evening hours and using lights that are skewed to longer wavelengths (i.e., closer to red) while avoiding lights that emit lots of shorter wavelengths (i.e., closer to blue) can help mitigate the issue. Research suggests that lights closer to red (including orange and yellow) may not inhibit melatonin production in the same way as our modern lights. This means that hunter-gatherers who stayed awake for a few hours past sunset using firelight and flame candles would not have impacted their melatonin production. Therefore, candles, lanterns, salt lamps with low-wattage bulbs, and light from a fireplace would be valuable illumination sources for times when bright lights are not needed (e.g., during night-time socializing with friends). Those needing to use computers late into the night would be advised to install f.lux, a free program designed to shift the color of the screen after sunset to help avoid eye strain and prevent disruption of sleep or wear blue-blocking glasses (and notice the word "needing" in this sentence, as opposed to "wanting"). While the harm of late-night computer use isn't alleviated by software or special lenses placed in front of our eyes, its effects can be lessened (technology is not the ultimate answer here, lifestyle is). It would be best to avoid the use of such media for at least 60 minutes (preferably longer) before laying down for sleep.

To help understand the value of melatonin (and the need for rewilded sleep), it will be useful here to discuss additional health implications of suppressed melatonin production. One of the important roles of melatonin is to increase nighttime levels of leptin. Leptin is a hormone that produces satiety—when leptin levels increase, the feeling of hunger decreases. Melatonin regulates leptin, helping to make sure we don't feel hunger at night (which would be a poor time to seek food on a wild landscape, and is not a good time to consume food, even for people that can walk to a refrigerator, for various reasons). Exposure to bright light in the evening, which decreases melatonin production, also decreases leptin production. As a result, we feel hungry and sleep duration can be curtailed (as preliminary research by Spiegel et al. in 2004 demonstrated).

A few paragraphs ago I alluded to the fact that our bodies do not have a single circadian clock, but multiple clocks. In fact, research has demonstrated that we have multiple clocks—one in nearly every organ of the body (and in our fat cells). Therefore, the need for light and dark exposure is to calibrate and synchronize the functioning of all these clocks. But, it is not just light and dark cycles that do this. If we engage in activities that would occur while we are awake late in the night (when we should be sleeping), we can disrupt the synchronicity of these clocks. For example, eating late in the night tells the pancreas that it must produce insulin, but the brain is preparing for sleep. This puts these two organs out of sync with each other. And with competing time cues, the stage is set for weight gain and various metabolic diseases (including type 2 diabetes). While it is clear that our body can recover from an occasional late night out and an infrequent flight to another time zone, frequent disruptions to the harmonic functioning of our circadian clocks is detrimental to our health.

Returning to the studies of sleep in hunter-gatherers, we can identify additional clues to creating environments and habits that support quality sleep. Sleep patterns in hunter-gatherers is strongly correlated with temperature—and temperature may have a role in the maintenance of circadian clocks in some portion of the body. Even though temperature fluctuations would have been lessened by the use of shelters, blankets, clothing, and fire inside of structures, there is still some variations that the hunter-gatherers experience that people living inside of thermostat controlled homes do not. Turning down the thermostat at night or, better, actually sleeping outdoors (even within tents) helps to expose the body to natural temperature cycles that can assist with better sleep duration. For me personally, I spend much less time awake in the early morning hours when I am outdoors—I essentially sleep all the way through the night in one block of time with only short interruptions. When in a thermostatically controlled setting, I am frequently am awake for long periods of time (sometimes hours) in the night before returning back to sleep sometime before sunrise. If you cannot sleep outdoors and others in your home want a constant temperature, consider closing the door to the room (to prevent heat from entering it) and/or opening a window so the room you sleep in gets cooler at night.

Hunter-gatherers also demonstrated a relatively consistent time of waking. In fact, establishing patterns of this kind, including pre-sleep routines, helps our circadian clocks to function better. Consistent waking time helps establish part of the approximately 24-hour cycle that governs the body—it essentially builds an anchor point that the body uses as a reference. Deviating from this destabilizes our circadian rhythms by adding inconsistency, forcing our circadian clocks to re-establish a rhythm of wake and sleep cycles. Consistent waking time (without using the snooze button for extended periods of time) is one of the many external clues our body uses to build daily rhythms (these external cues are called Zeitgeber cues). In this way, your body comes to learn that at 06:00 (or whatever time one wakes) is the time to initiate waking and alertness.

The amount of time spent sleeping has been hotly debated in recent years, with contradictory studies demonstrating the benefit or harm of different periods of sleep length. Honestly, I don't pay too much attention to these studies. I rely on various self-indicators to determine the amount of sleep I need to receive, including such things as my energy level at different points in the day, how alert I feel, and how easily I can perform cognitive tasks. And these things do change with the seasons and the tasks that need to be accomplished during daylight hours. One thing is certain, I do sleep more during the winter months (a pattern practiced by hunter-gatherers). And I don't nap often, except on the hottest summer days where escaping the heat in the shade of trees feels quite appropriate. Daytime napping for hunter-gatherers that have been observed was infrequent during the winter months (7% of the days), but more common during the summer months (22% of the days). This could reflect many things, including more efficient use of limited daylight hours during the winter season, a time when nighttime sleeping was generally longer (and naps would not be needed to recover alertness and vitality).

One item not examined in the research on hunter-gatherer sleep habits was noise. It was omitted because (very likely) noise was simply not an issue in non-industrialized settings where the wild humans lived. However, modern humans living or travelling in urban locations can be exposed to high levels of noise that can prevent sleep. We could go further and divide "noise" into three categories: environmental, mental, and physical. Environmental noise is the obvious kind of clamor that most people are familiar with and includes traffic, construction, jet airplanes, and similar kinds of sounds that can be disruptive to sleep. Mental noise is the assortment of thoughts we dwell on that prevents us from falling asleep. This kind of noise is often more intense when stressful events have occurred or are about to occur. Physical noise is something our bodies experience as a result of pain and discomfort from injury, upset stomach, or even the side-effects of prescription drugs. Essentially, if we are physically uncomfortable, it will be difficult to fall asleep. Collectively, environmental, mental, and physical noise are all an obstacle that must be overcome to fall asleep. When the noise levels are high, we will fall asleep only when we are very tired. Of course, if we have a quiet setting (which includes our mind), we can fall asleep easily. For many people, mental noise will be the most difficult noise item to overcome. Clearing the mind and using meditation and other practices can be of assistance here.

Humans spend approximately ⅓ of their life sleeping, but sleep seems to receive very little focus aside from the comfort of the mattress they lay on. It is often considered to be time we aren't productive, and so we want to sleep as short a duration as possible to get back to work and other projects. However, sleeping is profoundly important to our well-being, and improving the quality can make substantial improvements to our physical and emotional health. This means that the time we spend sleeping (or trying to sleep) influences the quality of life we have while we are awake. We need to make the places we sleep emulate features of outdoor living, which includes eliminating any artificial illumination, allowing temperature fluctuations, and curtailing loud noise. Moonlight and starlight do not need to be eliminated because their light intensity is below the threshold for stimulating alertness (as do many artificial light sources, especially smart phones, tablets, and e-readers that are held close to the eyes at night). I would go further and suggest that all sources of human-produced radiation (e.g., cell phones, Wi-Fi signals) should be turned off. While there is preliminary evidence to suggest that exposure to such things can disrupt sleep, there is not (yet) any compelling scientific data to suggest that such electromagnetic fields are disruptive to everyone's sleep. However, using the precautionary principle, I prefer to be bathed (as often as possible, and especially at night) in the radiation that humans have always been exposed to—that created by our earth. Putting cell phones on airplane mode and turning off Wi-Fi are easy tasks that I feel helps me attain a higher quality sleep. Sleep is more than just rest and recuperation. It is a time we visit other realms. The dreams we experience can be highly informative and have been used in various ways by all previous cultures on this planet. Perhaps reconnecting to natural patterns in regard to sleep also has the ability to increase the value of our dreamtime.

TOUCHING THE EARTH

Walking barefoot, sitting or lying on the ground, and even sleeping in close contact with the earth used to be common activities to all human cultures. As we have "matured" into a civilized species, we generally wear shoes for much or all of the year, primarily sit in chairs and on couches, and virtually never sleep on the ground. Industrial societies have, in a sense, created an additional level of separation from earth—a literal separation where their feet or other parts of the body are rarely in direct contact with the planetary body that supports their life. Our feet (along with our buttocks) are supposed to touch the earth. Certainly, there are times when we need shoes for protection from the cold or sharp items that could harm us—but we have taken this further than it needs to go. We now wear shoes so often that our feet are tender and cannot withstand the natural surfaces that we live upon. Think about that for a moment, our feet are designed to walk through the forests, across the prairies, and among the mountains, but we have pampered them for so long in our industrial living upon level and often carpeted surfaces that we can no longer be in contact with the earth without experiencing discomfort. This certainly cannot be described as a change that has made us more adapted to our environment, rather, it is an example of maladaptation. The fact that we rarely go barefoot has important implications for the strength and anatomical structure of our feet (which will be discussed in chapter 8). It also means that we are rarely exposed to an important source of healing energy.

While we could discuss (at length) emotional and spiritual reasons why people should be in touch with the earth, such reasoning might be lost on an industrial society who has created the disconnection people experience in the first place. Fortunately, there is emerging science and a number of preliminary studies that do support a real human need for direct connection to planet earth. I write "preliminary" because, to date, the studies have utilized relatively low sample sizes. I also write "direct connection" because I am meaning to convey the idea of human skin touching the ground (i.e., walking in shoes with rubber or polymer soles insulates those wearing such footwear from the ground). A little background is needed to help understand how our planet can be a source of healing energy that is supported by science.

White blood cells (also called leucocytes) are cells of our immune system that help to defend the body from infection and injury. There are five basic types of leucocytes: basophils, eosinophils, lymphocytes, monophils, and neutrophils. The last kind, neutrophils, are the most abundant leucocytes in the body and form an important part of the innate immune system that recognizes and responds to pathogens in an immediate and general fashion. Neutrophils are phagocytes, meaning they ingest foreign invaders and destroy them through one of several approaches. One of the approaches is the production of reactive oxygen species (ROS), which are chemically reactive molecules that include oxygen as part of their structure. Reactive oxygen species, while produced as a normal part of metabolism, are also produced to destroy microbial pathogens. Because ROS are chemically reactive, they steal electrons from other molecules, causing what is known as oxidative damage. This harms various components of cells, including membranes, amino acids, and DNA. Such damage can kill microbial pathogens. It is one of the reasons that neutrophils secrete ROS, so that foreign cells will be destroyed.

Anytime there is inflammation, including when the body experiences mechanical injury (such as hitting our shin on something hard), is burned, or is dealing with infection, the body undergoes a number of complex physiological responses to the site of damage. The redness, swelling, and warmth are the result of increased blood flow to the area. Increased pain sensitivity and (often) a loss of function also result from inflammation. During this process, neutrophils are released into the surrounding tissue and secrete ROS. This occurs to break up damaged cells so they can be removed and healthy cells can grow in their place. The ROS also destroy bacterial invaders if the skin was broken during the injury. While all of this is completely normal, ROS can and do harm nearby healthy tissue. These molecules act like free radicals in our body, damaging tissue and contributing to aging. Whether the result of acute or chronic infection or normal metabolic processes, ROS must be dealt with by the body (and quickly). A number of mechanisms exist for this. For example, the body produces endogenous antioxidants, such as the enzyme superoxide dismutase (SOD) to quench one of the most common classes of ROS produced by the body (called superoxides). We also ingest antioxidants as part of our diet. Antioxidants, whether produced inside our body or ingested in our diet, function by donating (or receiving) electrons to make the ROS chemically stable without becoming unstable themselves. Once transformed into stable molecules, the former ROS cannot harm healthy cells. An important item to note, as discussed in chapter 3, our modern diets contain many fewer antioxidants than that of our original diets. Fortunately, there is another way we can help compensate for the presence of ROS—free electrons.

Anytime someone sits, walks, runs, or plays on the ground, they have the ability to absorb free electrons from the earth. The planet we live upon is actually a mega-donor of free electrons. When we walk on sand, gravel, stone, or even lawns and other vegetated surfaces, electrons can be donated to the human body so long as there is nothing that prevents conduction, such as shoes with rubber or polymer soles, wooden floors, and foam pads. Walking on a wet surface, such as wet beach sand or a field that is damp with dew, improves the conduction and allows more extensive "earthing" to the occur (earthing is verb that means to be in direct contact with the ground). Remember, ROS and other free radicals cause harm by stealing electrons from other molecules. However, if a store of free electrons exists within the body, which can be donated to these free radicals and make them stable (i.e., chemically inactive), they will not contribute to oxidative damage in the body. In fact, it is likely that our bodies have used this mechanism of limiting damage from ROS for the entirety of human existence, and only recently has this mechanism been prevented through our lifestyles that limit contact with the earth.

One thing that is important to realize is that our mitochondria, the powerhouses of the cells, which produce the chemical energy our body uses to power various aspects of our metabolism, create ROS. This is a normal part of our metabolism and happens when we breathe, when we eat, and when we move. In fact, the more active we are, the more free radicals generated by our mitochondria. When the ROS are not "inactivated" by the body, they cause cumulative damage (to our DNA, our proteins, etc.). This cumulative oxidative damage contributes to aging and disease. The point of this paragraph is that even healthy people who are free of injury and infection produce ROS (and athletes produce even more, all things being equal). Therefore, neutralizing ROS is in everyone's best interest. And contact with the earth appears to help to accomplish this.

One of the interesting studies on earthing was performed by Brown and colleagues in 2010. They looked at delayed-onset muscle soreness. A small group of healthy subjects was subjected to exercise leading to muscle soreness. Half of the subjects were grounded while they slept using special conductive sheets and patches attached to their lower leg and feet that would allow the flow of electrons into their body. The other half of the subjects also slept using the sheets and patches but these items were disabled and were not connected to a ground. A number of white blood cell, red blood cell, enzyme, hormone, magnetic resonance, and pain markers were substantially different between the grounded and ungrounded test subjects. For example, total white blood cell counts were always higher in the ungrounded group. Further, neutrophils (which produce ROS) were always lower in the grounded group. Bilirubin, an important cellular antioxidant, was found in substantially greater amounts in the blood of the grounded individuals. This suggested that access to free electrons (through the grounding equipment) created a lower requirement for endogenous antioxidants to combat the free radicals produced during exercise leading to muscle soreness. The ungrounded subjects all reported greater levels of pain than did the grounded subjects (which suggests more rapid healing in the grounded subjects). While this research was considered to be a pilot study, it nonetheless provided a number of interesting results.

Another study looked at earthing and its relation to blood viscosity. This research was authored by Chevalier and colleagues and was published in 2013. Blood viscosity is a major issue for hypertension (i.e., high blood pressure), which is a significant risk factor for cardiovascular disease. Red blood cells (called erythrocytes) carry a negative surface charge that helps repel the blood cells so that they do not normally clump together. Clumping of cells increases their viscosity and requires higher force to move them through the human vascular network, which creates higher blood pressure. The researchers examined a small group of subjects who had just exercised and took blood samples before and after earthing. The earthing was accomplished with patches attached to the feet and hands that connected to a wire that led to a steel rod placed in the ground. Earthing was found to increase the surface charge of all red blood cell samples examined and significantly decreased blood viscosity and clumping of erythrocytes. While these results were identified in a laboratory setting (hence the need for patches connected to wires leading outside), it is possible to reduce blood pressure and lower the risk of cardiovascular disease by simply spending time barefoot outdoors.

Ghaly and Teplitz (2004) studied the effects of grounding on cortisol levels in the body over a 24-hour period with special attention to levels during nighttime sleep. Cortisol is a hormone that is produced in the adrenal glands in response to stress and low blood glucose levels. Elevated levels of cortisol have detrimental effects on the immune system, slow wound healing, disrupt sleep, promote anxiety and depression, and can lead to weight gain (especially when chronically elevated). Their work revealed that after grounding, test subjects demonstrated normalized cortisol levels (i.e., the hormone secretions were synchronized with the 24-hour circadian clock) and lower levels of this stress hormone at night. Research participants reported better sleep and less pain and stress. This research showed that connecting to the earth improved both objective and subjective measurements of health studied by the authors.

Spending time in contact with the earth ("earthing") is easily accomplished. It simply involves removing those items that insulate us (electrically speaking) from the planet. Walking barefoot, sitting or lying on the ground, and scrambling in steep terrain where the hands would be used for balance and to climb upward are all easy ways to reconnect. While grounding (dissipating static charge) can occur almost instantaneously, earthing is best done with extended time on bare ground (the longer the better). Getting at least 30 minutes a day when the weather allows would be very useful for many people, during which you could be doing things you need to do, such as foraging, weeding a garden, raking leaves, walking the dog, getting conscientious sun exposure, or whatever. Given that we are a technological society, we also have many tech options for earthing, such as grounding pads, sheets, and similar items that have a wire connected to a ground (which allows electrons to flow from the earth to the human). There are sandals and shoes with copper contacts that allow the feet to make electrical contact with the ground. There are even large cloth sacks that people can climb inside with silver threads running through them that allow grounding through a wire to the outdoors. For some people, such technology may be necessary. It does strike me that it has now become easier to manufacture a way to allow electrons to flow from the ground to our feet (while we sit indoors) than to just go outdoors and experience it. But, if I lived in a high-rise apartment, I might make use of this technology.

Preliminary research demonstrates that direct contact with the planet has a number of healing qualities for *Homo sapiens* (and likely other life as well). These including speeding wound healing, promoting better sleep, reducing oxidative damage, lowering blood pressure, suppressing inflammation, and improving various cardiac health issues. An aware person would likely understand all of this (on some level) without scientific study. Such a person would identify contact with the earth as healing, possibly even spiritually beneficial. Unfortunately, the awareness of most contemporary humans has been blunted, not necessarily by choice, but due to a life of living in constructed habitats away from the wild nature that fosters deep awareness of their surroundings—awareness that often transcends the usually discussed senses. Statements espousing that touching the earth may provide health benefits are simply, for some, not in the realm of science. In fact, these studies have been vehemently attacked by several sources who state they are exposing this topic as deception. And while there are valid criticisms of the studies, some of these were designed with double-blind methodology—and still identified positive outcomes. As a result, I remain open, even though this subject currently sits outside of most science work in the United States. Of course, science can effectively supply information only on topics that (a) have been considered for study and (b) the means exist to measure, record, or otherwise observe the phenomena of interest. In other words, if it cannot be measured, it does not exist. Of course, this statement assumes that the ability to measure some phenomenon has been appropriately devised. Can we truly make the statement that all means of assessing the benefit of contact with the earth have been devised? If we always wait for study to demonstrate what seems obvious (or should seem obvious), we may miss out on important aspects of health that could help us attain greater personal peace in our lives. Lack of contact with the planet is a kind of literal nature disconnection. It is a deficiency in elemental exposure, one that is easily corrected.

NAKED IS OUR NATURAL STATE

We hide ourselves today behind so many layers of protection that it is little wonder we have lost the ability to marvel at and function as stewards of creation. Living in cities and towns, within our homes, swaddled in clothes, enveloped in our modern worldviews—we are protected from the wild by layer upon layer of technology and domestication, all of which, we are told, is necessary to prevent the loss of our civility and halt the degradation into something more akin to a wild animal. But that is exactly what we are. We are animals, just those that have been changed by so many generations of taming that we are now completely infused with the idea that wildness is harmful to us. But if you have read this far, everything I have discussed to this point is a rekindling of our wildness and a return to a nature-connected lifestyle. This is not harmful to humans, rather it is rejuvenating to both the person and the landscapes they live upon. It is time to fold back the layers of defense and experience the world in a new and raw manner. Breaking the shackles of domestication sometimes requires something bold. I suggest that spending time in nature exactly the way you entered this world is one strategy for regaining our feral nature.

Our pervasive use of clothing now has certainly made it more difficult for us to receive the elemental foods our bodies need (such as sunlight and contact with the ground). It also makes it difficult for us to use the largest sensory organ in our body—our skin—because it is covered with fabric and dulled to the sensations found in the world. In industrialized countries, nudity is so often associated with sex that a suggestion we should expose more of our body to the environment might be interpreted as erotic or perverted (depending on the situation). Even if people could look past this and realize that nudity doesn't necessarily imply either of those things, we would need to contend with the fact that we have also been trained, since childhood, to be modest and fully dressed. Our modern societies equate clothed bodies with civilized behavior, and to go nude is to be uncivilized.

Clothing is a remarkable adaptation to the environmental challenges faced by humans. The advancement in early clothing, such as hide tanning and the invention of sewing, allowed *Homo sapiens* to move into cold environments and make use of extreme habitats that our bodies could not have endured without this protection. But clothing for domesticated people is more than just protection against extreme cold, intense sunlight, precipitation, or plants armed with prickles and thorns. It is also a way of demonstrating a profession (through use of a uniform) or demonstrating social rank through the clothing and their corporate logos. Doffing of clothing means the clear indicator of socio-economic status has been removed and people stand before each other with a kind of equality that nudity imposes. For some, who may have worked many years climbing the social ladder and are used to certain privileges provided by their status, such equality may be uncomfortable. However, for those who can be comfortable de-emphasizing this aspect of modern living (or gain comfort with time), this is shown to reduce stress that comes with low social status.

However, it is likely that our shyness and cultural modesty will be the biggest obstacle for some to overcome concerning nudity in the outdoors, even when they are completely alone. Many people are embarrassed of their physical form—which is a learned behavior. Young children, regardless of their height, weight, or shape, are comfortable running, playing, and just being nude. Further, they do not judge their parents and friends on their weight and lack of muscle tone. It is society that teaches them they are to have uncomfortable feelings about their physical body and criticize other's. This pathological modesty matures into a reluctance to share healthy, consensual touching with other adults, which has a host of emotional benefits. Overlaid on top of these emotions is the requirement that the body is to be covered for social or religious reasons. Eventually you end up with a person who feels uncomfortable without clothing even when the weather and other environmental issues (e.g., biting insects) do not require a person to be clothed. As such, modern humans miss out on wonderful opportunities to experience their world through their entire body.

This writing is not intended to persuade people to join a nudist colony or expose their children to nude strangers. It isn't attempting to have people roam nude through city streets as a protest against society. The words here are simply trying to express the point that nudity isn't a form of extremism. Being naked can be part of an important health strategy and a process of reconnecting to nature. It is also a way to escape culturally imposed restrictions on how we view ourselves. Nude sunbathing is a practice I use throughout the year when temperatures allow this activity. It exposes the maximum amount of skin to the sun so that my body can efficiently manufacture vitamin D_3-sulfate and cholesterol-sulfate. But there are many other benefits. It removes restrictive clothing (a good example is women's bras) that impede the flow of lymph and can elevate the risk of certain cancers. It allows one to use their skin as an effective sensory array when walking through the forest and other wild areas. It also generates self-confidence and reduces stress, thereby helping the body limit the detrimental effects of stress (e.g., hypertension, inflammation). There are many times when nudity isn't practical (even if appropriate); however, finding fellow rewilders who are comfortable with nudity can be an exhilarating experience. Shedding our societally imposed "textile tombs" has physical and psychological benefits for those who are willing to commit to the practice. It can also destroy the arbitrarily imposed social hierarchy based primarily, in many affluent countries, on physical wealth (or some other subjective standard that has nothing to do with true qualities of humanness).

THE PARADIGM OF CONTROL

Homo sapiens has been on a long march to control and improve conditions they experience and outcomes they have planned for. During this time, the ability of humans to modify landscapes (and damage them) has grown in terms of both the degree of modification and the extent of the world that has been modified. We are convinced these modifications are necessary and represent real improvements. We change, manipulate, alter, intensify, adjust, and control—without ever even questioning if this is the appropriate course of action (which is certainly true of many of human's inventions, simply because we can doesn't mean we should). Modern humans really do seem to be blind to the consequences of attempting to control nature. Every attempt to control our world using technological fixes only creates more problems that then require additional fixes. As Charles Eisenstein writes in the Ascent of Humanity[5]:

"Why is the technological fix so attractive? Because from the short-term perspective, it really does work. The first digging stick really did make it easier to obtain roots. A cup of coffee really does make us feel energized. A good stiff drink really does make the pain go away. Air conditioning makes us feel cooler on a hot day. Cars get us there faster. Fertilizer boosts the yield. With each stage of construction, the Tower rises higher. See, it's working! We're getting closer to the sky.

"Invisible at first is the fact that the fix is a trap. At the end of the day, the coffee exhausts our adrenal glands and makes us more tired, not less. The air conditioning habituates us to a narrow range of comfort, trapping us indoors. Cars inevitably bring more roads, more cars, and more time in transit. Food production technology brings population increases, and eventually less security and more anxiety."

We see this in so many of the ways we interact with the world. For example, in many parts of the United States, gray wolves (*Canis lupus*) were intentionally eradicated to make our landscapes "safe", protect livestock, and remove competition with hunters. Of course, eradicating apex predators from our landscape has resulted in some pretty unintended consequences. For example, deer (*Odocoileus* species) are now above the carrying capacity of the landscapes they live upon in many areas, causing extensive damage to the vegetation (both wild and cultivated). As a result of their number, State Farm (an insurance company) has estimated that over four billion dollars in vehicle damage is caused by collisions with deer species each year in the United States. This does not include the millions (usually tens of millions) of dollars of crop damage that occur each year in various states. Further, we must note that 200 deaths result from those accidental collisions with cars (annually). All of this to make the landscape safer, but it is clearly less safe now—human deaths from wolves are almost non-existent (since 1915, there have been a total of 39 aggressive encounters with wolves in North America and only 1 or 2 fatalities, depending on what source you read). But what about livestock? Certainly wolves would kill cattle, lambs, goats, and other domesticated animals and cause serious monetary losses for ranchers and the like. While this is true, the costs of gray wolf predation on livestock in substantially lower than the costs associated with large deer populations. For example, from 1996 through 2004, Wisconsin paid out a total of 380,518 dollars in compensation for wolf predation on livestock. While this figure does not include indirect costs to ranchers as a result of wolf presence (e.g., stress to domesticated animals leading to illness, increased herd surveillance costs), it pales in comparison to the 30,000,000 dollars of annual damage that deer do to crops in that state. We spent decades sterilizing our land of gray wolves, and, in doing so, made the country more dangerous for humans, not less. While we can't blame high deer populations entirely on the extirpation of wolves because there are other factors involved as well, such as the extirpation of other predators (e.g., mountain lions) and habitat alterations that favor deer, having large predators on the landscape would certainly help with this problem we created by trying to control nature.

The desire to control nature (and the resulting problems with this approach) is perhaps best exemplified in our manner of producing food. Agriculture relies on continued inputs to maintain

[5] Charles Eisenstain. 2013. The Ascent of Humanity. Evolver Editions, Berkeley, CA.

soil fertility for the growth of fruits and vegetables. In conventional agriculture, these inputs are industrially produced chemicals that do not stay put. For example, nitrogen is added to the soil in the form of ammonia, created through an energy intensive process that requires natural gas (a fossil fuel). Unfortunately, the nitrogen does not remain in place and enters ground and surface waters. In rivers and lakes, the fertilizer promotes the growth of algae that deplete the oxygen content of the water, creating biological dead zones that can be extensive when major rivers enter coastal bays and gulfs. Nitrogen fertilizer also contributes to climate change and ozone depletion. Conventional produce (which represents 99.5% of the agriculture in the United States by land area) also relies heavily on other kinds of chemical applications—herbicides, pesticides, and fungicides, which also do not stay in place. Our increasing use of GMO crops has also increased our use of certain herbicides (e.g., glyphosate), meaning we are polluting the soil and water with even greater amounts of chemicals. While proponents of chemical agriculture would dismiss this entire paragraph, there are a number of human health issues associated with agricultural chemicals, especially for those who work in this industry, including tumor formation, chronic and acute neurotoxicity, immunosuppression, hepatic toxicity, and developmental and reproductive issues (there are many, easily sourced articles in peer-reviewed journals for this information). Of course, this only discusses human health—we generally ignore the impacts to other-than-human persons. In summary, in our desire to control the production of food, we have also changed diets to be substantially lower in quality and much more devastating to the environment (which comes back to rob humans of their health). Industrial solutions always create industrial problems.

Our desire to control spills over into other areas of our life as well (i.e., it isn't just nature we are attempting to control). We want all aspects of our life to be regulated, and that includes our interaction with other people. We attempt to control the lives of people who are "below us", whether it be those with less seniority at work, those with less education in a topic, or those of younger age (especially our own children). Rather than considering all of humanity to have an equal standing, we erect a pecking order based on the possession of various traits that allow domination (in some form) over other people. It may be that the frustration people feel in trying to control certain aspects of their life that cannot be controlled spills over in social interaction. Rather than operate by consensus, we exert control over other humans and tell them what they can and cannot do and even what they should believe. Even certain credentials, such as a degree in a topic or a lofty designation, are now considered grounds for non-credentialed people to give up their sovereignty and follow the directions of those with "qualifications" without question. It is clear that industrial humans truly believe control is not only possible but is a necessary aspect of life. What if our desire to control only creates problems (as illustrated in the above paragraphs)? What if control creates a social delusion of the betterment of our lives that is not truly borne out when we examine all the information? Perhaps letting go of a control mentality could be useful for modern humans.

Abandoning a control ideology will be very difficult for people who have been raised with this mindset their entire lives. It permeates everything that our society attempts to do. More laws and regulations to correct the ambiguous ones from an earlier time that then harm some individuals and businesses because the laws are now too specific and are really designed only for giant corporations. More drugs to alleviate the side effects from the drugs that were being used for the initial symptoms of industrial living. On and on we go, as if we are trying to hold back more water with an ever larger dam while it clearly is beginning to crack and spouts of water are starting to appear. We simply decided that the earth was not enough and we must improve on her. Letting go of control, where possible, is perhaps exemplified in the idea of participation.

When we participate, we become part of the human and environmental communities (which are actually just one super-community). Our goal is then not to separate from these collectives and elevate ourselves above them in some fashion, but to join with them and function as a part of the whole. Participation involves flowing with ecological processes (i.e., mimicking them), rather than directing them to suit our own needs. We partake of and contribute to society. But rather than command, we suggest and offer alternatives by our own actions (i.e., we role model the change we wish to see). Participation puts trust in all that has come before us that our needs can be met (though not necessarily all of our wants) to produce healthy and rewarding lives. This mind set values long-term thinking and seeks to limit the harm caused by short-term decision making (which is epitomized by technological fixes). It also values cooperative partnerships—and not just with other humans—for which we can look to our wild landscapes for thousands of examples of this kind of interaction. Participation with our planet can take a multitude of forms. Instead of draining wetlands to create more agricultural fields, we learn to forage there in a manner that continues the lives of these valuable edible plants, a decision that supports the other beneficial values and functions of wetlands. Instead of channelizing the river and building dikes to attempt to control flooding, we recognize that some locations of the earth should not have permanent domiciles, or at least not the versions we construct in uplands. Instead of spraying more and more chemicals on the plants we eat, we could diversify the plantings, use crop rotation, and employ companion planting (among many other methods) to reduce the loss of crops to insects. Participation means that we don't always apply an unyielding industrial fix to our issues, but that we look into the ecological mistakes we are making and correct them with more biologically oriented solutions. Participation is the primary manner *Homo sapiens* has interacted with the world (until recently). It is not an approach we can completely abandon without long-term consequences. Unlearning domestication is very much about losing the need to control and engaging in participation.

SPIRITUAL AWAKENING

We are only seldom able to critically examine our actions and beliefs and see how these influence our health and interactions with the world (at least initially). Our upbringing in the civilized world has, in some cases, led us to believe in something or to act in a manner that can be detrimental to our being (even if only indirectly), but we are blind to this because we consider various views and actions to be normal. Modern civilization, as currently organized, is a relatively destructive entity in that natural resources (which is a euphemism for other life and the things life requires for survival) are used and/or degraded at an unsustainable rate. Why this occurs (unsustainable resource use) is the product of many different societal factors. One of which, which will be discussed here, is modern religion. It can be shown that contemporary belief systems contribute to various ideas that allow for ecocide and potentially interfere with a person's development into a more natural being.

Modern religion, in its multitude of forms, is a difficult topic of discussion for many reasons. It is a deeply personal issue to many people and the very definition of who they are is often related to their faith. This means that any discussion of faith between people of different belief systems frequently results in statements being interpreted as a personal attack, and emotions tend to interfere with any chance of a peaceful dialog. On top of this we must overlay two important issues: (1) religion is based on a conviction of the teachings of that faith and (2) there are differing interpretations of each religion's holy scripture (even by people within the same religion). The first issue creates a situation where no manner of argumentation (evidence-based or otherwise) can alter personal beliefs. It can even be stated that the level of conviction someone has for their beliefs is sometimes tied to their value as a religious person. The second makes possible for someone to be a Christian or a follower of Islam or any other religion and essentially condone any action they wish to take (or avoid taking). For example, members of the same religion may be accepting of homosexuality or consider it a form of sexual perversion and, in some cases, perpetrate violent acts on those who practice a different form of sexuality from that which they accept. Because of these two issues, religious discussion is almost without use in reforming how people view various topics. While this writing here is not to challenge anyone's belief system in any way, it is intended to point out that at least some modern religions actually stand in the way of rewilding and a society's transition to a more ecocentric worldview.

While it is certain that many people will disagree with the following four statements (and that is completely acceptable), both historical accounts and modern-day events will show that these four elements are common to many modern religions and are harmful to humankind and the world we live in. While some may appropriately respond with "that is not what I believe", the fact is that many use their religion to condone the four items I'm about to discuss. Whether or not they are correctly part of holy scripture and teachings is irrelevant because it is the interpretation held by different people that ultimately dictates the way they view and relate to the rest of the world. Therefore, I'm not discussing what is actually written in the Bible (or the Qur'an, Torah, etc.), or what all religious people believe, rather I'm discussing what a significant portion of religious populations actually have done and continue to act out on the world based on their interpretation of their religious instructions. All of these items below are contrary to an egalitarian, eco-centered, empathetic society that would value all of the planet's life equally. I ask that you read the following with an open mind and try to understand how I may have come to these conclusions. I also ask that you keep in mind I am not condemning modern religion and trying to suggest a more science-based approach. It would be easy to point out many examples where science has fostered a worldview and created objects that were not in humanity's long-term interest. What I am trying to accomplish is simply identifying aspects of religion that do not serve a rewilded human community. With all that in mind, below are four features common to many modern religions.

1. **Promote division**. The religion that one chooses erects an additional classification system that is used to distinguish different people, over and above the other ways we already classify humans (e.g., gender, age, ethnicity, country of origin, dietary preferences, sexuality, favorite sports team). The categories that people use to define themselves can generate strong pressures to avoid interacting with others who do not belong to the same category—a process that generates ignorance of the other and makes it easier to accept apathy for the fate of other people who practice different religions. Worse, it can foster hatred that can lead to the acceptance of violence against people of other belief systems. The United States has seen this in the past with its hostile taking of land from the Native Americans. The Doctrine of Discovery was used as justification for this theft. Essentially, this doctrine stated that the taking of land, property, and lives was acceptable because the indigenous people were not Christian (the difference in faith was interpreted as "they are lesser than us"). In fact, the Doctrine of Discovery has even been used in the Supreme Court (Johnson versus M'Intosh) to justify the actions of the European colonists here on this continent. As was stated in the not so distant past by one religious leader:

"We grant you [Kings of Spain and Portugal] by these present documents, with our Apostolic Authority, full and free permission to invade, search out, capture, and subjugate the Saracens and pagans and any other unbelievers and enemies of Christ wherever they may be, as well as their kingdoms, duchies, counties, principalities, and other property … and to reduce their persons into perpetual slavery."

While many would be quick to the claim "that was then and this is now", implying we do not view other humans in this manner anymore, it still continues in many parts of the United States concerning those that practice Islamic religion. Innocent Muslims, even women and children (i.e., non-combatives) are seen as an acceptable loss so long as known terrorists are targeted in attacks (whether or not the terrorists are actually present). Because of the current events of this world, we are now seeing a Christian versus Islam war where people of each background devalue the life of the other. While it may not be religion that created the tensions we are experiencing today, it is certain that religion (on both sides) contributes to the tensions. We are living in a time where unity is required to solve the problems faced by humanity. Any force promoting philosophical separation of humans is counter to a cooperative future. Rewilded communities may be composed of people with very different ethnic and religious backgrounds (but unified by place and intent).

2. **Further a human-centered worldview**. Many modern religions, especially those that fall under the categories of Judeo-Christian and Islam, are very much centered on humans having a very special place in the cosmos (this is referred to as anthropocentrism). This human-centered worldview often is taken to the extreme with the deities or single god having human-like qualities (or even a human-like form). While I do not dispute that humans are very special creatures with a unique ability to celebrate existence, I also recognize the value of all other life on this planet and each species' exclusive capacity to experience life in its own way. Some modern religions consider that other life (e.g., plants, animals) was placed here for humans to use and have dominion over. Said another way, the world was created specifically for human habitation, and life on the planet is merely to be seen as resources for human ventures. Further, humans are sometimes considered to be the only organisms to have "spirit" and an "afterlife" when the body has ceased living. In this way, the religions afford special privileges to humans that are not afforded to other-than-human persons. This consideration, that other life is less privileged than humans, allows all manner of horrible acts to be perpetrated on other-than-human life. In fact, such acts can be condoned by religion because humans are to have dominion over existence.

"Let us make man in our image, in our likeness, and let them rule over the fish of the sea and the birds of the air, over the livestock, over all the earth, and over all the creatures that move along the ground." Genesis 1: 26–27 (Holy Bible)

The Qur'an also has many statements espousing that creation was established specifically for people. This human-centered worldview actually allows for and promotes egocentric actions where things such as massive forest clearing and wide-spread pollution of rivers are not seen for what they are (i.e., ecocide, the extermination of other life on the earth). Ultimately, these practices come back to harm us with sickness and disease. We will not change our present course of action until we understand that we are part of a whole, and that whole is no more ours for the taking than it is for lions, kangaroos, or walruses. Without any empathy for the rest of the creation, we will destroy the very thing that gives us health in the first place—the natural world.

3. **Reduce the spirit content of world**. As alluded to in the previous paragraph, many religions consider that humans are the sole possessors of spirit. This stands in stark contrast to many indigenous religions (prior to the acculturation of native people) where they believed that much

of the world they interacted with was not merely imbued with spirit but was, in fact, spirit itself. We now live in a world where it is believed that other life and the abiotic elements that occupy this world (e.g., mountains, rivers, lakes, canyons, glaciers, oceans, ravines) are devoid of spirit. Whether or not this is actually true, it affects the way people view the earth. If you are a person who believes that the mountain near your home is a powerful entity that houses one or more deities that your religion recognizes, you will interact with that mountain very differently than a person who lives in a society that treats a mountain as an inanimate entity that houses nothing of value save for the metal ore contained within it (clearly, in this example, the mountains in each scenario will have different fates). As Charlene Spretnak presents in an interview about her book "Resurgence of the Real":

"It [the *Corpus Hermeticum*, an early spiritual and wisdom text] revealed that humans have a different source from nature: we were created directly by God, but nature was created by the Demiurge. Nature was newly understood, from the 1460s on, not as the holistic cosmos of divine creation but merely as raw material to be used by humans as we come into our true role of terrestrial gods on earth. The thing about such hubris, of course, is that it hates humility. Hence the respect and reciprocity with which nonmodern peoples, such as traditional agrarian communities and indigenous cultures, regarded nature was perceived as an affront, a "backward" vestige of history deserving of being crushed for the good of Progress. For generations upon generations, both groups were indeed crushed and assimilated by modern industrial states, whether communist or capitalist."

In many indigenous religions, the plants, animals, and certain geographic features were all important elements in their religions and served as central figures in their creation stories. Today, we live in a world largely expunged of spirit, which sometimes serves to reduce (in the minds of those that believe such) the specialness of this world and make for a mundane existence that is seemingly without purpose or significance. If we consider the world events to be nothing more than chemical and physical reactions, it allows for terrible actions that are injurious to this mega-organism we call the earth. If we were to consider the world to be filled with spirit (or something by another name that generated a deep respect), modern humans would approach each day with a very different perspective—and some events that we regularly witness today would not likely occur with any frequency.

4. **Endorse hierarchy**. Modern religions often possess a distinct set of bureaucrats and religious elites, each with a greater command of people below them. Often, those higher in the "church" (or whatever name is used in that religion) have a greater command of the holy scripture and are seen as closer to the creator. In the Catholic religion, it is organized from lesser to greater responsibility as Deacon to Priest to Bishop to Archbishop to Cardinal to Pope (though there is some overlap and in some instances a single person can occupy multiple roles). In the United Methodist religion, there are local churches who are arranged into districts that are overseen by District Superintendents, who are chosen from a pool of Ordained Elders that are appointed by the Bishop (and so on). It is sometimes claimed that Islamic religion does not have a strict hierarchy. However, there are religious leaders who are afforded various titles, such as Imam, Grand Imam, Ayatollah, and Grand Ayatollah, titles that command a greater degree of reverence than the other titles. Judaism also does not follow a strict hierarchy in the same sense of some religions but still there are titles afforded to different people and those titles come with different responsibilities and may require a greater understanding of the teachings (in this case, contained within the Torah). Regardless of the organization of the religion, there exist different roles within the faith. There is the laity, the general mass of worshipers who are guided through faith-based practices by the religious elites (e.g., priests, rabbis, ministers, bishops). The religious elites request or, in some cases, demand a kind of obedience—an unquestioning faith that their

teachings are correct. This places the elites between the laity and creation, in a sense, the elites act as intermediaries to the creator, establishing a hierarchy of:

worshipers→religious bureaucracy→god (or great mystery)

A religion without hierarchy would simply mean that people directly interact with creation. They would take personal charge of their spirituality and operate free of control (though they may request information and guidance from those more versed in the spirituality they practice). Domesticated humans are so accustomed to hierarchy and trying to ascend the chain of command that they often get caught up in the administration and governance of those below them, which may have nothing to do with the topic at hand (in this case, spirituality). Learning to think and operate for greater human and ecological good without requiring constant direction from leadership is a clear sign of a whole human.

We could go on. For example, some religions do not emphasize a quality of life on this earth but instead focus on reaching the afterlife where everything will be made right. Some religions do not believe that humans can harm god's creation (the earth) and, as a result, do not alter harmful practices. Some religions even consider environmental degradation as evidence of the coming apocalypse and choose not to act to prevent such dilapidation from occurring. While these may seem extreme, they are expected outgrowths of a nature-disconnected population practicing human-centered religion. While this may seem that I am condemning modern religion, it is simply not the case. Religion has many positive aspects that are not to be overlooked. To be clear, none of this writing is to encourage anyone to abandon their faith. I am attempting to promote awareness (nothing more). If we are mindful of the egocentric biases in our daily lives (including in our religions), we can openly confront these views and, hopefully, modify our practices so they are more in line with long-term decision making that protects the health of people and the environment. We do not have to believe that all of life is instilled with spirit to treat creation with respect. Call it something different (if you'd like), just realize that all life is animated and connected to each other by something very special. In doing so, we create the highest quality of life for all living things. We can change the way civilization operates because it is in the best interests of our children and their children. Historically, religions were based on nature and natural phenomena and deeply connected to place. Now, many modern religions seek to dominate nature and the humans that practice those religions and are often interested in expanding their influence (i.e., the amount of space is more important than the place). Through rewilding, we benefit from a willingness to expose all of the biases in our lives that promote separation from nature and further a domesticated mindset. Creation can be experienced, appreciated, and celebrated free of bureaucracy and hierarchy (which are elements of domestication). We can observe these things and be part of a group. We can be part of group that recognizes a need to participate in and fully embrace the wild.

NEOABORIGINAL STRATEGY FOR BEING WILD AND CONNECTING WITH NATURE

The nature divorcement that humans have experienced now pervades many areas of life and includes not just literal separation from nature but also a philosophical departure that creates a biased lens through which we view the world. Many people do enjoy spending time in the out-of-doors and may even prioritize time in nature. While this practice has innumerable benefits, this alone is only a step toward the rewilding of *Homo sapiens*. Even the very idea of a term like "nature" (or "wild") is usually seen from the vantage point of a lifelong immersion in constructed environments interacting with domesticated people. As a result, we are capable of capturing fleeting glimpses of connecting to a world that is rich in life but rarely do we get the entire picture. As Masanobu Fukuoka summarized in his work titled One-Straw Revolution[6]:

"Sickness comes when people draw apart from nature. The severity of the disease is directly proportional to the degree of separation. If a sick person returns to a healthy environment often the disease will disappear. When alienation from nature becomes extreme, the number of sick people increases. Then the desire to return to nature becomes stronger. But in seeking to return to nature, there is no clear understanding of what nature is, and so the attempt proves futile."

To reconnect with nature, we must define what "nature" is. Clearly, it might seem odd to define this important term near the end of the chapter. This was intentional. I wanted you (the reader) to travel through this chapter with your preconceived notion of nature and compare it against the one I will now present. Nature could be defined as a place, a collection of lifeforms, or even a process. It is this latter definition that I would have people consider—that nature is a dynamic process of cooperative interrelationships (i.e., at its core, nature is a verb, not a noun). While wild nature is often viewed as a struggle for existence and that only the fittest survive, this is (again) a highly biased viewpoint that does not adequately capture what is actually occurring in nature. Nature is about relationships, connections, and collaborations. The more connections an organism has, the more likely it is to survive. Even the act of predation by the Canada lynx (*Lynx canadensis*) on snowshoe hare (*Lepus americanus*) is a form of cooperation (through the generations) where the hares feed the predator and the predator maintains a strong population of agile, fast, and wary prey that do not overpopulate their landscape and, ultimately, devastate the vegetation they require for life. As such, natural areas are those places rich in collaborations where the effects of a single species of life rarely dominate the land—such as an inner city environment where the activity of one species (*Homo sapiens*) is virtually all that is present outside of a few organisms that can tolerate an urban setting. The cooperation among a myriad of lifeforms has been stifled in this constructed environment by a decidedly unnatural and very lopsided activity of one organism. Therefore, we can also define nature as a place where the effects of domesticated species are limited—the more the location approaches the constructed environment, the less natural it is.

While this definition of nature is not perfect and would be subject to problems of scale and usability in extreme environments (where few species at all can tolerate the conditions), I believe it still has merit because it allows people to find nature by searching for places with intact ecology (remember, ecology is a science of interrelationships). This definition also allows for an understanding of the degree of "naturalness" of a location. For example, a mountain forest that has been clear-cut will lose some of its subterranean life (due to death of the host trees and heating of soil that is no long shaded by the tree canopy). Many animals adapted to a forest may need to find another location to live (if it exists within range of the animal's ability to migrate). Further, the denuded slopes will supply silt to the streams below, increasing the turbidity of the water. Such a landscape is definitely presenting signs of disproportionate impact from a single organism, one that has lost a significant proportion of its former connections. However, there are still species of plants, fungi, invertebrate, birds, and mammals that can make use of recently cleared forests. While certainly impacted, this environment still contains some of its natural processes and is "more natural" than a city block. Likewise, landscapes occupied by hunter-gatherers were quite natural. Even though many groups applied various tending and

---

[6] Masanobu Fukuoka. The One-Straw Revolution. New York Review Books, New York, NY.

management practices to the landscape, such regions were still rich in a diversity of complex relationships—so much so that the western United States, when first explored, was thought to be a region that was without a trace of human impact (which was utterly untrue). Humans can exist in nature without skewing the natural processes and connections in an unhealthy manner (though it is to be seen if 7.3 billion people can accomplish this).

If nature is a process of complex connections, then to reconnect to nature would be to re-establish these connections and be an active part of this experience. Merely spending time in nature does accomplish this on some level. For example, in the later part of the growing season, our hair and clothing will pick up plant propagules, which we will transport to new areas, acting as dispersal vectors for these species. Just being outdoors walking, birding, and tracking will serve to move fruits, seeds, and spores—which benefits those plants. We can even deposit seeds after passage through our digestive system (if we can accept the fact that humans don't require toilet facilities for all of their bathroom needs). But deeper connection practices would involve more immersive activities, such as drinking wild water, foraging for wild plants, gathering medicinal fungi, stalking and hunting wild animals, and so on. These wild waters and organisms become part of our being as we imbibe and ingest them, altering the domesticated human in subtle and not so subtle ways. We give back by collecting truly sustainable amounts of wild plants (i.e., less than 1% of the population), and planting their seeds after we have dug the taproots or bulbs. When felling trees, we leave older individuals (at least some) that produce seeds, nuts, or other kinds of fruit for the wildlife in the area (including rewilding humans). We provide for medicinal fungi by not removing dead and dying wood from the forest, which serves as a food source for fungi that colonize decaying wood. We give back to animals by taking the least wary individuals and avoiding the usual selection of trophy animals (killing the largest and healthiest animals is a way to weaken the population). We release the largest fish we catch to maintain the fish community. We think and act beyond the near term so that we maintain a place where complex interrelationships can occur. We involve ourselves in this entire experience to the degree that we can (rather than sit afar in an indoor setting without any possibility of participation). Nature immersion is more than just being in nature, it is being nature.

Before we close this chapter with practical strategies that one can use to further nature connection and unlearn (to a degree) human domestication, let us remember that people on a rewilding path need to become active proponents of land conservation. Without wild places, we lose the ability (to a large extent) to rewild our lives. Nature immersion requires nature. Do everything you can to protect the forests, prairies, wetlands, water bodies, deserts, and mountains in your region from losing their numerous and diverse ecological collaborations. In becoming a champion for wild land, remember that you are part of the wild land itself (i.e., you are not protecting an area of land, you are protecting yourself). By promoting the idea that conscientious human use of resources is beneficial, we are more likely to garner favor with a broader array of people and succeed in conserving areas from urbanization. Conservation that precludes human interaction removes one of the possible connections a landscape can have, and furthers the idea that humans can't be part of wild ecosystems (which is incorrect). It also alienates humans from the wild, making it more difficult for people to appreciate the full value of natural places and more likely they will continue on a path leading to complete nature divorcement and hyper-domestication of the human race. With these items in mind, here are ten positive strategies that can bring oneself closer to wild nature.

1. Recognize that you have the capability of **being a wild human**. More than this, understand you need to have some part of your life that is free from hierarchy and dominion (these create an

invisible cell that robs people of some of their happiness, creativity, and enthusiasm). We also need to view other life from this same vantage (i.e., free from hierarchy and dominion). All of life benefits from a person who thinks from an ecocentric perspective.

2. **Spend time in nature** as often and as long as your situation allows. Push your boundaries in this area. For some, this may involve sleeping overnight in their backyard (for the first time). For others, it may involve spending weeks (or longer) in wilderness immersion, away from roads, fences, and buildings. Use this time to strengthen your body and reflect on your place in this world.

3. **Disconnect** yourself from technological media. Use your time in nature to do just that—let go of the desire to know every moment what your virtual friends are doing and writing. Live in the moment, experience nature first hand, and build your own experiences (rather than read about other people's experiences). You cannot build connections to the natural world while you are staring at a small screen that is displaying only modern human social interaction.

4. **Expose yourself to the elements** (when safe and legal to do so). Barefoot walking and even being nude (or meagerly clad) in wild settings is exhilarating when one has come far enough along on this path. Contact with soil, the earth, and direct sunlight all have immense benefit for our being. Taking in air in vegetated settings also has tremendous advantage (through our exposure to phytoncides).

5. Try to **establish natural rhythms** in your life following the patterns of light and dark (to the extent possible). Maximizing your use of natural sunlight (and minimizing your use of night-time lighting) helps to reduce use of fossil-fuel-derived energy for illumination and assists with the body's production of melatonin, which benefits sleep and cancer defense.

6. Set up your home to emulate **natural patterns of temperature**. We are not meant to exist in static state environments. Cool your home down at night to allow your body to experience temperature variation. Many find this is very helpful with promoting quality sleep, which is a necessary part of any strategy for healthy living.

7. **Let go of control ideologies**. We are accustomed to trying to control everything that is perceived to be beneath us (and being controlled by everything that is perceived to be above us). Remember, humans came from egalitarian cultures where equality was strictly practiced (i.e., hierarchy is not our natural condition). We also were integral participants on the landscape who did not need to commit massive resources to "improving nature" to bolster yields. We trusted in the world to provide (and it did, or we would not be present today).

8. **Practice spirituality** that is not controlled by bureaucracy. No human requires an intermediary between them and creation. While we can learn from our religious leaders, we do not need to yield our spiritual sovereignty to anyone. We can be part of an organized religion and still be an individual who celebrates existence free of hierarchy.

9. Build **connections to the wild**. Nature is a dynamic process (it is not merely a place one visits). The more time one spends in nature and the more interaction one has, the stronger those connections will be and the more likely one is to transcend mere survival and experience thriving. The more collaborations we forge (with all of life, including humans), the more likely

we will continue even in difficulty. This world is more complex than the survival of the fittest paradigm. Those who cooperate the most will endure the longest.

10. Express **gratitude** for natural places. These are wild citadels where people can interact directly with the earth and heal from too much time spent in situations that are harmful to our emotional being. Nature is a place where everyone is equal—there is no intentional malice directed at any being. Wild places are vital to our transcendence of domestication. Be thankful for them and do what you can to make sure they are protected from short-term, profit-driven ventures that destroy many of the natural connections that exist in those places.

8. Feral movement: humans in motion

Among the many changes modern humans have experienced as they transitioned from practicing a hunter-gatherer lifeway to that of an agricultural- and industrial-based lifeway, perhaps none are as dramatic as the changes that have occurred to the amount and kind of movement that contemporary people perform. *Homo sapiens*, especially in affluent countries, has converted from a species with a very active lifestyle spending large amounts of time in outdoor environments to a sedentary species that spends much of their time indoors in a seated position. Humans have amazing bodies that are capable of graceful movements, explosive actions, and endurance feats. We are (or, at least, were) adapted to moving over a diversity of terrain, from rock, to forest, to ice and snow, through water, and even underground in caves. We could even use our musculoskeletal system to remain perfectly still for hours (even in a standing position) to avoid being detected by animals that were part of our diet. The strength and stamina of the human body is simply remarkable. But we have changed that. Modern humans simply are relatively motionless for too much of the day. We have become maladapted to motion itself. In doing so, we have not only harmed our health and vitality but also have impacted the well-being of the next generation through heritable changes in genetic expression. Let me be very clear—our sedentary lifestyles make fundamental changes to our health, even at the level of our DNA. It is clear our lifestyles need change. We need to reincorporate principles of feral movement. But what is "feral movement" and how do we experience it?

THE CAPABILITY OF THE HUMAN BODY

If we wanted to discuss the amazing capability of the human body, we could fill volumes with descriptions of athletic prowess, stunning feats of strength, and dance that combines power, flexibility, and grace. But there would be more to describe than these acts alone. Some of the handmade baskets, ceramic vessels, and clothing made by traditional cultures represent perhaps the most intricate and coordinated movements humans perform that blend dexterity, art, and function (a demonstration of hand-eye coordination that surpasses that of any video game player today). With so many potential topics to discuss, this small space here does disservice to *Homo sapiens*. Using one example, we will feature the persistence hunt as a testimony to the physical aptitude of the human body.

The persistence hunt is an extreme feat of human endurance combined with a mastery of tracking. Wild humans using this form of hunting chase animals for prolonged periods of time until the animal is exhausted and can no longer flee from the hunter, at which point the animal is taken with hand-held or hand-thrown weapons (depending on the animal's size and potential to inflict injury). Hunters need to be able to distinguish the fleeing animal's tracks from others of the same species that may also be present—otherwise they pursue different animals through the course of the hunt and do not critically fatigue the original target of the chase. And this tracking is done while moving quickly over uneven terrain in (usually) minimal footwear or barefoot. Like many amazing feats that humans are capable of, the persistence hunt is a multidisciplinary activity, requiring more than just cardiovascular fitness.

To better appreciate the astonishing ability of those performing persistence hunts, it might be useful to present some figures obtained while anthropologists observed hunter-gatherers during this style of hunting (see Liebenberg 2006; Persistence Hunting by Modern Hunter-Gatherers). Of eight such hunts by the !Xo and /Gwi hunters of the central Kalahari region that have been observed, the estimated distance covered was 17.3–35.8 km (10.3–21.4 miles). These hunts lasted for 3 hours 35 minutes to 6 hours 38 minutes. What is perhaps most remarkable isn't the fact that these distances were covered while running over uneven terrain or in minimal (or no) footwear, but that these hunts occur during periods of elevated temperature. The temperatures recorded during hunts by these two groups ranged from 32 to 42 degrees C (89 to 107 degrees F), though most were over 35 degrees C (95 degrees F). In the case of these Kalahari indigenous, the temperature is a critical part of the success of the hunt. Humans, with their ability to perspire and with an upright posture—bipedalism exposes less surface area to the sun's rays—can remain within a core body temperature that allows high functioning. The animals being chased, despite being fast and powerful hooved mammals (e.g., eland, gemsbok, kudu, steenbok), are prevented from resting long enough to allow their body temperatures to return to an acceptable value. As the hunter approaches, the animal sprints away to presumable safety, using much energy and elevating the body core temperature. The hunter maintains a fast but efficient gait, overtaking the animal in a short time and forcing another sprint. After hours of running in the heat of the south African sun, the animal is unable to flee due to exhaustion and hyperthermia, allowing the tired (but not exhausted) human to successfully capture the animal. Imagine, if you can, running for hours in a wilderness setting with temperatures exceeding 35 degrees C and you will have an idea of the persistence hunt (at least as performed by the !Xo and /Gwi hunter-gatherers).

Another remarkable feature of the persistence hunt is that it was not confined to the Kalahari region. It has been noted in anthropological research from widely disjunct places. For example, the Tarahumara people, who now inhabit the mountains and canyons of northern Mexico, are known to have pursued deer in this fashion (which was noted in the book "Born to Run" by Christopher McDougall). The Diné (often called Navajo) and Paiute of the southwestern United States were reported to have hunted pronghorn (*Antilocapra americana*) by persistence hunting. Aborigines of northwestern Australia were documented to have used endurance tactics to acquire kangaroos for food. In northeastern North America, there are two groups who may have used persistence hunting (the confounding issue in this region is that this area was colonized by European settlers before careful anthropological work could document some of the natural history of these people, leaving some details of their lifeway to the realm of legend). The Penobscot, an eastern Algonquian group living in central Maine, was said to have had young men who could run swiftly and overtake moose and deer. These men were referred to (in the singular) as the k^{w}sih^{w}αpe, a word that also was used to denote a super man, a sacred man, and a pure man (the last because these men were prevented from having sexual relations). The Caniba, also an eastern Algonquian group, but long ago driven from their ancestral homeland along the Kennebec River and its tributaries, were also stated to have used persistence hunting during the winter by snowshoe, which they were described as being "able to overtake the swiftest of animals" in an 1887 writing.

Sadly, the persistence hunt is disappearing from the world. It is another aspect of indigenous lifeways that is being lost to industrial living (where convenience, comfort, and instant gratification are important). In the past 30 years, only two groups of people (living in the same region) have been observed participating in this style of hunting. While there are some people, such as Olympic athletes, who could physically perform the persistence hunt, they would not be able recognize and follow the tracks of the animals, may not be able to navigate back to camp without modern global positioning satellite equipment, and would not know how to fabricate the clothing, footwear, and tools used in the hunt. It is the capacity of people to perform astonishing feats while interacting with their environment and applying traditional skill sets that is perhaps the most amazing thing of all—all the while without athletic sponsorship to develop the conditioning needed for the persistence hunt.

MOVEMENT IN THE MODERN WORLD

Before we answer the question concerning the concept of feral movement, let's fully appreciate the kind of movement that is experienced in the modern world. First, to be completely open, there is simply not enough of it. While the overweight condition is not entirely the result of too few calories expended (because it is also the result of too many calories ingested and other complicating factors, such as endocrine disrupting chemicals), a sedentary lifestyle is a major contributing factor to overweightness. Here in the United States, a full ⅔ of the population is considered overweight (think about that for a moment). Half of those overweight are classified as obese (i.e., ⅓ of the American populace is obese). This is indicative of an epidemic of inactivity. A 2010 study reported that adult Americans took an average of 5117 steps per day (total activity). There are, for the "average person", 1309 steps in a kilometer; therefore, the average adult American walks approximately 3.9 kilometers (2.4 miles) a day. This number is well below other industrialized countries (Australia, Japan, Switzerland). It also falls very short of our wild progenitors (remember from chapter 2 that some extant hunter-gatherers who have been observed walked 8–16 kilometers (5–10 miles) a day). But these numbers don't tell the entire story because hunter-gatherers were walking this distance over uneven terrain with vegetation, streams, boulders, and other items that would have required turning, bending, stooping, leaping, wading, etc. to deal with landscape features. This would be in stark contrast to domesticated humans who primarily walk on roads, down hallways, and across rooms—all with uniform, often level, surfaces and requiring very little body movement except for that required for direct locomotion (save for occasionally opening doors and pushing buttons in the elevator). In other words, the movements experienced by the hunter-gatherers as they traversed the land would have required additional and more complicated movement (leading to more calories expended, and more lymph movement, which we will discuss shortly).

Movement, for most people, has really been replaced by sitting. Research on this topic suggests the many Americans sit more than eight hours of the day (e.g., a New York City study found the average time sitting was 8.2 hours a day, a study of full-time employees of large companies found the average time sitting was 13 hours a day). Review of similar studies from other affluent countries shows similar results that people from urbanized countries sit extensively. It isn't just office jobs that do a lot of sitting today. Let's keep in mind that many professions that used to expend a lot of calories in physical work, such as the timber industry, now have many sedentary jobs where workers sit inside of the climate-controlled cabs of heavy machinery and operate controls with their hands and feet. Research also shows that those who sit a lot at work often do not make up for their movement deficits at home (i.e., they tend to also be sedentary out of work, engaging extensively in behaviors like television viewing, gaming, and the like). Prolonged sitting is associated with significant increased risk of cardiovascular disease, depression, stress, diabetes, obesity, muscle/joint problems, and a reduced feeling of well-being. Cancer rates are also considerably higher in those who sit prolonged periods each day. The amount of research that can't be summarized here on the health-robbing effects of prolonged sitting is staggering. Instead of poring through endless reams of data on this, let us summarize this idea by mentioning a study published in 2012 in the British Journal of Sports Medicine. The authors calculated that every hour of time spent sitting (e.g., watching TV) reduces a person's life expectancy by 21.8 minutes compared with the 11 minutes of estimated loss of life expectancy for each cigarette smoked. In some ways, the amount of time one spends sitting each day is a more important factor in determining the health of the individual than the time they spend in activity.

It is often helpful to think of sitting in this way: when we sit, we ask chairs and other kinds of furniture to do work for us. Instead of sitting in a way that we support our body (especially the upper portion), which occurs when we sit or squat on the ground or the floor, we use seats to hold us in a position where it requires our body to hold less of our body weight load. Essentially, the chair is a kind of splint for back, hips, and upper legs. Given how much time we spend in this position—modern humans are more practiced at sitting than any other activity—our body adapts (in a way) to this low force environment over time by losing muscle and skeleton mass, changing the length of connective tissue, and altering blood vessels. It costs our body in metabolic energy to maintain features of the musculoskeletal system that we do not need. So, in a sense, modern bodies are so weak, in part, because they are adapted to sedentary behavior in which furniture holds their weight. Additionally, holding one position for hours and hours each day has additional ramifications. We lose range of motion because our bodies are not being used to their full potential. You can easily identify this for yourself: simply feel how stretched the muscles and tissues are in your calf when you stand, and then sit with your legs bent approximately 90 degrees and notice how much looser they are. Sitting in chairs shortens some groups of tissue and lengthens others (but not just temporarily). This is one reason why doing a flat-footed squat as an adult is difficult for many people because the Achilles tendon and the muscles in the calf have lost flexibility from infrequency of certain uses (more on this later). But not only do we lose range of motion, we lose function. Joints that are chronically maintained in common position gradually become adapted to that position—and those tissues that have been chronically shortened or lengthened are unable to provide the full functionality of the joint. This means that if we use those parts of the body in ways different from the usual day to day activity, other tissues adjacent to them must compensate (to a degree). This places additional stresses on these compensating tissues and can lead to injury.

The problem (regarding movement) for contemporary humans is that they have spent tremendous creative efforts to build a convenient life that is without "too much" movement. They start in the morning with automated technology to prepare morning beverages and end in the evening with universal remote controls to change stations on the television without leaving the chair or couch. They have found ways to take all of the movements they used to perform, including those involved with food preparation (e.g., grinding, mixing, stirring, sorting), and have them performed by kitchen machines and laborers in distant lands (who sort, peel, slice, blend, and powder foods for purchase in supermarkets). At every turn, we seek to build in convenience, creating an ever greater movement deficit in our lives. Sedentary jobs are on the rise in affluent countries, despite the fact they are linked to a variety of health disorders. On the weekends, pushing a lawnmower became too much work (and, now, a symbol of lower status), so a riding lawnmower became a must, allowing the user to remain in a seated position for more of the day. Walking up stairs or down hallways also became too much effort, so escalators and moving sidewalks became commonplace in some settings. While our current version of industry spews toxins onto our landscapes (in part as a direct result of the lack of movement we engage in), we put our imaginative talents to work to create new ways to sit more of the day. Is this really the best use of our ingenuity? This topic seems to support the idea that we have lost an ability to determine what is really important in the world. But this is a digression; let's get back on topic.

It is recommended by the United States government that its citizens experience 2.5 hours of moderate-intensity aerobic exercise each week (that is 30 minutes a day). In place of this, a person could perform 1.25 hours a week of high-intensity activity (that would be only 15 minutes each day). In addition to one or a combination of these activities, Americans should engage in strength training (e.g., weight lifting, calisthenics) twice a week. A very large study with over 450,000 participants performed by the CDC found that only 20% of the people included in the study met these basic exercise requirements. And of those 20% who did, what kind of movement did they engage in? Many may have visited a gym to use various pieces of equipment (e.g., elliptical trainer, stationary bike, tread mill), or may have had such equipment in the house. Or perhaps they walked or ran on a street or track, or rode a bicycle. In any of these cases, they performed a repetitive motion or a small set of repetitive motions—in fact, they would have experienced a tiny fraction of a percent of the possible kinds of movement and positions the body is capable of. Such exercise would lead to a deficiency in essential movement that would have (in a sense) "nourished" the musculoskeletal system. Remember, movement is a particular type of activity that humans must experience (i.e., it is part of the experiential food group).

Keeping in mind that domesticated humans spend a great deal of time in constructed settings, which are geometrically depauperate compared with natural settings, our bodies simply do not need to work through the same range of movements as those moving (or living) in wild settings. This means that certain portions of our musculoskeletal system fail to receive the movement nourishment they require for health. This has a myriad of effects on the human body. One of those is movement (or lack of movement) of lymph. Lymph is the fluid found in the interstitial spaces between the cells of our body and in our lymph vessels. An adult has approximately 10 liters (2.9 gallons) of lymph fluid (compared with about 5 liters (1.5 gallons) of blood in an average-sized adult). Lymph serves several important functions, including managing fluid levels in the body, immunological defense, and lipid absorption. Lymph is a critical part of our immune system because as it picks up some of the cellular wastes (i.e., metabolites) found in the interstitial fluid, it also collects bacteria and metastatic cancer cells (when present). These are transported by a system of vessels (called lymph vessels) to various locations (e.g., spleen, lymph nodes) where they are destroyed. The lymphatic system does not have a centralized pump like the cardiovascular system. Instead of a heart, it relies on two primary mechanisms for movement of lymph: (a) a thin layer of smooth muscle cells adjacent to the vessels that contracts in a peristalsis-like fashion and (b) contraction of adjacent skeletal muscles that compress lymph vessels. Both of these processes are facilitated by a series of valves in the lymph vessels that prevent backward flow of lymph; therefore, lymph fluid generally moves from body tissues to lymph nodes and ultimately back into the vascular system.

The movement of lymph fluid is highly dependent on our body's movement. As our muscles contract and push on the lymph vessels, the squeezing action moves the fluid along. When we are sedentary, the lymph does not move efficiently and collects in low places where gravity draws it. In fact, a sedentary lifestyle is reported to reduce lymph flow by as much as 94%. Too little movement is, for example, the reason why some elderly people who sit for long portions of the day have substantial edema in their feet and ankles. This edema is not merely unsightly, it is indicative of a serious health issue. Cellular wastes need to be removed for the effective functioning of our cells. Further, proteins need to be appropriately returned to the bloodstream and foreign organisms (e.g., bacteria) need to be cleaned from interstitial fluid. All of these are accomplished (at least in part) by our lymphatic system. When bacteria (or macrophages that have engulfed bacteria) are not removed, our adaptive immune system has no way to generate specialized white blood cells (such as B-cells and T-cells) that can attack the specific bacteria at the site of the infection. The reason for this is that the specialized cells are not made at the site of infection but in lymph nodes; therefore, lymph (with the offending bacteria) must move from the site of infection to the lymph nodes so that the body can produce a more precise defense. Our adaptive immune system has a stronger response than our innate immune system (the latter is what operates initially at the site of infection). The point of the last two paragraphs is that movement turns out to be critical for the functioning of our immune system. The more diverse and frequent the movement, the better the transport of lymph through the lymph vessels. A small set of repetitive movements, what now constitutes much of modern movement, is not going to efficiently move lymph in all locations of the body.

While lymph movement is well-known to be driven by bodily movement and associated contraction and relaxation of skeletal muscles, many do not realize that our blood is also dependent on this same movement. In other words, the heart organ is not the sole mover of blood through our vessels (except when we are motionless). It turns out that the usual (and vastly over-simplified) model of the cardiovascular system is simply not accurate. Muscle contraction causes blood vessels to be compressed and then relax, pushing blood from areas of high pressure to areas of low pressure—though not randomly but in a coordinated fashion. Muscle contraction works with the heart to move blood into the capillaries and out of them so that the cells of our tissues can be perfused with oxygen. Without movement, our cells are poorly perfused with oxygen (and without a regular supply of oxygen, our cells die). This "skeletal muscle pump" is a critical part of cardiovascular system, especially when we are standing and engaged in movement. Here is the critical piece of this you must understand: only those muscles engaged in movement help supply oxygenated blood to the tissues adjacent to the capillary beds. Therefore, muscle groups you do not use (or do not use frequently) do not assist in the movement of blood. This is another critical reason why a diversity of movement is necessary for the health of our entire body.

Movement in the modern world is plagued by a number of issues. There is not enough of it. There is not enough diversity of it. And we tend to think about it incorrectly. Movement doesn't have to all be high-intensity training. Walking to visit a friend, crouching to pick up sticks in the yard, reaching to pick apples from a tree, and crawling beneath low hanging branches in the forest are all examples of low-intensity movement that is highly valuable for the body (i.e., it is part of the holistic movement needs we must satisfy). When we structure our lives to have too little movement, physical motion becomes that which we do to offset the calories we have ingested. Instead of celebrating (through practicing) what are bodies are capable of, we seek excuses to remain relatively motionless. Movement becomes penance (in a sense) for eating too much. Therefore, we approach movement not with excitement but with dread. Katy Bowman said this very well in her book "Move Your DNA"[7]:

"Our current model sets both food and movement as a negative. Eating food (a biological imperative) makes us feel guilty, and we turn movement (also a biological imperative) into punishment. Atonement for diet through exercise. It is no wonder so many people feel unable to begin moving (and eating) in a way that honors both food and our innate ability to move. We've got it all backwards in our minds."

Modern humans have gone to great lengths to make sure that movement (and exercise) is done on their terms. We have created convenient lives that require very little motion. Then, after work, we drive to a gym and "work out", trying to acquire the movement needs of our body because they were not met in our daily living. Instead of active lives that provide a rich variety

[7] Katy Bowman. 2014. Move Your DNA: Restore Your Health Through Natural Movement. Propriometrics Press, United States.

of physical motions being performed in different positions, we structure our living to be comfortable and convenient. That way, we exercise when and for how long we wish to. Unfortunately, this approach to movement (i.e., limiting the motion to a short period of the day), while far better than being completely sedentary, has some major drawbacks for our health. **Research shows that being sedentary most of the day is not compensated for by a short duration of exercise** (see the article by Biswas and colleagues who published a review of 47 studies in 2015). In other words, a long period of sitting outweighs the benefits we get from a brief period of workout. Of course, this kind of activity does not emulate the movement patterns of our ancestors—movement patterns that our physiology and anatomy require for health.

THE GYM IS NOT WILD

The gym membership has become synonymous with a healthy lifestyle. Many people would consider the gym a place to strengthen the physical body. And while it may do that, the gym can also be described as another thermo-regulated environment under artificial lighting that utilizes unnatural and/or isolated movements, which is to say, it is much like other venues that make up domesticated human living. This probably sounds like a strong statement against gyms. It isn't meant to imply that the gym setting never has application and that it should be avoided but we must understand its limitations if we are to truly identify why it might make sense to use our local landscapes more and the gym less.

One of the major problems with domesticated humans is that we are divorced from nature and are not reaping the benefits of exposure to the elements. Gyms do nothing to address this serious issue (but it is entirely possible to change the setting we use for physical conditioning and correct this problem). Elemental foods, which we discussed in chapter 3, are not found inside the gym. Clean (or at least cleaner) air, sunlight, contact with the earth, and exposure to natural settings are all benefits obtained while moving outside. Outdoor settings require us to accommodate for uneven ground and angled terrain, which generates awareness of our surroundings and greater balance. Further, we can potentially get a wider range of movements (especially when off trail), benefitting our musculoskeletal and lymphatic systems in ways that gym equipment can't. While gyms can have net benefit for people using the equipment in those settings, there are many health reasons why it makes sense to seek movement (or at least some proportion of the movement) outdoors.

When we examine the kinds of exercise that are utilized in the gym setting, we can identify further limitations of that environment. Many of the exercises are unnatural, forcing the body to do movements that are not required in natural living. Isolating one or more muscle groups to build large muscles is a common practice in gyms, again, something that would rarely occur or even need to occur in a more nature-connected lifestyle (and is this practice actually health-driven or ego-driven?). Most physical tasks require multiple muscle groups cooperating together in an intelligent and complex way while the body is balanced to avoid slipping or falling. While machine weights are easier to learn and use (especially when working out alone), they sometimes have a very unnatural arc of motion. Further, the machine actually does some of the most important work for the user—the technique involved in balancing and stabilizing the weight is done by the machine. Equally important, most gym equipment involves highly repetitive motions done from the exact same position. Natural movement is frequently different in some facet (or facets), especially given that movement requirements change as tasks are performed toward completion (e.g., construction of some particular structure, whether it be for shelter, food storage, or ceremony, involves placing, holding, and securing materials at a variety of heights).

Due to the repetitive nature of some gym equipment and the fact that that equipment may isolate muscles that rarely (if ever) operate independently from other muscles, valid criticism has been waged that such equipment contribute to creating injury, rather than protecting the body from it.

Gyms are enclosed settings that come with a wide range of indoor environmental hazards. It would be sensible for gym users to be aware of these threats, which are sometimes significant, that are routinely found in this setting (the following is only a partial list). Visiting a location to benefit one aspect of your health while harming other aspects might not be the best use of time or personal resources. Gym owners and managers that attempt to address the following features are to be commended.

• The pools are often disinfected with chlorine, a chemical that kills bacteria. However, when chlorine combines with organic molecules, such as microbes and sweat and urine (from the swimmers), it forms toxic disinfection byproducts (e.g., chloroform) that can produce allergic reactions in some people, such as asthma, skin rashes, and irritated eyes, and are known to be carcinogenic (recall the discussion from chapter 4).

• Gym surfaces, such as exercise equipment, showers, and changing rooms, are disinfected with various chemicals that can be quite harmful. For example, triclosan, a common ingredient in antibacterial soaps, has been linked to suppressed immune system function, endocrine disruption, allergies, and thyroid issues. Other cleaners, including those used in the showers, can contain formaldehyde and glutaraldehyde, chemicals that are known to produce allergic reactions, headaches, and cancer.

• The air quality in most gyms is quite deplorable. In addition to the volatile organic compounds (VOCs) that are off-gassing from the paint on the walls, the carpets, the carpet pads, and the adhesives that hold the carpets down, there is also an abundance of phthalates found in body and hair sprays used in the changing rooms. These chemicals, often related to the fragrances found in spray products, are also known to disrupt endocrine function.

• The mats that people use in gyms for comfort while stretching, for yoga, and other purposes are often made of polyvinyl chloride (PVC). PVC products require additives to produce the desired qualities in gym mats. These additives include phthalates (which cause endocrine disruption), dioxin (a very harmful and carcinogenic compound), and lead and cadmium (toxic heavy metals). Other additives contribute to the off-gassing that occurs in gyms, further adding to the poor air quality found in most of these facilities. In fact, air quality indoors is usually much worse than that outdoors (frequently with 2–5 times the total pollutants found outdoors, sometimes much more). Of course, it is noteworthy to mention that PVC mats do not biodegrade, and often end up polluting ground water or air (depending on whether they are placed in a landfill or incinerated, respectively). Remember, when products like this are "disposed of", that phrase is merely a euphemism for "let someone else deal with the health issues this product causes", an unfortunately reality of these items.

• Ethylene vinyl acetate (EVA) is another material that gym mats are made from, and it is also used for the protective foam padding on gym equipment. EVA includes many toxic compounds, including ammonia and formamide, which are corrosive. EVA also off-gasses, further contributing to the poor air quality and known to produce eye and skin irritation, respiratory problems, and (potentially) cancer. Further, exposure to EVA can impair proper fetal development.

• Gyms are usually very poor locations if you are trying to limit your exposure to human-created electromagnetic fields (EMFs). EMFs are produced by the Wi-Fi, mobile phones, and powered equipment that are used for cardiovascular conditioning. High levels of EMF are known to be found in gyms. Though most people do not concern themselves with this form of radiation, increasingly studies are being published that demonstrate EMF affects sleep patterns, mood, and memory in some people (and may even alter genetic expression in individuals exposed to high levels).

All of this certainly makes it sound as though I'm condemning gyms. That isn't the case. But to neglect mention of these items in a book attempting to reconnect people with nature would be inappropriate. While gym exposure to the aforementioned items, alone, is not likely to cause health issues in a relatively healthy person, the fact that many people already have abundant exposures means the gym contributes to the body burden of these chemicals. Further, those with sensitivities may wish to limit their time in this setting. The gym certainly has a place in our movement regime, but to make it the core location of physical motion has significant limitations. If you have a choice, I would encourage you to spend at least some of your time moving in the outdoors. This setting has innumerable advantages, some of which are reaped just by being in a natural setting (e.g, reducing stress, benefitting mood, assisting with creativity, connecting people to their landscape).

Modern people need to find ways to spend more time in nature, not less. Even more than this, they need to find ways to do more natural things, which constructed environments don't always support. For example, lifting weights off the ground, setting them down, and then repeating this motion for the duration of the strength training is not natural (while lifting some heavy items for an actual purpose, such as shelter construction or stacking firewood, is). Domesticated people use energy to drive to the gym, spend time in a setting that requires energy to make it semi-hospitable, only to use more energy to power the treadmill or make possible reading the digital display on the exercise machines. Moving and exercising are supposed to use energy stored within the human body (not versions of energy stored within the ground). Rewilding our movement provides us with solutions to many of the problems discussed in this section.

THE PROBLEMS (PLURAL) WITH MODERN SHOES

Footwear has been an important item of clothing for humans, allowing our species to move over more kinds of terrain with safety. Hazards that footwear protect from include plants with spines, prickles, and thorns (which are collectively are referred to as "armature"), sharp stones, hot surfaces warmed by solar insolation, and cold surfaces and substrates (e.g., snow, glaciers) in areas closer to the poles, high in elevation, or during the winter season. Indigenous footwear was designed to deal with the specific hazards of their landscape—though it should be noted that no group wore shoes throughout the year. So there was plenty of barefoot time for everyone. With that written, indigenous groups from different regions made different kinds of footwear. Clearly, the Inuit (from northern North America) made different footwear than the Diné (southwestern United States). The former dealt with extreme cold, walking on snow and ice for a large part of the year and even navigating frigid water and slush in their footwear. The latter needed to deal with hot temperatures, scorching sand and gravel, and a variety of plants that produced armature capable of piercing the bottom of the foot. Despite all these differences, most indigenous footwear had a remarkable number of similarities—and stark differences from many kinds of modern footwear. Let us start there (with the modern footwear).

Modern footwear comes in a vast variety of forms, making it impossible to generalize among all of these kinds. Running shoes are different from leather boots, which are different from dress heels, which are different from flip flops. However, all of these shoes (and I repeat, all of them) have one or more features that can (and often do) create problems for the musculoskeletal system. To initiate the discussion of modern footwear, we must first understand that what we do to our feet, we do (to some extent) to much of our body. As Katy Bowman points out well in her book "Whole Body Barefoot", our bones, cartilage, tendons, ligaments, and muscles form an interconnected system. When we adjust the angles on one part of this system (such as when we bend over at the waist), we cause lengthening and shortening of various tissues through the length of our body and cause bones to be positioned (with respect to one another) differently. Therefore, changes we make to our feet (through the shoes we wear) have effects on the rest of our body.

One universal part of shoes (of any style) is the sole. This is the bottom of the shoe that protects us from sharp objects or a ground surface that is either too hot or too cold for prolonged contact with our feet. Modern footwear, largely, has relatively rigid soles. While certainly some portions of the sole flex or hinge, much of the sole is quite inflexible. In fact, some shoes also utilize a metal (historically), fiberglass, or Kevlar shank to increase rigidity of the sole. Modern soles act like a splint for your feet—meaning that the 33 major muscles of each foot do not need to perform as they were designed to. As a result, they atrophy, to the extent that some people are no longer able to walk barefoot for any length of time without the "support" provided by shoes. Further, given that there are many thousands of nerve endings in the foot, it is clear the nervous system in the foot is designed to sense the environment we walk through. However, a thick sole takes complex terrain with various macro- and micro-surface details and converts this to almost the exact same stimulus on the bottom of the foot each time we take a step. We should be receiving information from the nerves in our feet, which would be used to answer questions like what is the angle of the terrain, what is the substrate like, are there items beneath my feet that are loose and can shift, are their objects or depressions that require the feet to adjust for balance, what is the temperature of the ground, how slippery is the ground surface, and so on. Much of this information is lost with modern footwear—which amounts to another form of nature disconnection. This loss of information means that our proprioception is affected. Proprioception is the ability of the body to understand where it is in space, which allows us to keep ourselves oriented and perform multiple physical tasks at the same time. Thick-soled shoes rob our feet of some of the proprioceptive ability because we are unable to sense some aspects of the environment we move through.

Most modern shoes are designed with a raised heel. It is such a common feature of contemporary shoes that footwear lacking a raised heel looks unusual to many people. The heel, you may be surprised to learn, serves no verified beneficial purpose with regard to our foot, leg, hip, and back health (remember, what happens to the feet happens to the rest of our body). The heel was designed primarily for cultural reasons (e.g., attractiveness, style) and not with a protective purpose in mind. Certainly, the heel found on historical horse riding shoes helped to make sure the shoes would not slip out of the stirrups (so it did have a functional purpose); however, it was not designed to protect the foot while walking. But what about running shoes, aren't the heels of those shoes designed to protect the foot from repetitive impact on the ground? Let's hold that question for a couple of paragraphs. For the most part, heels serve only to raise the rear end of the shoe (sometimes substantially) when compared with the front end of the shoe where the toes are located. This changes the angle that the foot is normally positioned with respect to the ground. With the heel raised further from the ground than the toes, it essentially creates the situation that people wearing such shoes are constantly walking downhill, and the problem is exacerbated with taller heels, a taller person, or a shorter foot (all of these features make for a more pronounced angle of compensation by the body). But is this really a problem? Well, no, not when we walk downhill some of the time because our bones and tissues in our feet are designed to do this, as are our knees, hips, and back, which all must make adjustments when we walk downhill (without these adjustments, which amounts to leaning backward, we would fall forward). However, when we walk in shoes our entire lives that are pitched forward (due to a raised heel), our body doesn't make temporary adjustments, it begins to make ones that are more permanent (note: different people make slightly different adjustments for this forward cant of the shoes).

There are several problems with heels. First, we begin to lose range of motion in our ankle because it is effectively lifted a slight bit (relative to the toes). Instead of feet being parallel with the ground (when on a flat surface), they are set at an angle, which keeps the foot in a position called plantar flexion instead of neutral (see Figure 8.1). Therefore, natural positions like flat-footed squat, are difficult to establish and hold for many people. Second, all of those adjustments in our legs, hips, and back change the way our body carries this load. This can create ankle, knee, hip, and back problems because the loads experienced by the body are shifted backward in a way that we are not meant to experience on a continual basis. Third, heels can create a chronic situation of a slightly bent knee, which shortens muscles in the calf and those on the back of the thigh. This prolonged knee flexion can, over time, pull the pelvis into a slightly tilted position, which then subsequently pulls on the lower vertebrae in the spine. Therefore, some lower back problems can be created or exacerbated by our footwear and the way we move in these shoes (read compensate for the continuous raised heel and the resulting forces applied to our musculoskeletal system).

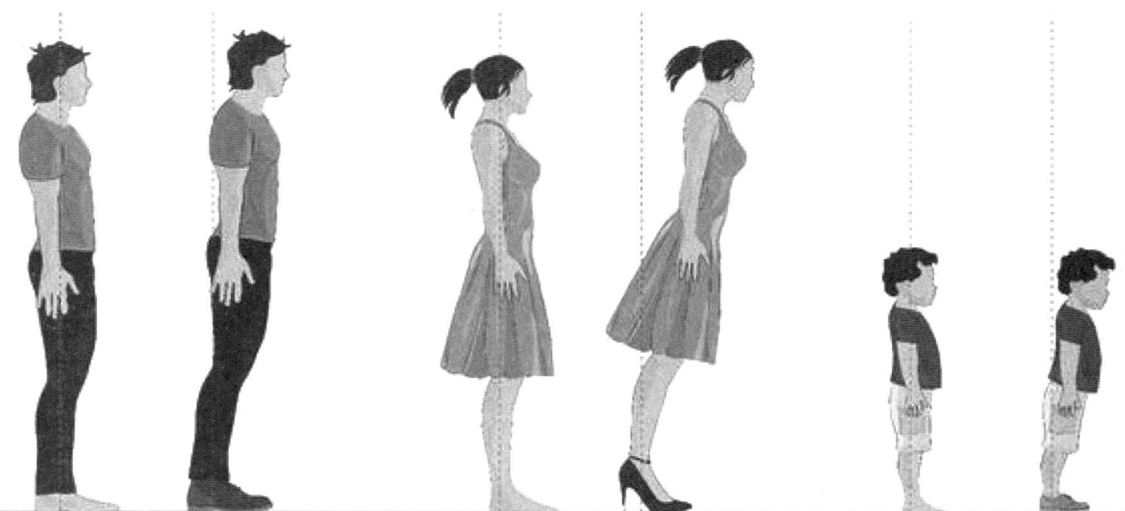

Figure 8.1. The effect of heels on footwear is to tip the body forward (as if one was walking down an incline), forcing an adjustment in the ankle, knees, hips, and back to compensate for this downward-tipped angle of the foot. All of this chronically distributes the loads on various joints differently than someone standing in a neutral position with their heels on the ground.

Most of us believe that a thick, cushioned heel (which is raised) on running shoes is designed to protect the foot from excessive impact. The fact is that the cushioned heel on running shoes was designed without careful science (making those running in such shoes unknowing Guinea pigs—sound familiar?). A 2009 review by Richards et al. in the British Journal of Sports Medicine failed to identify a single example of original research demonstrating that a cushioned heel and features in the shoe to prevent inward rolling of the foot (i.e., pronation) benefit distance runners. The thick heel of the running shoe changes the gait from one that lands more toward the front of the foot (as seen in hunter-gatherer runners) to one where the heel contacts the ground first and then the forward part of the foot slaps down onto the ground after this. This running gait is so common today—due to the use of running shoes with heels—that most people believe it to be the "natural" running gait of humans. There are several problems with this unnatural gait. Perhaps most importantly, it shifts the footfall impact from the more forward part of the foot, which allows the body's shock absorbing systems to operate, back to the heel where the foot forcibly impacts the ground. You can identify this for yourself. Try thumping your heel on the floor or ground and then do the same with the ball of your foot. You will notice the heel strike is quite abrupt and jarring, while the ball of the foot is softer because there are more tissues (including those of the ankle joint and muscles of the calf) flexing to absorb the footfall. The heel strike completely changes the mechanics of running and the resulting forces experienced by the body. For example, when someone runs using the heel strike method, their toes are pulled backward (a position called dorsal flexion) and the heel takes the impact. Then, the forward part of the foot flaps forward (into plantar flexion) and the arch receives very little of the load (at this point—the arch will be loaded, but not until the knee begins to move forward of the foot during the running stride). Contrast this with a forefoot strike, where the foot lands in plantar flexion (the toes are pointed down slightly) and then the ankle bends so that the toes are no longer pointed downward (i.e., the foot begins to enter dorsal flexion). While this happens, the arch begins to stretch and flatten as it is loaded. This analysis could continue to discuss additional details of the foot and ankle, demonstrating tremendous differences in the biomechanics of these two running styles.

Despite all this, one can still point to the cushioned heel of running shoes and assert that this must provide a protective padding that limits excessive force to the feet (and the structures connected to the feet). However, this assertion would not be correct. While a human who is running will strike the ground with an amount of force, the style of running can change how rapidly those forces are experienced by the body. Research on heel-strike running demonstrates it to present much more abrupt forces to the body than forefoot-strike running, which presents the same total force but in a more gradual fashion (for those who can visualize this, the force curve is much steeper in heel-strike running). The best analogy I've seen to describe the differences in the force equate the foot to a rod (not a perfect analogy but the point will be made). Heel-strike running is similar to dropping the rod from a given height perpendicular to the ground so that the rod strikes perfectly on its end. Forefoot-strike running is like dropping the rod at an angle to the ground so that it strikes on end and then the rod continues to move until the other end also strikes the ground. The nearly instantaneous force applied by heel-strike running is completely unnatural and, in part, responsible for the large number of injuries seen in people who run frequently (studies indicate that 60–65% of runners experience injury over the course of a year). The forces experienced by the feet and the rest of the body during heel-strike running are more abrupt whether or not the runner is wearing a modern running shoe. In other words, it is the style of running that produces the more instantaneous forces, and this style of running is usually seen in runners with heeled shoes (i.e., the contemporary shoe promotes this kind of running).

Moving on to the problems with modern footwear, let us look at aspects of the upper, the part of the shoe that is connected to the sole and wraps over the top of and behind our feet. While there are several issues with the upper, one of the important ones to discuss is the toe box. This is the forward region of the upper that encapsulates the toes on each foot. Many, many shoes hold the toes together in slight (or severe) compression, not allowing them to spread out and articulate independently of one another. Such a toe box limits the functioning of the foot and contributes to atrophy of the muscles involved in moving the toes, which weaken because they are not allowed to move inside of most modern shoes. Further, the toe box of some shoes has a shape that does not match the shape of our foot. This shape disparity is perhaps best exemplified in some women's shoes where the front of the shoe comes to a point near the centerline of the shoe but feet are asymmetrical, with the point of the foot positioned at the big toe or the toe adjacent to this one (i.e., not near the centerline of our feet). The pressure created by such an upper compresses the foot in a highly unnatural way. As a result of years and years of being compressed inside of a shoe's toe box, many people have difficulty spreading their toes apart (a movement called abduction). This is indicative of another loss of range of function of the foot due to the footwear we have chosen.

Given all these problems (and more not discussed here), the obvious question becomes: what should we be wearing on our feet? The answer to this is, unfortunately, not simple. Assuming that someone has spent a fair amount of time barefoot during their life so that their feet are not debilitated from being confined to footwear, they may be able to easily transition to more time barefoot or (when bare feet are not allowed or appropriate) minimalist-style footwear. Such footwear has a relatively thin and flexible sole that both allows the user to sense the ground beneath them and protects the wearer from sharp plants or human refuse (e.g., nails, broken glass, metal edges). For those who have spent excessive time in modern shoes, such an immediate transition may not be possible. The feet (and the structures connected to them), including the musculature and connective tissue, are simply too weakened and inflexible. They have not needed to support themselves because they have been contained within footwear that not only has prevented their proper function but also has caused them to atrophy. The ability of the feet to prevent excessive rolling of the ankle inward or outward (for examples) is too difficult for the feet to perform on anything except perfectly level terrain. Which is another good point—many people who do spend time barefoot do so inside the home, on level lawns, and other such terrain where the feet are simply not stressed (in a beneficial way) to perform the tasks that wild feet are capable of. For those who cannot immediately transition to barefoot walking, both strength training and flexibility work may be necessary to rebuild the full function that feet are capable of (see Whole Body Barefoot by Katy Bowman for exercises designed to transition to barefoot walking and an extensive bibliography of scientific articles that support statements made in this section).

Minimalist shoes are a good option for those who are in places where bare feet are not appropriate (due to terrain hazards) or allowed (due to legal issues). Such shoes not only have thin soles, but also lack heels (i.e., the heel of the foot is not raised on cushioning higher than the toe). Further, such shoes should have a spacious toe box that does not compress the fore portion of the foot. Lastly, minimalist shoes should have some kind of upper or lacing/strapping system so that the foot does not require a special movement or position to hold the shoe on. Toe-gripping is necessary with many flip flops and some slippers, a position that should not be held for long periods of time by the foot, which can affect the muscles of the toe and the strength of the arch. Examples of minimalist shoes include moccasins (excluding some new styles with a raised heel and supportive structures around the heel), Vibram Five Fingers, Vivobarefoot Shoes, and Soap Box Shoes (for children). For those wanting something like a flip flop or sandal, check out Unshoes Minimal Footwear. And for those needing something warm (where a thick sole is necessary to provide insulation from the cold ground), look into Arrow Moccasin Company (made to order), Steger Mukluks, or Soft Star Shoes. There are lots of companies out there making minimalist shoes now, so it is not difficult to find lots of options. Of course, one could make their own footwear (using many kinds of indigenous patterns). That would be the "wildest" option if it were a contest (which it isn't), but people living in a consumer-based economy rarely consider making things for themselves.

Undoubtedly some of you reading this section have heard some controversy regarding barefoot running and minimalist shoes. First, there was a lawsuit. Second, there are all kinds of injuries occurring to people wearing minimalist shoes (suggesting these are not a good idea). Let us begin with the lawsuit, which involved the Vibram brand called Five Fingers (a minimalist shoe with separate compartments for each toe on the foot). The litigation was not because these shoes damaged people's feet. The suit occurred because of the way the shoes were advertised. The company made claims that could not be upheld by the way some people used them. Some people continued a heel-strike running gait after transitioning to Five Fingers, but such shoes really require a forefoot-strike running gait. In any case, minimalist shoes do not guarantee that people will not receive injuries due to their use. For example, a study by Ridge and colleagues in 2013 demonstrated greater bone marrow edema in the feet of 10 of 19 experienced runners who made a transition to minimalist shoes. Making a rapid transition from modern heeled shoes to minimalist shoes is, for most people, simply not a smart move. Their feet are not prepared for the use they are about to receive, and those making the transition are unfamiliar with walking and running in un-heeled shoes. It can take people months or even years of barefoot walking to undo the harm caused to their body by contemporary shoes. There are many weak parts of the foot that require strengthening and mobility work (or else the stronger portions of the foot attempt to make up the difference and damage can occur to those overly stressed parts). Further, many people who run on hard surfaces expect shoes to protect them, but such surfaces (like pavement) were never meant to be run on for any appreciable distance by human feet. An expectation that any footwear will prevent injury on such a surface is erroneous.

The writing here in this section is not a call to abandon all modern footwear and walk barefoot all the time (though I do not discourage people from intelligently trying to reach this goal). Some professions require specialized or protective footwear to prevent injury from equipment, heavy objects, heat, etc. However, if I were to work in such a profession that required (for example) steel-toed boots, I would spend as much time as possible out of these shoes when not working to prevent loss of function, misalignment, and atrophy of my feet (and the tissues connected to them). It is pretty clear that modern shoes make substantive changes to our musculoskeletal system. We even walk and run differently as a result of these shoes. Domesticated humans simply believe that thick-soled, heeled shoes that compress the toes together are normal. When discussing this topic, I like to present the following question: if we were part of a society that wore a design of shirt that caused us to lose muscle mass in our arms, lose range of motion in our shoulders, and force our body to compensate for the shirt by misaligning certain joints, would we continue to wear said shirt simply because it has been a tradition for a few generations? Well, quite possibly, but it would be no more logical to wear this kind of shirt than it is to wear the styles of footwear found in affluent countries. Our bodies can benefit through rewilding our footwear (or discarding them altogether) and regaining full function of our feet.

AN OVERVIEW OF FERAL MOVEMENT

Feral movement (or natural movement) can be described as a suite of physical skills that would be required for accomplishing necessary living tasks throughout the year for a nature-connected human. Essentially, a person must be able to perform all of the movements that a particular environment demands. These physical abilities can grouped into categories and require different fundamentals to accomplish them in a capable and efficient manner. Much like how in chapter 3 we described various aspects of hunter-gatherer diet and presented ways to emulate that diet, even when wild food was not available, we must now do the same for movement. Essentially, if we can paint a picture of how wild humans moved and how much they moved, we can figure out how to mimic this movement in our life for greater individual health.

Clearly hunter-gatherers had a great many physical tasks that needed to be accomplished. And without fossil-fuel-powered machines or migrant laborers, they needed to do all the tasks for themselves. Therefore, physical activity was not an option but a necessary feature of life. Our physiology and underlying genetics are based on this necessity of frequent movement. Let's take a small bit of space to describe typical hunter-gatherer activities. First and foremost, walking was a core human activity. While the famous book title suggests we were born to run, the reality is we (humans) were born to walk (and are also capable of running). Wild humans covered great distances in their yearly travels (refer to the section "skeletal structure and physical fitness" in Chapter 2 for some figures). Further, almost everything they travelled with was carried on their person or sometimes dragged or sledded behind them; therefore, other muscle groups beyond those needed for locomotion were being used, and the skeleton was often loaded with additional weight. In addition to walking (and running), they also sometimes needed to climb, jump, crawl, and stalk. Frequent daily activities included the search for food (i.e., hunting and gathering). Hunting involved a range of motions used in travel, stealth, and use of hunting weapons. It sometimes also required the rapid pursuit of prey. Gathering included various movements, from digging, to cutting, to picking, to additional specialized movements (depending on the plant food being obtained). Both kinds of food procurement involved carrying the harvests back to the campsites and villages, where cutting, butchering, pounding, and stirring would be needed to prepare the foods for consumption. Fuel wood was a very important resource, and gathering, lifting, and transporting it back for cooking, heating, and tool manufacture were reoccurring activities (in fact, fuel wood was so important that sometimes camps were moved on the basis of the availability of this resource). Many tasks requiring the hands (and sometimes also the mouth and feet) were needed for clothing, container, fiber, and tool manufacture. Shelter construction involved chopping, cutting, scoring, lashing, lifting, holding, and other kinds of activities (beyond the collection of materials used to fabricate the home). Stooping and sometimes crawling were needed to enter and exit shelters (depending on the style of the structure). Personal interaction involved (depending on the people) ceremony, dancing, intimacy, and play fighting. And so on. Hopefully the point is made that our ancestry involved a life rich in a variety of movements, some of which were moderate to high intensity.

However, we shouldn't paint a picture that suggests every day was a marathon because it wasn't (far from it). Hunter-gatherers had plenty of leisure time (remember, they worked far less time each day than we do now). While they didn't nap that frequently (more in the summer than in the winter), there was plenty of very light intensity movement that didn't boost heart rate (e.g., making and mending clothing, weaving branches and other plant material for baskets, wrapping fibers for cordage, socializing). Research actually suggests that some groups expended about as many calories a day as we do. For example, the Hadza of Tanzania expended about as many calories a day as do people living in the United States or Europe (after adjustment for body size differences; based on research by Pontzer and colleagues published in 2012). Even though the Hadza were more physically active, it turns out that our bodies use most of the energy obtained from food for maintenance costs (e.g., cellular activity, digestion, moving blood through vessels, organ function). The authors of this study explain that when humans burn extra calories on physical movement, the body compensates by adjusting calorie usage (prioritizing essential functions), so that we ultimately burn relatively similar amounts each day. This result, that a modern-day hunter-gatherer group and domesticated humans living in industrialized countries burn roughly the same number of calories each day, was quite unexpected. It is one (of many reasons) why I do not personally attempt to estimate the number of calories burned each day.

Of course, we should not extrapolate too much from the results of a single study (despite the fact the results of the Hadza study were extremely interesting). Other studies exist for hunter-gatherer energy expenditure and suggest they do expend more calories (see Cordain et al. 1998, Physical activity, energy expenditure and fitness: an evolutionary perspective). For example, !Kung hunter-gatherers of southern Africa use almost the same total calories (2169) as office workers in the United States (2247, these figures for males). Except that there are two confounding factors. First, the !Kung spend a greater proportion of their daily energy expenditure moving than Americans (41% vs. 27%). Second, the !Kung are smaller than Americans (an adaptation to their local place), and smaller bodies need less energy to move them around. Therefore, the 899 calories a day used for physical activity would actually, once adjusted for body size, be significantly more than this for an American (if they were to do the equivalent amount of work). Said another way, if an American walked 1 km, using the same number of calories, the !Kung hunter-gatherer would walk 2.2 km (based on calculations by Nigel Barber). Clearly, they are more active than people working in a common profession in the United States. Research on the Aché of Paraguay confirms these conclusions. They use more total calories per day (3314 for a male), use a greater proportion of these daily calories for physical activity (53%), and the 1771 calories used for physical activity would again be greater because these people are also smaller than American office workers (who use only 614 calories each day for physical activity).

Let us not forget that sex (as in intimacy) is a valuable form of movement with many benefits beyond the actual movement itself, including decreased feeling of stress, increased feelings of well-being and bonding, increased longevity, reduced incidence of cardiovascular disease, enhanced immune system function, and improved production of certain sex-related hormones (e.g., testosterone, prolactin). Sex is an important form of movement that can require exertion and significantly raises the heart rate. Thirty minutes of spirited sex has been likened to walking approximately 3.2 km (2 miles) in terms of its energy expenditure. Depending on the positions utilized, sex can involve major groups of muscles and associated tissues (e.g., pelvis, upper legs, back, arms). In fact, variety of position can add to the overall movement diversity experienced by couples (or groups) with the resulting benefits of actuating certain muscles and connective tissues that are quiescent for much of our public lives. Safe, consensual sex at least twice per week can contribute to a healthy lifestyle and bolster our time spent engaging in feral movement.

Knowing that hunter-gatherers moved more (on average) than those in western societies, it is sometimes helpful to break movements down into categories. This is done here to help the reader determine that they are experiencing a wide range of movement. Kinds of movement can be grouped into categories (as conceptualized by Erwan Le Corre[8]):

Mobility. This group of movement accounts for the ways we physically move from one place to another on our landscape. Distance covered is not an important part of the definition. Walking, running, jumping, crawling, climbing, snowshoeing, skiing, paddling, and swimming are all ways we effect locomotion from point to point (some, of course, happen only at certain times of the year).

Manipulation. Manipulation involves touching and holding fast or moving other objects. Anytime we perform work of some kind, we are manipulating objects. Movements that include lifting, throwing, reaching (for something), gathering, cutting, chopping, digging, pushing, dragging, carrying, and steadying are all manipulation-type skills. But this also includes activities like sewing, weaving, wrapping, binding, tying, pouring, stirring, and so on.

Self-defense. Combat-oriented skills are the ways we defend our physical bodies from an aggressor, whether it be a human animal or an other-than-human animal. These movements are a blend of mobility and manipulation skills—similar to carrying a loaded pack on our backs (we are both moving ourselves and moving an object). Self-defense is a critical (and often neglected) aspect of movement skills that can include striking, blocking/parrying/covering, throwing, tripping, joint manipulation, long bone breaking, choking, wrestling, restraining, stance, and footwork. Protecting your person (or people in your care) is of paramount importance and is one way we maintain our health through prevention of injury by aggressive animals (human or otherwise).

Each of these kinds of movements require fundamental movement skills in order to be able to perform them correctly and for as long as we need to.

Strength. Physical strength is the ability to do work with our bodies. More exactly, it can be described as the amount of force we can apply to objects in our environment. Pushing, pulling, lifting, and heaving are all movements that benefit from greater strength (though strength alone is not all that is required for these movements). Free-weights, body-weight exercises, and performing tasks that require power are ways we increase our strength.

Coordination. Our ability to manage our movements in a dexterous fashion is one way of describing physical coordination. Coordination is what allows some people to move in a graceful manner while performing physically challenging movements. It is an ability to direct our trunk and limbs to perform different functions at the same time. At its core, coordination is training the body, moment by moment, to contract and relax the muscles in the correct sequence and to the precise degree. Coordination relies very much on balance (i.e., our ability to be stable while performing tasks) and timing. We improve our coordination by training specific movements and improving other movement fundamentals.

Endurance. A person's ability to maintain a level of physical exertion without fatiguing describes their endurance. There are different kinds of endurance (e.g., aerobic, anaerobic), and these are based on a suite of physiological characteristics, including our metabolism and how efficiently our body can supply muscles with energy (there are several pathways our body uses to

---

[8] Erwan Le Corre. 2014. MovNat Certified Level 1 Trainer Manual, version 4.2. MovNat, LLC.

supply energy where it is needed; e.g., creatine phosphate, glycolytic, aerobic). These pathways require different training methods to optimize their functioning (not all kinds of endurance require focus on the cardiovascular system). A variety of medium- to high-intensity movement training can improve our overall conditioning (which is technically different from endurance, but that is another topic).

Balance. Our ability to prevent ourselves from falling or collapsing when performing various actions relies, in part, on our balance, which is an ability to understand our position in space and our position or movement with respect to gravity. Balance relies on three separate systems to coordinate this fundamental skill, including the somatosensory system, the vestibular system, and the visual system. All of these function together to help us maintain balance (and when we turn one of these systems off, such as by closing our eyes, balance becomes more difficult). Balance and strength collaborate with each other to create stability. Balance is an easily practiced movement fundamental that is often neglected.

Flexibility. Some movements we wish to perform require that our tissues be pliable enough so that they can allow the necessary range of motion through a joint (or series of joints). While most people believe that we maintain flexibility by stretching, the reality is that our movement patterns (or lack thereof) make a huge impact on our limberness. Maintaining movement (so that our joints don't adapt to a common position and lose flexibility) and practicing a diverse set of movements (so that our connective tissue and muscles are stretched beneficially) are ways we can promote flexibility, even in age.

Timing. Movement requires a specific sequence through time in order to be successfully performed. Some actions have a relatively long window within which a motion can be completed (e.g., reaching for a handhold from a position of balance), while others need to be achieved within a very narrow time period (e.g., grabbing a handhold during midflight of a dynamic leap). The ability to correctly time movements is an important movement asset, especially for certain kinds of environmental demands that involve interacting with fast and/or agile lifeforms, such as the capture of prey species for food or successfully defending oneself from an aggressive person. Coordination and timing are related, though the former is more about managing different portions of the body simultaneously whereas the latter is about managing movements through time.

Motivation. Movement requires motivation. If a person is not motivated, they will remain sedentary. Historically, the will to move was provided by hunger and thirst (or by a need to defend themselves from harm). Today, it is often guilt for having eaten. For the neoaboriginal, motivation for movement will come from a variety of places, including the desire to celebrate human capability and their unique expression of this. Ultimately, restructuring our lives so that the motivation for movement is provided by things we need to accomplish with our bodies will be desirable (because we have shed some technology that had allowed us to be sedentary).

These are the core movements and their movement fundamentals. I find it extremely helpful to think of movement in these terms as it provides me with a way to analyze why I may be having difficulty performing a given action—which then allows me to formulate a plan to address my movement deficiencies in order to successfully perform the action of interest. More than this, thinking of movement in these ways also means these are the "vitamins" of movement and that I need to incorporate all of these movement fundamentals into my daily living. They are all inter-related. For example, failure to stick a landing while leaping from a rock may be interpreted as a lack of strength in the legs to prevent the body from falling forward but it may easily be a deficiency in balance to land in a more neutral position. Throughout the week, I need to focus on all these fundamentals, not just strength or endurance. Fortunately, natural living accomplishes most of these movement fundamentals without a need to do movement for the sake of movement (which is what most people do when they exercise).

Before we leave the topic of defining feral movement and its core parts, it is important to note that not all movements need to be considered exercise. Said another way, all movement does not have to be high-intensity activity—in fact, most of it should not be. Don't get trapped in the idea that if you are not sweating profusely and gasping for breath that your movement isn't doing you any good. This is a very common (and erroneous) belief that only serves to stop people from engaging in beneficial movement. There is more to movement than just building muscle mass and increasing endurance. Remember, we need to move lymph and blood around (which can be done with light intensity activity). We also need to maintain joint mobility. While certainly we should have (or acquire) the ability to perform some high-intensity exercise, there is much more to moving the human body than this.

Equally as important to this entire topic, when you are not moving, use positions other than sitting in a chair. Our positions we use at rest also affect our health, especially when we chronically use one position. There are a multitude of body postures used by indigenous people when they are at rest. These include a flat-footed squat, which they could maintain for long periods of time. They also placed their buttocks on the ground and varied the ways the legs were positioned, including cross-legged, sole to sole, knees bent with feet on the ground, both legs outstretched, or one leg outstretched and the other folded (among other variations). They also knelt, with one or both knees touching the ground. Even the ways they stood provided evidence for diversity of posture, with one leg often being held off the ground in some manner. These are all ways we can increase the diversity of the positions we experience each day (which aids with joint mobility and keeping muscle groups strong that we rarely use when seated in chairs). But (and a big but), don't switch one chronic position for another. For example, using a standing work station helps to stop us from sitting in chairs too much, but chronic standing (in one position) will ultimately lead to some of the same outcomes as chronic sitting. To assist with all of this, stop using some of your furniture for a portion of the day (or even get rid of some of your furniture). While it may sound, at first, silly to sit on your floor when you visit with guests, remember that doing so strengthens your body and gives you additional movement variety because you now have to get down to the floor and stand back up again each time you do so (i.e., you are adding squats or variations of this to your daily movement routine). No one is stating it has to be uncomfortable—use a blanket, towel, mat, or animal hide (whatever) below you to provide some padding from a hard floor. There is no doubt that this strategy (of avoiding use of furniture) will add diversity to the positions we experience each day. Variety is the key with our movement and our positions of rest. Change them constantly throughout the day.

Feral movement is diverse, it is not a prescription for the same level of movement day after day throughout the year. Rewilding humans require variation in their movement—don't seek to walk 10,000 steps each day. Some days do less, some days do LOTS more (and then rest the next day). And disperse the movement throughout the entire day (not all in one block of movement/exercise). Just like with barefoot walking and running, some people will need to incorporate feral movement gradually into their life. The long-term sedentary behavior and movement on perfectly plane surfaces has created a condition of weak bodies that are accustomed to a highly reduced amount and diversity of movement. Strengthening and mobility exercises may be needed to rebuild the body so it can successfully transition to wild terrain. Finding a natural movement coach to facilitate this process may be a wise idea (i.e., needing movement coaching is not a sign of weakness). Injuring your body only serves to keep you from experiencing the movement humans are designed to engage in.

BENEFITS OF MOVEMENT

We have already discussed some of the important benefits of movement for human health. This section will go a bit deeper and help you understand how critical movement is for the proper functioning of our physiology and expression of our DNA. Engaging in physical activity is not just for muscles and cardiovascular system, but it improves many issues that we might face as a result of troubled physiology. Movement benefits our bodies down to the cellular level. Following are some examples of how physical activity awakens ancestral health.

There are many studies showing that movement positively affects mood. Those who maintain a regular regimen of activity are, on average, happier than those who do not (interestingly, depression is often greater in those who used to move regularly and then stop for some reason). There is so much evidence supporting the mood-enhancing effects of movement that some psychologists are now using physical activity as a method of treating depression. The fact that moving our muscles plays an important role in our overall disposition demonstrates how interconnected seemingly separate aspects of our physiology actually are. Researchers have suggested that movement helps to treat depression through one of several mechanisms. Physical activity increases levels of serotonin (a neurotransmitter), endorphins (neuropeptides that help ease pain), and endocannabinoids (substances that can activate pleasure circuits in the brain), all of which collectively reduce feelings of sadness and anxiety, thereby benefitting overall attitude. The endocannabinoids, cannabis-like substances produced within our body, are especially interesting because they readily cross the blood-brain barrier (unlike endorphins) and promote a number of beneficial actions that serve to assist with intense activity (such as promoting blood flow by dilating blood vessels). Movement also increases body temperature, which can have a calming effect. Further, movement is known for its ability to assist with beneficial sleep (which has a protective effect on the brain). The mood-enhancing effects of movement are likely related to all of these items (and some not yet discovered).

Movement is also known to increase brain-derived neurotrophic factor (BDNF), a protein the supports the growth of neurons (also called nerve cells). It is hypothesized that the brain releases BDNF to protect neurons from the expected effects of potentially intense activity (such as chasing, fleeing, or fighting). However, BDNF does more than simply protect neurons, it also encourages the growth and differentiation of neurons and the connections between neurons (called synapses). Research indicates that exercise that boosts production of BDNF improves long-term memory and bolsters cognitive function (including faster processing of information). While high-intensity movement (e.g., sprinting, weight lifting, wrestling) is known to increase production of BDNF, light- to medium-intensity activity that can be sustained for long periods of time (i.e., aerobic exercise) also has a beneficial effect here. Through BDNF (and other endogenous compounds), movement translates to greater neuronal activity and enhanced communication between neurons. This is why some people experience a sense of calm and ability to work through difficult issues after exercise.

Another benefit of movement is that it improves a process called methylation. This is a metabolic process that happens throughout our body at a frequency of over one billion times each second. Technically, methylation is the transfer of a methyl group (a fancy term for a carbon atom bonded to three hydrogen atoms) from one molecule to another. The transfer of methyl groups is an important aspect of human physiology and is involved in detoxification, energy production, cell and DNA repair, inflammation, production of endogenous antioxidants, and immune system response (among other processes). The important item here is not that you understand exactly what methylation is but that you understand that this process occurs very frequently and is critical for health. Physical exercise improves methylation. This means that exercise upregulates cellular repair mechanisms, improves fatigue, lessens inflammation, and helps detoxify the body. More than just improving methylation, exercise actually changes gene expression (beneficially) with regard to inflammation, insulin response, and metabolism. A recent study (see Lindholm et al. 2014 in the journal Epigenetics) showed that exercise four times a week over a three-month period actually altered expression at over 5000 sites on the genome of muscles involved in exercise (and many of these changes, including those affecting methylation patterns, were in regions of the genome called "enhancers" because they can boost function). Therefore, movement augments our epigenetic function (and that of our children).

Physical exercise also benefits our epigenome in other ways, especially in regard to cancer. Even regular moderate-intensity movement (which includes walking that generates an elevated heart rate) is known to lead to expression of genes that suppress cancerous tumors. More than this, exercise decreases the expression of oncogenes. Oncogenes are genes that have been altered in some way (such as mutation or abnormally high expression) that now have the potential to cause and sustain cancer cell growth. For example, old or damaged cells that would normally undergo a programmed cell death (called apoptosis), a normal process in the body that prevents altered cells from replicating, can be "turned off" by oncogenes (thereby letting cells with potentially damaged DNA to proliferate). When exercise decreases the expression of oncogenes, this is another way of saying it turns them off so that they can't alter other genes that contribute to cancer.

Exercise helps protect us against cancer in more ways than just changing the expression of genes and oncogenes. Physical activity, especially the kinds that cause large groups of muscles to contract, utilizes glucose that could be used to fuel cancer-cell growth. Exercise can increase glucose uptake in the muscles 20- to 100-fold (this accomplished by the hormone insulin, which promotes absorption of glucose circulating in the blood to the muscles). Essentially, exercise "disposes of" blood glucose, helping to maintain a metabolic homeostasis (i.e., it helps regulate our metabolism to remain within beneficial parameters). High levels of circulating glucose (which can occur in relatively sedentary people, especially after meals) is a risk factor for various cancers and low survivability after a cancer diagnosis.

There are many additional topics that could be discussed here. For example, exercise has been shown to change the abundance of certain bacteria in our gastrointestinal system, indicating that physical activity may have significant benefit to our microbiome. We could go on at length describing the benefits of movement (which includes a broad-array of activity, some of which is moderate- to high-intensity exercise). At this point, I'm hoping you have been convinced of the need to move on a frequent basis. What might be the hardest thing to acquire is the motivation (at first). Each person has what motivates them to remain active. No matter who you are, finding a group of like-minded individuals will keep you moving more—our community keeps us accountable so that we don't get too many "free days" from feral movement. I urge you to find people (or animal friends, such as the domesticated dog) who like to move with you. This will keep you from spending too much time sitting in a chair.

NEOABORIGINAL STRATEGY FOR REWILDING OUR MOVEMENT

Hunter-gatherers had a biological need to move, for if they did not they would starve (or die of thirst). We still have a biological need to move but this is not because we need to secure food (or water) from our landscape but because our physiology requires it. A sedentary hunter-gatherer would face death in the near term. Modern humans, in contrast, suffer shorter lives and decreased quality of life when they are sedentary (i.e., lack of movement creates chronic, rather than acute, issues for city builders).

Equally important, hunter-gatherers engaged in a wide variety of movement. Consider this passage by Robert Kelly describing (very briefly) the yearly travels of the Newe (Shoshone):

"The Great Basin Shoshone, for example, spend the winter in villages in the piñon and juniper forests of the mountains. As spring came, they moved down to the valley floors and gathered tubers, bulbs, and the first seeds of spring; later, they moved upslope as seeds ripened there. In the summer, they might move to a river where trout were running, or to a marsh where they could hunt waterfowl and gather bulrush seeds. In the early fall, they would move back into the mountains, establish winter camps, and collect piñon nuts while hunting deer and bighorn sheep."

Consider the vast variety of activity and terrain that the Newe encountered as a result of living in a natural habitat. Now contrast this with the habitat we typically encounter (e.g., inside of our homes, offices, and supermarkets). Our problem is that we have modified our habitat (just like we modified our diets) to something that does not support physical health. We have multiple ways we can solve this dilemma. One, we can interact with natural habitats more frequently. Two, we can change the habitat of our home to better reflect our movement needs. Even better, we can do both. The point is that we need to step outside of the usual patterns that have been established by domesticated people in affluent countries. This lifeway, while physically easy, it robbing us of our movement potential and the health that comes with engaging in feral movement.

Movement is critical for human health. Without movement, a human is a sedentary organism not living up to their potential. While we experience thirst and hunger as reminders of the need to drink and eat, movement doesn't work in that way. We discover that we needed to move by feeling fatigue and soreness when we try to engage in activity that should not produce discomfort in a fit individual. While these sensations are the body's way of telling us we need to move more, they sometimes have the opposite effect (i.e., they cause people to avoid moving), which only compounds the problem. Keeping all these ideas in mind, following are ten ways you can rewild your movement for greater health and fitness.

1. **Walk** at least eight kilometers (4.8 miles) on most days. For the average person, this would equate to walking 10,472 steps (very close to the 10,000 steps guideline recommended by many authors). Try to find areas that allow you to walk for some or all of the distance off road, such as along hiking trails and overland. Although walking or hiking for the sake of the activity (or a view) is a perfectly appropriate reason, consider using walking to replace some car travel (e.g., trip to store, post office, bank) when it is possible. In other words, use your movement to accomplish tasks that you normally use fossil fuels for. But use walking for other wild activities as well. Roam your landscape to find edible plants and fungi, or to locate animal tracks and den

or nest sites. Rather than walking this distance all at once, break up the day (i.e., the periods of sitting) with several walks.

2. Spend as much time as your setting and your physical health allow for you to **be barefoot or in minimalist shoes**. No one is stating you have to run on hard surfaces in these shoes (hunter-gatherers certainly didn't). Walking off trail where the soil, leaf litter, or vegetation absorbs foot falls is a perfect way to get the benefits of barefoot walking without overly impacting the feet and supporting structures of the leg. This benefits many aspects of foot and leg health/strength when done properly.

3. **Running** two or three times a week for at least 20 minutes will provide high-intensity activity that is in line with our ancestry. If you are unable to run a significant distance or length of time, run as far as you can. As weight is lost and the body is strengthened, the distance and time will increase. For those who can, replace some of the running with sprinting (or alternating intervals of sprinting and jogging). High-intensity activity of this kind is excellent for conditioning the body (when it is not overdone).

4. Some form of **strength training** or, better, actual activity that stresses your musculature and accomplishes a necessary task, should be practiced two or three times a week. Strength training does not have to be consist of lifting weights up and putting them down, then lifting them again, then putting them down (you get the idea). Rock climbing (even if in a gym) and wrestling are examples of activities that stress the muscular system and do not involve overly repetitious movements. The main issue is that the strength training should be diverse so that it incorporates different muscle groups and different motions. Focus on body weight exercises (which cost no money to perform) and free weights over machines weights.

5. Keep the **movement fundamentals** in mind as you develop your strategy to recover a wild body. A strict focus on one fundamental (for example, strength) may create imbalances that lead to injury. All of the fundamentals are important: strength, endurance, coordination, balance, flexibility, and motivation. Try to build a lifestyle that engages all of these core nutrients of feral movement.

6. **Recovery and rest** are more than just acceptable, they are necessary. After a long day of activity (e.g., hike in the mountains, athletic contests, long-distance run, physically strenuous projects), it is perfectly appropriate to have an easy day (or two) for recovery. This helps your body heal and prevents injury from overuse. Likewise, being still during the day (if not for too long a period) is also valuable. Spend daily time that is without movement in a diversity of positions, including standing, sitting, cross-legged sit, flat-footed squat, etc. Being in one position too much of the day has long-term negative consequences.

7. Spend as much time as possible **moving outdoors**. This is our ancestral habitat and it provides the best training ground for our bodies based on the variation in angle, surface features, obstacles (e.g., trees, downed logs, streams, boulders), and elevation. Outdoor movement in a variety of settings (and seasons) will best provide the challenges to our body for building a strong human that is capable of feral movement.

8. Change your **indoor environment** to better accomplish your body's movement needs. Avoid using furniture to support your weight for part of the day. Perform some activities standing that you normally do in a seated position (make alterations to your work station or kitchen to allow

this). Grind grain and other food-stuffs by hand using a manual grain mill rather than purchasing flour. Put natural objects on the floor that you can walk safely over or stand on to keep your feet and ankles strong and flexible (e.g., cobbles, small logs). Instead of using stairs each time to reach another floor in the home, consider arranging the household so that you can use a ladder some of the time. For more physically fit people, build a pole or hang a rope to climb upstairs or slide down to the floor below (or even install monkey bars on the ceiling to traverse the room when emptyhanded). These are just examples—your creativity is the only limit here to building a better habitat within your home.

9. Move with a **community** of like-minded people. Your community helps provide motivation (a movement fundamental) on days you are feeling unenthusiastic. There are numerous benefits to engaging in communal activities—it is an inherent human way of doing things. Do not ignore your family (especially your children) as part of your community. While including them may require one to tone down the intensity or duration of activity, it will profit them immensely now and later (by establishing good movement habits).

10. Have **gratitude** for the movement your body is capable of. Celebrate this as often as you can. You will have days due to injury, sickness, or schedule that will force you to be sedentary. Therefore, take advantage of every opportunity to express movement in your personal way. For too long, domesticated humans have marveled over their technological innovations that allow them to be sedentary for long periods of the day. It is time for us to change this and give thanks for the amazing physical ability of the human animal.

9. Hormesis: expanding comfort zones

One of the major obstacles to modern humans reconnecting with nature is an ability endure the conditions presented by their local environments. Humans experience physical stressors when they enter wild landscapes, including heat, cold, physically demanding terrain, wind, precipitation, biting insects, extremes of humidity, and/or intense sunlight. While many locations in the world have periods of the year in which weather and temperatures may be very mild, most places have at least some period of year (or most of the year) when the conditions are demanding. Humans, until recently, have always spent a great deal of time outdoors and were acclimated to their homelands. It was, in fact, imperative that people be able to function outside of the home, sometimes during extreme conditions. Today, humans are still adapted to their environment but their environment is the domesticated setting (i.e., indoors). Given that such settings are typically climate-controlled to a large degree, modern humans have lost (in large part) an ability to endure the outdoor setting where their homes are located. While it is certainly true that even wild people required protection from and needed to avoid certain aspects of their environment (e.g., frigid temperatures with driving wind, high temperatures coupled with intense sunlight), there is no doubt that they were capable of enduring environmental extremes that would cause many people today to suffer tremendously. If *Homo sapiens domesticofragilis* is ever to fully understand the value of wild places, she or he must be able to spend long periods of time in such areas. To do so, for many, will require a method of building a much greater tolerance to the stresses they encounter. Such a method exists, and it is called hormesis.

WHAT IS HORMESIS?

Hormesis is a term that describes a beneficial biological response to stresses. More accurately, it is usually considered to be a biphasic response—the body responds favorably to minor or low-dose stresses but can be overwhelmed and harmed by major or high-dose stresses. Most everyone is familiar with hormesis, they just may not be aware of this term. Strength-building exercise is one of the most common forms of hormesis that is practiced. When a person lifts weights that they can safely control, they put microscopic tears in the muscles, which, upon healing, actually strengthen the body in multiple ways (i.e., strength training accomplishes more than just increasing the size of the muscles). In essence, the weight being moved by the person is stressing, but not overwhelming, the musculoskeletal system. The body responds by increasing the mass of the muscles and the strength of bones and connective tissue involved in the activity. Additionally, strength training performed on a regular basis can increase metabolism, build anaerobic endurance, and protect against physical injury. However, if the body is overwhelmed, due to excessive weight or training too frequently, then injury (in some form) results. This form of hormesis (strength training) shows the biphasic dose response because training with appropriate resistance (i.e., the weight used during exercise) at the correct frequency creates a beneficial response (several in fact). Too large a dose of strength training creates a detrimental response.

Continuing to examine strength training, it would be important to assess the effect of this hormetic activity on the body at the appropriate time. Why? Because if one had the diagnostic tools to examine the body shortly after strength training, a number of seemingly deleterious items would be detected. Exercise boosts metabolism, and as a result, increases oxidative stress. Oxidative stress is caused by the production of free radicals, chemically reactive molecules that are produced as a result of normal cellular physiology. The more intense the activity, the greater the production of free radicals and the greater the degree of oxidative stress. Free radicals, like reactive oxygen species (ROS), can damage cells and create other free radicals, contributing to a host of chronic and degenerative diseases. Cortisol, a hormone released from the adrenal gland in response to physical or emotional stress, would (most likely) be measured as elevated post exercise. While cortisol is an important hormone that has vital functions, elevated levels are associated with poor outcomes in many areas. Various markers of inflammation would also be measured as elevated in the body after exercise. Inflammation, especially if chronic, can exacerbate many health conditions. Of course (as mentioned in the previous paragraph), if you had a method of looking microscopically at the muscles used during the strength training, one would observe minute tears indicative of stress caused by a resistance to movement (e.g., the weight being lifted). All of this would look very bad if someone were to present these results on a continual basis.

Fortunately, after strength training, assuming someone allows the body to rest and recover (followed by more exercise with additional rest and recovery), the body adapts to these stresses and becomes stronger. Even some of the responses to exercise, like inflammation and oxidative stress, are, ultimately, beneficial to the body. Inflammation is crucial to the repair and rebuilding, and growth of damaged muscles because it signals a complex series of processes that ultimately creates stronger muscles. The oxidative stress, caused by free radicals generated as cellular by-products during the strength training exercise, conditions the body to respond to this threat. Ultimately, regular exercise boosts endogenous mechanisms of dealing with free radicals (like ROS), thereby protecting against cellular damage that would occur from repeated workouts if the body failed to adapt. Hormesis, the application of a beneficial level of stress to provide a positive outcome (often an increase in the body's ability to cope with that stress), is a natural mechanism for building a stronger and healthier body. The trick for the neoaboriginal is to learn how to apply hormesis to a wide variety of environmental stresses in a way that promotes natural strength.

GROWING OUR TOLERANCE OF TEMPERATURE EXTREMES

There is little doubt that wild animals are very adapted to their climates, in part because they have resided in that place for a long period of time, allowing their various physical, physiological, and behavioral adaptations to become very refined for their environments. Indigenous people are no different, and there are many credible reports of their tolerance of extreme climates. The Yámana people (also called Yaghan) of extreme southern South America are exemplars of wild people's ability to endure and accept cold. These indigenous people live in a region characterized by cool, humid, and rainy weather with strong winds for much of the year. Summer temperatures in much of their historical range (Tierra del Fuego) typically don't often surpass 9 degrees C (48 degrees F) and winter temperatures average around freezing (i.e., 0 degrees C or 32 degrees F). On some of the islands in this region, the climate can be described as sub-Antarctic climate, and while moderated by the proximity to the ocean, it is still too harsh for tree growth to occur. Early sightings and anthropological records of the Yámana are barely believable, not because they exceed the ability of humans, but rather because most modern people are simply incapable of doing what they did, leading people to believe the stories were far-fetched. Observations of the Yámana in the 1800s and early half of the 1900s described them as a people who wore relatively little clothing (though this apparently changed after prolonged contact with Europeans). In fact, they were sometimes observed sleeping in the open without shelter or covering (e.g., hides, blankets) of some form—temperatures that were causing substantial discomfort to the shivering European explorers. Perhaps even more impressive was the swimming by the women in waters measured at 9 degrees C (48 degrees F) for the gathering of shellfish (part of the diet of the Yámana). The tolerance of cold possessed by the Yámana clearly left a lasting impression on the explorers who observed them.

Of course, there are people living in even colder environments than the Yámana. The Inuit of Nunavut (north-central Canada) experience some of the coldest temperatures on a regular basis of any people in the world. For example, average daily high temperatures range from -23 to -33 degrees C (-10 to -27 degrees F) during the month of January (and no, those aren't typos, those are the truly the mean daily maximum temperature experienced by these people). Of course, clothing, shelters, and various adaptations by the people allow habitation in such a cold part of the world. Imagine using snow shelters (iglu or using the English spelling, igloo) where the internal temperature cannot rise too much above freezing (i.e., 0 degrees C) or snow begins to melt and drip on those inside. While this might sound horrible to those accustomed to "room temperature", with the outside being -50 degrees C (-58 degrees F) on some days, slightly above 0 C represents a significantly more hospitable temperature. Most people in affluent countries cannot envision sleeping close together on a raised bed made out of snow covered with the hides of caribou (*Rangifer tarandus*). These conditions may not sound pleasant, but the Inuit make use of the cold in their daily lives, as it allows for creation of winter homes, hunting of seals, and transport by sled (i.e., it is not considered to be a detrimental feature of their environment). Nunavut truly classifies as a polar region and traditional people lived there and experienced health and happiness (though that is changing today with the loss of their traditional lifeways).

Whether we were to write about indigenous living in cold or hot environments, the story would be relatively similar. The indigenous are exposed to very different temperatures from those experienced by many people living in affluent countries. Moving from one climate-controlled interior habitat to another, many of us spend little time immersed in our outdoor settings. We leave our heated (or air-conditioned) homes, get into our vehicles (which may have been remotely started), and quickly bring the temperature of the automobile cabin to a comfortable level. We park as close as we can to our place of work or where we will shop, making a quick dash to another indoor environment that is kept at a comfortable temperature. We concoct all manner of reasons to remain indoors—it is too cold, it is too hot, it is too humid, it is too dry, it is too rainy, it is snowing too hard, it is too "buggy", the sun is too bright—all the while our bodies and metabolism adapt to a very narrow range of conditions. In other words, we become more and more maladapted to our planet. The constant pursuit of comfort is weakening our ability to be spend time in the outdoors (along with consuming more fossil fuel energy). It is taking away our capacity to be wild.

Throughout the day, we actively seek to limit the time we spend in conditions outside of our thermal neutral zone (TNZ). This refers to a temperature range that a creature can inhabit that requires no regulatory changes in their physiology. In other words, there exists a temperature range at which each organism is comfortable and is not expending additional energy to keep their bodies within an optimal setting. When an animal finds itself outside of this temperature range, it must use energy to warm or cool its body. Shivering, constricting veins to keep heat closer to the core, boosting metabolic rate (and the heat generated by the body), and piloerection (i.e., lifting hair and feathers to capture more warm air) are examples of physiological responses to conditions below the TNZ. Likewise, perspiration, panting, and dilating blood vessels (to facilitate heat loss from the core) are responses to conditions above the TNZ. The TNZ varies for each form of life that we might examine and even changes throughout the year for that being. A moose (*Alces americanus*), a large member of the deer family that inhabits north-temperate and boreal forests, has a lower TNZ than a nine-banded armadillo (*Dasypus novemcinctus*), an insectivorous mammal of south-temperate to tropical regions that is adapted to relatively warm environs. A species' TNZ is an indicator of climate it experiences over the course of its life, and some wide-ranging species that can be found over a large range of latitudes will show different TNZs when southern members of the species are compared with northern members of the species.

The important thing to realize about TNZ is that it can change. While humans do not have the same ability as do many wild animals to make substantial changes to this temperature range (who, for example, can change the density of their fur or feathers), we do still have an ability to acclimate to our surroundings. And coupled with appropriate clothing, food, hydration, etc., humans can do more than simply function in harsh climates; they can actually enjoy a degree of comfort. However, people cannot become accustomed to the temperature and weather of the season without a willingness to experience discomfort. Adapting to a specific set of conditions requires experiencing those conditions or something that mimics them. The point is that if we always seek continual comfort, spending the vast majority of our daily living within a narrow range of mild temperature, then we will have a difficult time dealing with more extreme conditions and, as a result, will seek to avoid those conditions even more. This is a poor strategy for people to follow for several reasons, including the fact that people are sometimes forced to deal with inclement conditions (e.g., extreme weather, wild fires, flooding, earthquakes, terrorism). These are things that even those living in affluent countries sometimes have to contend with. It would be prudent to be able to function when conditions are not ideal.

How can we acclimate to the cold or the heat? The simplest answer is that we just spend more time in those environments. This is exactly what indigenous people did to become accustomed to the seasonal temperatures of their homelands—they lived in those temperatures. Understandably, this would be a difficult challenge for most people because of time constraints due to modern living. Fortunately, it does not require full and constant immersion in outdoor weather to gain a good degree of acclimation to it. We can intentionally subject ourselves to cold or heat for short periods to allow our bodies an opportunity to experience these environmental conditions. For example, acclimating to cold can be facilitated, in part, by dressing too light for the weather when we intend to be outside for a brief period of time (e.g., carrying firewood from the wood shed to the home, getting an item from the vehicle parked in the driveway, walking to the mailbox to check for deliveries, taking the family pet outside for a bathroom break). Doing such tasks as these while barefoot or with ungloved hands (even in the winter) helps to further the acclimation process. Going further (for those who can), wading into ponds and streams or brief plunges in these water bodies during the colder portions of the year will assist with conditioning the body to cold weather. All of these actions alter the physiology of the body, allowing it to conserve or produce more heat, thereby keeping the body at a safe temperature despite cold ambient conditions. Young and colleagues in 1986 published a method of accomplishing cold acclimation using cool (not cold) water (the paper is called "Human thermoregulatory responses to cold air are altered by repeated cold water immersion"; though I would assert the title is misleading, because 18 degrees C, barely below room temperature, should not be termed as cold, it may still be of use to some readers). There are innumerable ways to accomplish a cold challenge (for example) that helps to harden our bodies against environmental stresses.

Acclimating to heat challenges is, in many ways, similar to acclimating to cold. Exposing your body to safe periods of heat stress, especially over consecutive days, helps the body to boost its physiological mechanisms to deal with high temperatures (e.g., increased sweating, decreased heart rate, higher plasma volume to deliver more blood to the surface capillaries). Heat stress can be generated by ambient temperature or through exercising at an intensity that challenges the heat-relieving mechanisms of the body. Experiencing heat challenges for one hour (or more) each day appears to be most effective at acclimating the body. Over a course of acclimation to high ambient temperatures, gradually increase the level of physical exertion so that the body has an opportunity to change its TNZ and adapt. More extreme heat stresses can be achieved through heated environments, such as sweat lodges and saunas (though it is important to not overwhelm the body in these situations, using common sense, good hydration, and paying close attention to the body). Acclimation has been found to take place over the course of 10–15 days with consistent exposure. It is also lost (without exposure) within a couple of weeks.

When some people read the preceding few paragraphs, they might interpret them as a call to shun all comforts and live a life of suffering. This is not what is being recommended—in no way am I suggesting a masochistic life that is filled with uncomfortable physical experiences. I am proposing that we should experience temporary discomfort now and then so that it does not cause us to cease functioning on a relatively high level when we find ourselves in such situations. I am also recommending that we change our attitude about temperatures outside of our comfort range. A poor mental approach to experiencing temperature extremes is a sure way to create a barrier to understanding how such conditions can actually provide us with benefit (see below). Constant complaining about the weather simply serves no purpose. A rewilded human makes every effort to embrace his or her world and the tremendous diversity found on this planet, including the diversity in temperatures. Modern humans miss so much of what happens on this planet by hiding from weather and remaining in their homes—satisfied to see wild animals on game cameras and You Tube videos. However, it is much more rewarding to generate our own experiences (rather than watch those that others have lived). It requires us only to accept that permanently living in comfort is interfering with our ability to lead more natural lives.

Need more convincing? Understandably, we all come from a society where comfort is a driving focus of our innovations. Be assured there are many reasons why experiencing extreme temperatures (in a safe manner) is a benefit to your health. Let's start with cold. Exposure to cold, especially after exercise, has been shown to boost immune system function in several ways. Increases in specific kinds of white blood cells (e.g., monocytes, leucocytes, tumor necrosis factor-α, interleukin 6) have been observed, which aid the body's ability to fight infection and disease. Some immune cells not only increase in number but also in activity, such as natural killer cells. Cold exposure, especially after vigorous movement, also raises adiponectin levels in the body. Adiponectin is a protein hormone that regulates glucose levels (by moving glucose into the muscles) and facilitates the break down of fatty acids, which facilitates weight loss. This also has a muscle repair and recovery effect, helping people who use cold hormesis to recuperate faster post workout. Interestingly, cold exposure appears to promote cell longevity through increased autophagy—a natural process that disassembles unnecessary and/or poorly functioning cellular components, essentially allowing cells to clean out various components and recycle them. Enhanced autophagy can create healthier cells, thereby allowing them to live longer. Cold exposure also can raise metabolism and lower blood glucose levels. All of these benefits of cold hormesis (including some not listed here) are supported by research published in peer-reviewed journals.

Now, what about heat exposure? Is there also a suite of benefits for heat hormesis? The answer is yes. Engaging in exercise that causes a rise in body core temperature or using tools such as a sweat lodge, sauna, and hot spring, which subject the body to short periods of heat exposure, people can reap a number of advantages for their health and performance. While some of the following has been identified from dry sauna use at 79 degrees C (174 degrees F) for at least 20 minutes, two times per week (or even hotter, longer, and more frequent), it is very likely that some of the results (at least to some degree) can be realized by other forms of heat hormesis. With that in mind, let's begin with the benefits. First, heat exposure of this kind, especially in conjunction with exercise, can improve muscle endurance and inhibit muscle loss during times of disuse (i.e., when one isn't being active and participating in muscle-building or muscle-maintaining movement). The mechanisms for this include the fact that heat exposure increases blood flow to the skeletal muscles, which brings more glucose to them. It also increases blood flow to the heart, benefitting cardiac function. Second, heat exposure helps to build muscle mass through a variety of means, including an increase in molecules called heat shock proteins. These are proteins released in response to stressful conditions, which includes heat but also includes cold and ultraviolet light. Heat shock proteins can repair damaged proteins and prevent oxidation that can harm muscle proteins. Heat shock proteins also boost growth hormone levels, thereby increasing muscle growth. Third, heat exposure, which leads to heat acclimation, helps the body adapt to the increased ambient temperature by more effectively dissipating heat through sweating and increased blood flow to the skin. Fourth, heat exposure improves insulin sensitivity by increasing glucose receptors in the muscles. This is beneficial for everyone, but especially diabetic and prediabetic persons, as it helps cells to recognize insulin and lower blood glucose levels. It also benefits muscle growth because insulin helps to prevent muscle degradation. Fifth, heat exposure promotes longevity, in part through the production of heat shock proteins. Significant reductions in cardiac arrest and all-cause mortality have been observed with regular exposure to heat stress. And sixth, heat hormesis increases brain-derived neurotrophic factor (BDNF), a protein we discussed in the chapter on movement (Chapter 7) that stimulates growth of new brain cells. Through BDNF and other molecules (e.g., norepinephrine, prolactin), heat exposure has been documented to improve memory, learning, and focus and repair brain cells. I direct the reader to the work of Rhonda Patrick for extended discussion of the effects of heat hormesis (which she refers to as "hyperthermic conditioning"). All of these benefits (and more) are available through a willingness to step outside of our comfort zones and practice hormesis.

It is clear that the body isn't merely capable of tolerating temperature stresses but actually benefits from hormetic exposure (i.e., one that stresses but does not overwhelm). *Homo sapiens* has all of the physiological mechanisms for becoming adapted to the conditions found outside of the home. Humans become stronger and enjoy health benefits by experiencing nature—including the full spectrum of weather and being active in that weather. Nature disconnection, which is exemplified by spending the vast majority of our waking time inside one or more temperature-controlled structures, is weakening the human species. It is also contributing to greater pollution because we use more fuel of various forms to keep our interior habitats (whether that be our home, office, or automobiles) within a fairly strict temperature range all the time. Humans, like most wild animals, have a remarkable ability to acclimate. We simply need to abandon the "always comfortable" mindset and embrace infrequent temporary discomfort.

PHYTOCHEMICAL HORMESIS

Phytochemicals, plant compounds, were discussed in detail in chapter 3. Now, we will examine them in a new light—from the perspective of hormesis. Plants concentrate various defensive chemicals in the roots, stems, leaves, and fruits. These chemicals are designed to protect the plants against various pathogens and herbivores, such as bacteria, fungi, and insect larvae. Other compounds protect the plant against oxidative stresses. Upon ingestion by humans at appropriate doses—as derived in a traditional diet through a diversity of both raw and cooked plant foods—the phytochemicals subject cells in the body and the entire organism to a mild to moderate stress. This stress leads to an adaptive response in the body that ultimately makes the human organism more resistant to greater levels of similar stress. Interestingly, the body also becomes more resistant to other stresses because the body's mechanisms of adaptation often confer generalized resilience to a suite of stressors.

For example, chalcones are a group of polyphenol compounds in a variety of plants that serve several purposes, one of which is to act as an antifungal chemical. Thirteen different chalcones are found in the Japanese plant ashitaba (*Angelica keiskei*), a perennial herb that is part of the local cuisine. These are considered to be hormesis-inducing phytochemicals by Son and colleagues (in their 2008 paper called "Hormetic dietary phytochemicals") and activate a number of pathways that confer greater strength to the body. For example, chalcones have anti-inflammatory action, due to their ability to regulate aspects of the immune system (e.g., nitric oxide production, cytokines in macrophages) and their ability to suppress production of cyclooxygenase-2 (also known as COX-2), an important enzyme in the inflammation process. High levels of COX-2 stimulate the production of other compounds in the body that promote several aspects of cancer that are deleterious to human health. In fact, chalcones have been shown in multiple studies to possess anti-tumor activity. The potential health effects of chalcones go beyond inflammation and cancer. Some chalcones have been shown to protect the brain against ischemic injury, which can occur when blood flow is restricted due to clots, resulting in a brain tissue with reduced perfusion of oxygen-rich blood. These examples demonstrate how a particular plant chemical can provide protection against several different stresses the body might experience.

Another example of phytochemical hormesis may prove useful. Phenethyl isothiocyanate (PEITC) is a phytochemical found in some members of the mustard family (the crucifers), specifically in species of watercress (genus *Nasturtium*). It belongs to a group of compounds called isothiocynates that function as deterrents to herbivores but are damaging to the plant itself. Therefore, they are stored as harmless compounds called glucosinolates and are converted to the active defense compound by the enzyme myrosinase (which are kept separate from each other in plant tissues but brought together upon injury caused by feeding on the plant). Multiple animal studies demonstrate that PEITC has anti-tumor activity and is able to provide protection against tumorigenic effects of some carcinogenic compounds. So, in effect, a feeding deterrent found in plants can protect the mammalian organisms from cancer and cancer-causing substances.

One of the major obstacles that people with domesticated palates will experience is the fact that some wild plants, with their rich diversity of phytochemistry, present stronger tastes and flavors than the cultivated produce they are accustomed to. While eaten by indigenous people, there are wild species of plants that are considered too bitter, acrid, or astringent to be enjoyed by most modern people. Clearly, the plants do not like to have their leaves, stems, and roots consumed—so they protect them with an array of polyphenols, terpenes, glucosinolates, and alkaloids (among other types of phytochemicals) to discourage herbivores, including *Homo sapiens*, from consuming them. Of course, these plant compounds have been well studied and offer a wide array of benefits (through their hormetic actions), some of which have been summarized by Drewnowski and Gomez-Carneros in their 2000 paper on bitter taste and phytonutrients. As they noted:

"Sensitized to the bitter taste of plant alkaloids and other poisons, humans reject foods that are perceived to be excessively bitter. This instinctive rejection of bitter taste may be immutable because it has long been crucial to survival. The food industry routinely removes phenols and flavonoids, isoflavones, terpenes, and glucosinolates from plant foods through selective breeding and a variety of debittering processes. Many of the bioactive phytonutrients currently studied in the laboratory have long been treated by industry and consumers alike as disposable bitter waste."

Of course, the problem is that what is now considered "too bitter" (or "too acrid") is a subjective categorization. If you have grown up in a civilization consuming plants that have had some of their original phytochemistry (which is still found in the wild progenitors) muted by various processes, then any bitterness experienced might be regarded as too bitter. What is of importance here is that bitter is not simply a method of detecting plant poisons but also a method of detecting antioxidants. Much like we perceive sour to identify organic acids, and sweetness to detect sugars, and saltiness to recognize salts, we are capable of identifying some antioxidants through their presentation of a bitter taste. For example, the bitterness found in brewing the seeds of coffee (*Coffea arabica*) belong to antioxidant compounds. Another one, the bitterness experienced in dark chocolate, made from the seeds of the cacao tree (*Theobroma cacao*), comes from a higher concentration of polyphenol antioxidants than that found is milk chocolate. In fact, in certain portions of plants, especially nuts and fleshy fruits (and their seeds), the primary contributors to bitterness are flavonoids, which are potent antioxidants. If we consume a diet bereft of bitters, we are also consuming a diet with reduced levels of free-radical scavenging compounds that likely contributed to the cancer-free condition experienced by hunter-gatherers living their traditional lifeways. But, it is important to keep in mind, as mentioned previously, with many hormetic compounds, there are additional benefits to other areas of the body. Flavonoids also combat inflammation, benefit the cardiovascular system, improve aspects of detoxification, and support nervous system health.

There is no doubt that the definition of "too bitter" has changed. There was an abundance of bitter foods in indigenous diets. For example, the Ivilyuqaletem of southern California (often called Cahuilla by others) consumed the leaves and flowering stems of a native dandelion (*Taraxacum californicum*) in the spring and early summer, greens that would be considered bitter by American palates. The Iñupiat of northwestern Alaska ate the emerging, bitter leaves of diamond-leaved willow (*Salix pulchra*), a species they referered to as "kanuŋŋniq" in their language. The Iroquois of northeastern North America consumed the young shoots of common milkweed (*Asclepias syriaca*) after cooking, a wild food that varies from mildly to moderately bitter. The examples could continue. Bitters, which derive from an array of different phytochemicals, have several minor benefits that many in affluent countries don't get to experience on a regular basis. Bitters stimulate the production of gastral enzymes and fluids, helping to facilitate the process of digestion. One of these is gastrin, a hormone that promotes secretion of gastric acid in the stomach. Gastric acid (also called stomach acid) helps to break down food in the stomach and acts as a barrier to certain pathogens (which are killed by the low pH). For some, acid reflux can be the result of too little gastric acid (a condition called hypochlorhydria). Bitters help to ensure adequate levels of stomach acid. Bitter foods also stimulate the production of bile from the gall bladder, which aids in the digestion of lipids and acts as a mild laxative (helping to prevent constipation). Bile contains some very beneficial components, including bile salts (which are necessary for the conversion of pro-vitamin A to the active forms) and lecithin (an emulsifier that aids in the absorption of fat-soluble vitamins). As a result, bitters ultimately help in the digestive process and ensure we recover vitamins in the food we consume.

Like the temperatures in our homes, which we have limited to a specific range, we have also purged certain tastes and textures from our diets, limiting our meals to a somewhat smaller range of tolerated flavors. The different gustatory experiences from the diversity of wild foods are an indication of the varied phytochemistry that is now lost from our nutritional intake. Expanding our palates, practicing a phytochemical hormesis, is a way to recover our ancestral exposure and tolerance of beneficial plant compounds. A rewilded palate learns to appreciate the stronger flavors that some wild foods present, while maintaining the common sense rationale of avoiding extremely bitter, acrid, and burning plants—all sensations that have been developed from a very long relationship with plants to protect *Homo sapiens* from accidental poisoning due to ingestion of an excessive dose of specific plant compounds. Phytochemical hormesis, when practiced in a manner that emulates hunter-gather diets, has significant advantages for the neoaboriginal.

THE VALUE OF CALORIE RESTRICTION

Hunter-gatherers generally experienced less famine than food-producing communities (see Berbesque et al. 2014). However, that does not mean that food scarcity didn't occur—as it did for some groups, and may have even been a routine experience for a short period during each year. An example would include late winter and early spring in north-temperate regions of North America, where food supplies may be exhausted and animals being hunted have also depleted their fat stores. Another example would be dry seasons in some tropic and subtropical areas. Although, it is important to note that some hunter-gatherer cultures apparently did not experience food shortages on any regular interval. The Hadza of Tanzania (as reported by Marlowe in 2010) do not lose weight during anytime of the year, even though the foods consumed can change substantially. However, regardless of the group, our hunter-gatherer ancestors had lean days when hunters were unsuccessful and conditions may have prevented foraging for available plant foods. The point being: there was an occasional day (or days) when people received lower caloric intake and would have experienced hunger to some degree. In fact, even in a day to day pattern of successful hunting and gathering, food was not immediately available from the refrigerator or at the 24-hour shopping center located a couple of blocks away. Keeping in mind that some gathered foods required cooking or some other method of processing prior to consumption, hunter-gatherers could not immediately satisfy hunger in the way most people living in affluent countries can. And, as it turns out, this hormetic experience of occasional hunger has substantial health benefits for those who experience it.

Many residents of affluent countries experience food abundance on a scale never before witnessed on this planet. Literally, at any moment they wish, "food" can be ingested—or it may perhaps require 2 minutes in the microwave oven to be ready. Shipped, trucked, and flown from all over the world, various fares are available, many out of season, to the modern consumer. Certainly, we don't want to overlook the fact that even in wealthy nations food insecurity does occur for some people for various reasons (e.g., poverty, inefficient distribution systems, waste). However, in a country where approximately ⅔ of its residents are overweight (the United States), calorie abundance (as opposed to nutritional abundance) surely must exist on a fairly broad scale. Americans, similar to their dislike of temporary discomfort from cold or heat (or whatever), don't want to be hungry (ever). To satiate their mild pangs of hunger between meals, they reach for all manner of snacks. Many of these mini-meals are highly processed, contain an abundance of simple carbohydrates and/or oxidized lipids, and ultimately use some of the body's stores of nutrition to deal with the health insult they create.

But there is a much bigger problem than this. Constant satiation of hunger often has serious implications for health. One of these is that the body never needs to utilize any of its stored fat. By providing the body with a constant supply of fuel, the body is constantly needing to deal with an influx of calories (rather than tapping into some of the stockpiled fuel). It responds by producing insulin, a hormone that has many effects on the body. The one most people know about is to remove excess glucose (a sugar) from the blood and store it in some fashion (one of which is to store it as fat). But there are other roles that insulin serves, such as storing excess nutrients, retention of sodium, controlling growth hormones, and increasing cellular proliferation. Because of these and other roles of insulin, a constant supply of high insulin in the blood is a risk for factor high blood pressure, obesity, congestive heart failure, osteoporosis, and cancer. Therefore, it is actually quite healthy to experience short periods of hunger.

There are a fairly large number of studies looking at the effects of brief periods of food shortage—which translates to intentional, short-duration fasting in a society with tremendous food abundance. These studies have been done on both humans and laboratory animals and generally demonstrate very positive effects. As might be expected, intermittent fasting can reduce weight and body fat. But it goes further than that. As Klempel and colleagues published in 2013, alternate day fasting produced lower weight and reductions in body fat, but also decreased LDL cholesterol and triglycerides, which are important measures (when elevated) for risk of coronary heart disease. These results were seen regardless of whether the dietary regime utilized a low-fat or high-fat diet on non-fasting days. Other studies support these conclusions and demonstrate that these results are experienced in overweight and normal weight individuals.

Intermittent fasting has other benefits as well. For example, it has been shown to reduce various markers of inflammation. Keeping in mind the chronic inflammation is, for lack of better words, a really bad thing for human health, strategies that decrease inflammation and decrease expression of inflammation-related genes (which intermittent fasting does) can be a huge benefit. A 2007 study by Johnson et al. demonstrated that those conditions that include inflammation as part of their symptoms, such as asthma, show significant improvement with intermittent fasting. A really important piece of this story is that the decreases in inflammation were also seen in the brain. Considering that inflammation in this part of the body (i.e., neuroinflammation) is associated with various degenerative diseases and mood disorders, intermittent fasting appears to have a protective effect on the brain.

One of the more exciting studies on intermittent fasting looked at the effects of calorie restriction on age-related neurological decline. Using middle-aged laboratory rats, the researchers (Singh and colleagues) studied a variety of brain-function markers after 12 weeks of intermittent fasting. The results, which very likely apply to humans, were quite positive. The authors of the study reported increases in motor coordination and learning response with a decline in observed oxidative damage to proteins (a normal part of the aging process that can be hastened by various aspects of modern living). Ultimately, the study suggested that some forms of calorie restriction can slow (or, in some cases, prevent) age-related mental decline. Other studies support this work, demonstrating that fasting is beneficial for the brain, and such a practice can even assist in supporting the growth of new neurons or other cells. This makes intermittent fasting, a form of dietary hormesis, a very powerful tool for maintaining health.

To summarize this section, intermittent fasting, a pattern that emulates calorie procurement in hunter-gatherers, has a wide range of benefits. It has the ability to improve insulin response (along with other hormones, such as leptin), decrease inflammation, lessen oxidative damage, protect against neurological decline, drop weight while maintaining muscle mass, lower triglyceride levels, and increase human capacity to resist stress (one of which is hunger). Subjectively, some people also report mental clarity, calm mood, and a more uniform feeling of energy (i.e., no crashes) as a result of intermittent fasting (and there are valid reasons for these anecdotal reports). The problem is that people don't like to be hungry, and as a result, restricting calories each day is a difficult strategy to maintain. This is why the common approach, called "dieting", in general, is such a monumental failure in permanently reducing weight—people ultimately stop restricting calories (and gain back the weight they lost initially). Further, limiting calories on a continual basis is not the usual pattern experienced by wild humans. Typically, there were periods of food abundance punctuated by short periods of food scarcity or absence, which was then relieved with a successful hunt or foraging event.

Intermittent fasting is a more realistic way to restrict calories and, it turns out, to be easier for people to maintain. The general idea is to eat a normal (healthy normal) amount of food for five days of the week and then "fast" for two days of the week (this is similar to the popularized 5:2 Fast Diet). The fasting days should be non-consecutive (i.e., avoid back to back days of fasting), which allows one to time the non-fasting days to best match planned periods of high activity or celebration (where restricting food intake would be difficult). Given that leaping into abstaining from eating for a day can be difficult, I'm an advocate of a graduated approach where on two days of the week (you choose which days) you simply cut caloric intake to ¾ of normal. After some time (as one acclimates to feeling some hunger), this becomes half of the normal caloric intake. Ultimately, this becomes ¼ of the usual calories needed for one's particular lifestyle (for most people, this would be in the range of 500–600 calories). Remember, hormesis is about gradually pushing boundaries, not leaping into the fire on the first day. Much like most people do not immediately attempt to lift a massive weight on day one, but, rather, build to this effort slowly through weight training (which is a form of physical hormesis). The great thing about this approach is there is no real need to completely eliminate food as restricting calories to below ½ of the usual amount appears to offer some benefits similar to actual fasting (though not eating at all once in a while is a good practice for a healthy adult). Further, there is no need to use intermittent fasting all the time. Do it for a month and then take a month off. Do it for eight weeks and then stop for a while. Variety in this version of intermittent calorie restriction is completely appropriate and, again, emulates actual patterns of seasonal abundance and scarcity for most hunter-gatherers. To make this even more accurate compared with ancestral patterns, on some of the fasting days, omit animal foods completely and eat only plant foods (still aiming for about ¼ of your optimal caloric intake). This is not intended to be a step toward vegetarianism but rather a recognition that hunting and fishing forays were not always successful and it was the women, the primary foragers in the indigenous cultures, who solely fed the families on some days with their harvests. On some days, it would have been underground storage organs (e.g., tubers, rhizomes, bulbs, corms) that would have formed the bulk or the entirety of the day's meals—days when hunters were unsuccessful and other, more preferred plant foods, such as nuts and fleshy fruits, were not available.

Many people eat, not because they are hungry, but because they are bored or want something to do while socializing. Therefore, plan the fasting days (more accurately "calorie restriction days") around times when the mind and body will be busy (so that food isn't always on the mind). Of course, intermittent fasting isn't for everyone (or at least not for everyone at certain stages of their life). For example, most infants were protected from short-term food shortage by their mother's breast milk. Therefore, infants and breast-feeding mothers (along with pregnant mothers) shouldn't intentionally fast. Further, diabetics and others with blood glucose regulation problems can get into serious problems with fasting (until they learn to regulate their insulin better). The idea here (as with everything presented in this book) is to take personal responsibility for your actions, which begins by thoroughly researching and understanding practices you are about to embark on.

THE NEOABORIGIANL STRATEGY FOR STRENGTHENING THROUGH HORMESIS

Hormesis has many advantages for human health, and it is an effective strategy for promoting longevity. While seeking well-being might seem like a selfish pursuit, in actuality a person in a state of healthiness has the capacity to use less of the world's resources. While this is not meant to read as a judgment on people experiencing illness and chronic disease, the fact is that sickness can be incredibly costly (in time and resources) for the people suffering and those who care for them (including the society they are part of). This point makes "health" a very eco-conscientious choice; that is, assuming the person uses their health to live in a nature-connected manner. Taking this idea even further, we can directly tie an inability to endure any discomfort (or at the very least a strong desire to always avoid it) by many modern humans as one important reason they will not alter civilization's practices or detach from civilization altogether. For example, knowing, at least to some extent, the ecological costs of crude oil production, transport, and use (in one of its many forms), we continue to use it to fuel our cars, heat our homes, and produce electricity because the other options are not as comfortable—walking more places (sometimes in cold or rainy weather), letting the home be cooler than usual on occasion, and reducing our use of electrical appliances. The argument being posited here is that society's inaction to lessen the ecological damage it is creating can, in some cases, be clearly tied to the comforts its citizens enjoy. Hormesis provides an answer to this dilemma. It suggests that living through occasional discomfort not only is possible but also has profound beneficial effects.

As a final thought on hormesis, many people need to apply a philosophical hormesis to their daily living. What is meant by this term (philosophical hormesis)? Essentially, people need to push their accepted boundaries in terms both of what they are comfortable with accepting and what they are comfortable with doing. Given that members of affluent societies have had a lifetime of exposure to certain ideas and ideals, thoughts and principles that are very different from those growing up in a more eco-centric culture, we need to come to the understanding that our way of life has, along with some wonderful qualities, some serious drawbacks in terms of how we view and treat the other life we share this world with (which has manifest ramifications for future generations of people as well). Only through a willingness to embrace uncomfortable and sometimes grief-producing ideas can we push forward and break through the veils of domestication. We need to turn a critical eye to our own actions (rather than just those of people living in different countries). We need to have exposure to very normal things that we ask other people to do for us, like killing and butchering animals. This is something we need more comfort with, at least in time, because it will put inhumane methods of taking domesticated animal life in the spotlight and force a reformation of these practices (but only if we get involved in this aspect of animal husbandry). This is but one example of topics we need to broach as a society, there are a multitude of others that we need to shed our complacency for, such as affluent countries role in perpetrating ecocide in undeveloped countries to fuel rampant consumerism, real gender equality that is based on historical models (discussed in the next chapter), and the need to remove wealth as one of the necessary qualifications for our political representatives (we could on at length here). Believe it or not, the problems we face in each one of these aforementioned topics is based on a disconnection from the natural pattern of wild humans. Through confronting the ideals we hold as necessary truths (i.e., practicing philosophical hormesis), we can ultimately see through these "ideals" as falsehoods that ultimately benefit a small proportion of society.

Hormesis is a natural mechanism for increasing human vitality. It can often be practiced without any financial cost. For example, gradually increasing your length of exposure to sunlight is a form of hormesis (in addition to all those discussed in this chapter). As one experiences more sunlight, the body adapts by producing more pigment, and the person can remain in the sun longer without burning. This increased exposure to natural light benefits other areas of human health (e.g., vitamin D production). The point being made here is that many kinds of hormetic exposures are free of cost. Following are ten ways a neoaboriginal can use hormesis to strengthen their mind and body.

1. Understand that the **human organism can adapt tremendously to natural stresses**. Hormesis isn't just a theoretical process but an actual human trait for acclimation to our environment. It has a large body of evidence supporting it, all of which states the human body can expand its tolerance of various stressors and benefit from that stress (sometimes in seemingly unrelated ways). Hormesis offers humans a way to transcend their domestication and recover their wild strength.

2. Resistance and free-weight training are forms of **physical hormesis** that most are familiar with. So too are endurance activities like running, hiking, and swimming. Engage in these activities in a way that you push personal boundaries to build a strong body. Physical strength is one of the important components of skillful movement (not to be focused on at the expense of other movement fundamentals). Most people can practice physical hormesis anywhere they are located because they have their body as a free weight to use in resistance training.

3. **Increase your tolerance of cold** by safely experiencing cold stress (i.e., do not overwhelm your body). You can (for example) be cold for some time on a winter outing and have spare clothing (and a friend) along with you when it is needed. You can also walk barefoot in the snow for a short distance (gradually increasing those distances) or take cold-water plunges. Embrace cold not as the enemy to be confronted but simply a natural feature of our landscape that must be experienced for health.

4. **Increase your tolerance of heat** by safely experiencing heat stress. High ambient temperatures and long-duration activity are methods of experiencing heat challenges that can strengthen the body. Remember that heat stress (as well as cold stress) improves cardiovascular and neurological function.

5. If you are in an urban setting and have little exposure to non-climate-controlled settings, consider **artificial hormetic expsoures**, such as a cold shower or bath (cold) or a sauna (heat) to allow your body to reap the advantages of these practices.

6. Recognize that **beneficial phytochemistry** is lacking, to a degree, in all modern diets (see the section "plants and their nutritional elements" in chapter 3). This can be recovered through exposing the body to safe amounts of edible wild plants and stronger-tasting heirloom cultivated species.

7. Improve your **acceptance and appreciation of bitter-tasting plants**. Bitterness is often tied to antioxidants in food plants. Avoiding bitterness in the diet serves only to reduce an entire

class of plant chemicals that were part of our ancestral diets. While extreme bitterness is not to be ignored (as it may be an indication of toxicity), many bitter compounds promote health when they are ingested as part of a diverse diet.

8. Practice **intermittent fasting** to better emulate hunter-gatherer diets in today's world. Through restricting calorie intake on two non-consecutive days of the week, there are a host of benefits that can be gained, some of which pertain directly to the brain and cognitive function.

9. **Push your philosophical boundaries** by critically evaluating aspects of modern living that have hidden (or not so hidden) costs. Examine the arguments that modern people use to maintain unhealthful living. Be cognizant of the fact that most statements to maintain the current mode of living are, in actuality, a plea to continue the tremendous comfort and convenience that citizens of affluent countries enjoy.

10. Have **gratitude** for our ability to tolerate and grow stronger from various forms of stress. Humans are remarkable animals and have incredible bodies that are capable of much more than we ask of them in our daily, domesticated living. Be thankful for hormesis.

10. Communal organisms: experiencing real community

Homo sapiens is a communal species. It has lived in communities connected by more than just relation for its entire existence. And before humans arose, their hominid ancestors lived in communities. This way of life and manner of interacting with one another is a fundamental part of our being. Real community (to be defined in the next section) is something that people need for health and happiness—it is a kind of nourishment that must be experienced. In the modern world, dysfunctional municipal divisions and virtual communities (i.e., social media) are the most frequent forms of communal interaction that most people are involved in. These contemporary versions of community, while not entirely negative, touch upon only some of the social needs of people and fail (utterly) in providing an actual community that is in line with our evolutionary exposures. In order to maximize our "nutritional benefit" of social interaction, we need to examine traits of original human communities and find ways to emulate these in our daily living. Community is one of the most overlooked aspects of healthy living, in part because domesticated humans have not experienced healthful versions of this for so long that they appear to have forgotten what it looks like (or, more accurately, what it feels like). It is also one of the most difficult to attain, as real community stands in stark contradiction to the very manner in which our civilizations are organized and administered. Community will be the greatest challenge for the neoaboriginal, and also the ultimate inspiration that will provide the precise catalyst needed for people to fully engage in a truly immersive rewilded lifestyle.

COMMUNITY DEFINED

Community, a term today that is used to describe almost any group of people who share one or more cohesive traits, is a word that is used far too loosely for the purposes of this book. In fact, nearly all modern communities in affluent countries do not have the fundamental traits that defined the original human communities (i.e., hunter-gatherer communities). Defining community here sets the stage for understanding why society fails to produce emotional health for such a large proportion of its members. For example, a recent poll (2013) found that only 33% of Americans considered themselves very happy. For a country that is doing tremendous ecological harm to the world, it is unfortunate that only ⅓ of its members are happy (i.e., it would be desirable for more good to come of the lost biological resources). With clinical depression affecting 1 in 10 Americans at some point in their life, no amount of healthy eating or fresh air is going to generate health for these all these people. And while depression is a complex disorder with various root causes (including nutrition), healthy community function could go a long way to supporting those with depression.

Hunter-gatherer communities are egalitarian, highly cooperative, and practice extensive food sharing. Whether we are discussing riverine people in the Amazon River Basin of Brazil, who rely on different species of fish, or arctic populations of Iñupiat, who depend heavily on bowhead whale (*Balaena mysticetus*), caribou, fish, and bearded seal (*Erignathus barbatus*), the pattern is very similar—widespread sharing of hunted and gathered foods with both kin and non-kin in the community. The food sharing helps to promote food security within the group and serves to provide access to nourishment for those who have limited mobility (e.g., young, elderly, infirm, injured). The distribution of food in this manner builds strong social ties and these collective ties comprise one of the most important sources of well-being reported in indigenous people (during surveys performed by anthropologists).

It is important to mention here that most first contact and anthropological accounts of hunter-gatherers practicing their traditional lifeways report happiness, contentedness, and a positive outlook on life. These observations are supported by the fact that many people in agrarian societies will migrate to urban centers (when they arise) to take part in industrial living because they believe their situation can be improved. However, this is not true of hunter-gatherers. So long as their land base has not been degraded and they have not been pushed into marginal habitats, they often require substantial coercing to leave their lifeway. Given that intact hunter-gatherer communities did provide happiness and equality, we need to understand the elements of these communities in order to identify how to emulate them.

While there were differences and some exceptions among the different hunter-gatherer groups, there were also a number of commonalities regardless of what part of the world one visited. It is here, with the definition of community, that we must begin because the meaning in use today does not uphold the core values of this critical aspect of tribal living. If we examine aspects of hunter-gatherer communities, we will identify most (or all) of the following traits among the different groups. While on the surface some of these may not appear as important aspects of community, they all contribute to the nature of the communal experience of indigenous people. Some of these aspects will be discussed in greater detail within this chapter.

1. **Place and commons**. They inhabited a specific place and it was within that particular area that they could apply their ecological knowledge and wisdom—especially as it pertained to food, a defining characteristic of different communities around the world. There was a geographic definition to each community, and each community was bound to a specific part of the planet (e.g., the Inuit of northern North America would not be adapted to the desert of the southwestern United States). Their place influenced the songs they sung, the legends they shared, and the creation stories they passed down through the generations. Further (and equally important), that place was held in common by all of the people of that band. Therefore, the land belonged to all the people (not to individuals).

Today: People are less defined by their place, and are free to move and take up employment in distant areas because industrial living is less tied to a specific landscape. The specific details of the landscape, such as the species of fish in the rivers or the kinds of oaks in the forest, are simply not meaningful details to most contemporary people (people who consume a somewhat homogenized industrial diet). Their creation stories often originate in another place. The land itself is divided up with substantial private ownership and restricted access for people to some properties.

2. **Nomadism**. Hunter-gatherer bands were nomadic to lesser or greater extents, with weekly or seasonal movement (depending on the group) to different areas based on the availability of critical resources (such as food, shelter, fuel). The number of movements per year ranged mostly from 2 to 80, with the majority of groups moving 3 or more times. Exceptions to this occurred only in extremely resource-rich environments (e.g., Pacific Northwest).

Today: People are sedentary in nature and the only movements are generally when someone takes up residence in a new city or town. In other words, people today don't move their place of residence on a continual basis within a specific home range. Those who do (such as wealthy persons who own one or more homes) do not move residence for ecological reasons.

3. **Small group size**. The communities were relatively small, and most bands reached an upper limit of around 30–50 people, though there usually were several to many such bands that comprised the greater tribe. Further, these bands would congregate with others who spoke similar language on a periodic basis. Within such a community, everyone knew each other and cooperated with those people for survival, even having shared child care with other members.

Today: There is hardly a village that contains as few people found in a hunter-gatherer village, with our larger cities containing many millions of people, most of whom don't know each other and actually compete amongst one another for resources.

4. **Low population density**. Hunter-gatherers lived in low population densities with much more land per person than agricultural and industrial societies. Differences existed among different groups because some lands contained more biological abundance than others (e.g., a rainforest contains more macroscopic animals per unit area than does a desert). In general, hunter-gathers existed at population densities of 0.005–2.5 people per square kilometer (very rarely did groups exceed this number, such as some in the Pacific Northwest, but most were below 1 person per square kilometer).

Today: While clearly there is a great variety in the average number of people per square mile in different regions of affluent countries, it is often significantly higher than in hunter-gatherer populations. For example, New Jersey (the most people-dense state in America) has approximately 467 people per square kilometer and the United States as a whole has approximately 34 people per square kilometer. These numbers escalate the probability of conflicts occurring.

5. **Political structure**. Indigenous cultures lacked political bureaucracies and extensive hierarchical structure (i.e., all members of the group were sovereign and equal). This not only included men and women but also the children of the hunter-gatherer groups. There was consensual decision making within the group.

Today: Modern societies are highly organized along hierarchical lines, with members of different posts having authority over other people. Almost no one is sovereign (especially children) and equality is lacking, especially for some people of a certain economic status, skin pigmentation, gender, or social class. Decision making is primarily by political elites (i.e., a small fraction of the society) who attain their position by appointment, election, or heredity.

6. **Equal wealth distribution**. There was little or no wealth differentiation among the people in each culture. Even the elders or sachems, when present in a particular group, did not have more material wealth than other members. Affluence within hunter-gatherers could be described as an ability to acquire and make everything that was necessary for living from their landscapes.

Today: There is currently a massive wealth disparity around the world (i.e., it is not restricted to the United States). According to Oxfam, the lower 80% of humanity (as defined by annual income) has only 5.5% of the world's wealth and earn, on average, 1/700th of what the top 1% of people earn. Affluence is defined by the amount of material wealth that has been accumulated, not by someone's ability to perform necessary tasks for themselves and their community.

7. **Division of labor**. Hunter-gatherers possessed substantial division of labor along gender lines, with men and women performing different tasks—though (a) the specific tasks often differed

between groups of different regions and (b) both genders were equal (in terms of respect). Division of labor allowed each gender to provide their specific gifts to the community.

Today: Division of labor exists in some fields and is not present in others but, in either case, there is not equal respect for the genders as evidenced by less pay for women in the same role as men and fewer women in elite positions.

8. **Sharing**. Hunter-gatherers possessed an indirect reciprocal gift economy that resulted in a compulsory sharing of resources. As such, the efforts of hunting and gathering were distributed to the group. This sharing helped to protect against failed hunts or lean foraging forays experienced by different members of the group and strengthened the social bonds. It was so ingrained in their values that, in many groups, the children ate food with the people they happened to be with (who may not have been their parents or even their aunts, uncles, etc.). Very key to this concept is that people within the group did not compete for the common resources.

Today: There are a variety of economic systems in place, and while different ones do redistribute some portion of the wealth at varying levels, it is an enforced redistribution by taxation of the members that many people would opt out of (if the choice existed). In other words, it is not a cultural pattern of sharing to ensure the survival and continued health of all members of the group. Further, members of the same community compete with each other for material resources, land, and employment.

9. **Cohesion**. There was a strong sense of cohesion in most groups because there were a number of common forces holding them together, such as the risks they faced and their strategies to overcome them. The survival needs of all members of the community were similar because they inhabited the same landscape, and they frequently overcame these pressures with similar methods. But, it went further than this because they also shared common beliefs and a common intent.

Today: People are fractured along ethnic, political, religious, educational, financial, gender, and philosophical lines. Even within a small rural town, there are a multitude of beliefs concerning how things should be accomplished, what should be allowed, who should do it, how it should be paid for, and what the end result will be. While any civil district can come together for certain causes, there are still underlying differences that cause friction and clashing over many issues.

So what does all this mean? Does it imply that we must practice nomadism and move around within a geographic region for happiness? Well, no (however, it was another way that people became familiar with their landscape and related to it). What it does suggest is that a community must participate together in some substantial activities in order to really connect with one another (i.e., singing in a choir, while producing some positive benefits, may not be significant enough). Without sharing in important aspects of life, a community may not have enough purpose to form or survive. To boil down these nine traits into a more cohesive definition of community that fits with the ancestral pattern, I would suggest the following:

A community is a small group of people who reside (sometimes loosely) on a given landscape, share common resources, experience equality and similar affluence between the genders (even though they may each do different tasks), and can operate by consensual

decisions due to similarities in beliefs, for the benefit of the group, to accomplish living in their place.

To contrast this, I would posit that a society operates quite differently:

A society is a large group of people who often live over an expansive area, compete amongst one another for the common resources, experience inequality and wealth disparity between genders (or other social classes), often can't operate by consensus due to dissimilar beliefs and goals (rather, decision making is by majority or minority rule), and often move forward on actions that benefit only a small segment of the people.

Certainly, this writing is not meant to suggest that all aspects of society are inherently damaging. After all, our friends and families are a part of society, and societies are able to accomplish tremendous things by pooling resources (though they also damage the land base at the same time). Some societies do attempt to produce equality, such as through the creation of laws that try to provide equal benefit for all. However, the very fact that laws are required to force equality is the tell-tale feature of the failure of modern society and speaks to the fact that certain people are in a greater position of influence and may have more privileges than others. This aspect of society is another excellent example of nature divorcement because most wild people were able to experience equality, and they had varied ways of producing equality. For example, the Ju/wasi of the Kalahari region used a special system of sharing important animal harvests. When larger animals, such as greater kudu (*Tragelaphus strepsiceros*), gemsbock (*Oryx gazella*), and common eland (*Taurotragus oryx*), were successfully harvested during hunts, most of the animal was transported back to the encampment where it would be shared. Animals such as these were extremely important because they could feed many families, providing not just calories but also deep nourishment, especially for the developing members of the group. The one responsible for dividing the kill was the owner of the arrow responsible for taking the animal's life. You might think this would always be the hunter, but it was not so. The Ju/wasi would give, share, and trade arrows quite frequently. The arrow sometimes belonged to those who were not often successful as hunters for various reasons (e.g., because they had experienced an injury that would prevent them from the swift movement needed to track the animal after an accurate arrow shot). This group of people had a manner of removing the recurrent privilege of harvest sharing from a successful hunter, who would have a disproportionate amount of attention and influence if they routinely took large animals during hunting and others did not. This distribution of the role of harvest sharing through arrow ownership (and not the one who shot the arrow) was one manner of providing equality within the group.

Going further with the differences that can be observed between an actual community and an industrial society, we can see that the fundamental definition of community is violated in a modern society. The word "community" comes from the Latin *communis*, which refers to things held in common. In a hunter-gatherer community, the land is the primary item held in common (i.e., it is not owned by any individual member, though certain groves of trees or sections of a lake may be used by specific families). In a modern society, the land is not held in common, except for specific parcels that are arranged as public lands and parks. Most of the land is held by either private individuals or corporations, who are free to use the biological resources on those lands in a way that benefits the individual and not necessarily the entire society. In fact, some individuals and corporations actively degrade the quality of the lands through practices such as unstainable use, irrevocable alteration, or pollution, so that the land is not available for future generations in the same quality as it was to the previous owner. Acting for short-term individual benefit rather than long-term communal benefit is a defining feature of contemporary people—a trait that arises because society values wealth accumulation over the health of its members.

Without laboring the point, society, and even those groups of people called communities within it, rarely provide many of the commonalities of ancestral communities (which we are evolutionary programmed to live within). Some people understand that our agricultural diet, something that has been practiced for around 11,000 years or less (depending on the region) is a very new diet when considered in an evolutionary context. We have practiced a very different form of nutrition for so long that the heavy reliance on agricultural foods simply has occurred too quickly. Likewise, we have existed in communities that are very different from the civilizations we now experience. The shift from relatively small groups of people operating by consensus to larger chiefdoms, where few people represented many, began only 7500 years ago. In other words, we have had even less time to adjust to societal living than we have had to adjust to our new diets. Therefore, it is worth critically analyzing our social experiences in the context of how long we have existed differently. Those who wish to experience actual community will need to find a way to engage in as many of the following features as possible. These items, which I call **Necessary Features of Actual Community**, allow a hunter-gatherer community to be emulated in the present-day setting.

1. Connect to a landscape with others and let that landscape shape your community. A group of people living in Maine will have differences from one in living in California. These landscapes have different problems to solve and require different approaches. They also provide different kinds of foods and, as a result, will shape nature-based communities in dissimilar ways. This means there is no one simple strategy for any community that will meet the needs of all people across a continent. Place is an important identifier for a community. While science would attempt to observe the characteristics of place (e.g., the rock, the snow, the plant life, the water) without bias, it simply introduces a special kind of bias that attempts to observe creation free of emotion. Communities of people will interact with the elements of their landscape in a distinctive manner and observe creation through their own unique emotional lens of "connection to place". This lens creates subjective reactions to the same phenomenon that are all equally valid. For example, northern people may celebrate a snowstorm for its ability to assist with travel, while southern people might experience snow as a threat to their lives. (Science simply states it snowed for X length of time resulting in Y accumulation.) Without a place, the community is unanchored, such as in a virtual community found online on social media—these communities lack physical interaction between members and the land; therefore, they can experience only a fraction of human social communication and connection. Even if your community is primarily about singing, let the land shape the way you express the songs.

2. Keep your community small. This is not about being exclusive; others are free to create their own communities in their area as well. Further, communities can interact with one another. This is not a call to abandon all ties with other people not belonging to your community. However, if the close community becomes too large, personal familiarity becomes compromised and restrictive laws and regulations are often required to maintain unity—such procedures always go too far and impact personal sovereignty. In keeping the community small, also attempt to keep the group small in relation to the available land (i.e., have a low population density). Ample land on which to roam and the ability to find private locations allow people the space to be alone and unwind from any social tensions that may arise.

3. Share resources, or some resources, or something of value to the community (such as information, ways of doing things, methods of constructing items). Without sharing, it isn't a community. The more one shares and more people that share, the stronger the bonds and the more durable the community. Food sharing is perhaps the most powerful way to create lasting social connections. Sharing builds positive feelings towards members of the community and helps to promote equality. Sharing needs to also transcend material things (to the extent possible) and include items such as intent, ceremony, responsibilities, and chores. Nothing makes tedious work go by like sharing positive community practices (e.g., talking, joking, singing, storytelling). Joint action (a sharing of work and experiences) fosters coherence and community identity. The sharing of rituals will further strengthen social bonds, which are important to the maintenance of community.

4. Treat genders (and ages) as equal. More than this, deeply respect the gifts of all members of the community. Even though the genders may do different work for the community, it should be clear that without the collaboration of all the people, the community won't function. The hunters are not more valuable than the gatherers (to use a historical example). Likewise, those who cook are not less valuable than those who build homes. Very importantly: equality doesn't mean gender doesn't or shouldn't exist.

5. Operate by consensus, which is to write that a few individuals shouldn't dominate decision-making. This is not to say that some members of the community won't have expertise that makes their contribution to a particular topic extremely valuable. This is exactly what being an elder is about (at least in that topic) and it is wise to listen to them. But everyone needs some involvement in the process so that they feel empowered and valued.

6. Do not let a hierarchy form, rather operate in an egalitarian way. Hierarchies are artificial constructs imposed upon the group (i.e., they exist only when the society erects them). If you are able to succeed in numbers four and five, preventing hierarchy will occur naturally within the community. This ensures that certain privileges aren't afforded to some and not to others, which averts one source of social jealously and bitter feelings within a community.

If you currently experience only some of these components of actual community, then it is likely you are living in the modern, industrial world (a time when and a place where people generally experience only fragments of healthy community). Compounding this problem is the fact that some features of civilization are so prevalent and ingrained that we do not see them as a problem or even sense the harm they can do—we might, in fact, even view these features as necessary elements of human interaction. The supporting of unhealthy communal practices is not unexpected given that most humans alive today have been raised within dysfunctional communities (to lesser or greater extents) and do not realize that humans have lived differently for most of their existence. Take hierarchical social structure for example, it leads to social privilege, which is perhaps exemplified by the fact that wealthy people serve less time in jail (or none at all) for the same crimes than do lower income people. Further, social privilege is almost always abused, as evidenced by the many recent examples of police brutality, where people who were not being aggressive were beaten or killed by officers of the law. These examples (of many we could discuss) generate social strife that creates stress and feelings of unease, ultimately weakening social bonds and leading to fractured community. This is clearly borne out in the United States with social disunion along economic and racial lines. To contrast our current situation with that of a healthy community, someone afforded greater respect (what we might call a higher title) would only experience greater obligation. Those who truly labor for their people do not request or require greater privilege because it is the health of their community that motivates them (not greater financial compensation).

Of course, there are many logistical aspects of community that are necessary for it to function well. Communities must be tied to a meaningful purpose (otherwise they may disband for lack of intention). Meaningful purpose will encourage commitment to both attend and participate in the community. In hunter-gatherer cultures, the meaningful purpose was long-term survival and health of the group. That can still be a goal of contemporary community (or another important one can be chosen). For a community to survive, people must learn how to communicate honestly, effectively, and without prejudice. Inflammatory language, assuming one's viewpoint is the only correct way forward, and always assigning blame are excellent ways to block effective communication (hence, carefully chosen language, respecting all viewpoints, and working toward resolution without assigning blame are good practices). Undeniably, all members must participate in functions that benefit the entire community. That means that sometimes we must do things we don't enjoy doing. It also means that all members must share and be part of the reciprocal gift community (though, as stated earlier in the book, reciprocity doesn't have to be as simple as A gives to B and B gives back to A).

BENEFITS OF ENGAGING IN COMMUNITY

Community involvement isn't an optional activity for humans. Much like eating, drinking, and breathing, community has a large impact on our health (positive or negative) and overall outlook on life. After all, humans are innately pro-social, and removing healthy social interaction certainly is a detriment to emotional well-being. Humans respond favorably to being part of a group that engages in positive activities. Is there science to support this? The answer is yes, though the majority of studies looking at this have focused on volunteering (an optional activity). In an affluent society where people work a substantial portion of their waking hours, time is, in many ways, one of the most valuable commodities they have. Therefore, when they give their time, they are giving something of great worth.

We might think that volunteering within and outside of our communities would primarily benefit those receiving the support. Research demonstrates, that in many circumstances, this is not the case. For example, one study in 2005 found that those who received social support had no health improvements as a result; however, those who provided the social support had lower rates of mortality than those who did not give (these results were identified after controlling for a number of variables, including socioeconomic status, marital status, ethnicity, gender, and education). In another study, published in 2003, older married adults who provided support to others had lower rates of mortality five years later than those who didn't. Further (and more to the point), longevity was correlated more strongly with those who gave than with those who received support.

Volunteering and providing support to one's community is especially beneficial for older adults because it often offers some physical activity (especially important in a sedentary society) and it provides a sense of purpose. Study supports that volunteering moderates the sense of lost purpose felt in retired persons who no longer earn a wage as a result of regular employment (see Greenfield and Marks 2004 for one example). Community service has been associated with a greater experience of life satisfaction in older adults than if they were to continue employment. Meaning and purpose in life is an important aspect of psychological health in humans. Community involvement is shown to help in these areas, as well as alleviate social isolation and reduce stress, especially in older adults who are not regularly interacting with coworkers (as they did before retirement).

Volunteer studies often demonstrate greater benefit to older adults than younger adults, in part because younger adults see the community engagement in a negative way (i.e., as obligatory), which detracts somewhat from the benefits it could provide. As a result, some studies that have examined a range of adult ages find greater benefit for those later in life. For example, in one 2000 study, volunteers reported greater life satisfaction and better physical health than those who did not volunteer, but older volunteers testified to greater benefits than did younger volunteers. An interesting point is that while depression is often an obstacle for middle-aged adults engaging in volunteer activity, it is not in older adults (depression has even been described as a catalyst for volunteering in this age group; see Li and Ferraro 2006).

However, before one assumes that they should wait until later in life to engage in healthy community practices, the 1992 study by Moen and colleagues suggests otherwise. They examined data from interviews conducted in 1956 and 1986 of women in an upstate New York community who had volunteered occasionally from the time they had married until the age of 55. These women scored higher in functional ability and were more likely to occupy multiple roles in later years (a measure of community integration) than those who had not volunteered. These results were seen even after controlling for socioeconomic status and previous illness. They suggest that volunteer work throughout life has positive outcomes for people that are expressed to a greater degree when people reach their elderly years.

Volunteer activity is routinely associated with longevity and improvements in health, even after controlling for obvious variables (such as personal health at the onset of the study). Several studies demonstrate that those who volunteer on a regular basis have lower mortality rates than those who do not. The positive feelings generated by helping others make improvements in several important health parameters, including blood pressure (keep in mind that high blood pressure contributes to cardiovascular disease, stroke, and premature death). Those suffering from chronic pain experience decreased levels of pain, disability, and depression when they begin volunteering compared with those who do not (as reported by Arnstein and colleagues in 2002). A 1997 study by Sullivan and Sullivan found that those people who volunteered after experiencing a heart attack reported declines in depression and feelings of despair—two important risk factors for increased likelihood of mortality in coronary artery disease patients. In fact, states with higher volunteer rates experience lower mortality rates from and overall less incidence of heart disease. Clearly, community engagement benefits physical and emotional health.

A well-known example of the role of community in health and mortality was presented by Eric Klinenberg, who authored "Heat Wave: A Social Autopsy of Disaster in Chicago" in 2002. He studied a late-July heat wave that occurred in Chicago, Illinois, in 1995. Medical examiners showed that there were 739 more deaths than normal during this particularly hot week. The interesting part of the story (and what is relevant to this chapter) is what the US Centers for Disease Control identified as individual-level risk factors after the heat wave had occurred. For example, Latinos represented 25% of the city's population but were only 2% of the heat-related deaths, a group of people who lived in densely settled neighborhoods, a busy commercial life, and lively public spaces (i.e., they experienced some functional aspects of community that provided protective measures). This contrasted with most of the African-American neighborhoods that endured high deaths as a result of the heat—most had been abandoned by employers, stores, and residents in the previous decades and had experienced a decay in social support systems. While the high death toll was considered a natural disaster by some, hundreds of city residents were found dead, alone, behind locked doors and sealed windows, isolated from neighbors, family members, and friends, and without assistance from public agencies. As Klinenberg asserts, there is nothing natural about that (i.e., humans are meant to form communities, within which members can support one another during times of stress).

Studies demonstrate that volunteering and being a member of an active community contribute to positive health outcomes. Greater happiness, increased feelings of life-satisfaction and self-esteem, lower levels of depression, and greater physical health are experienced by those engaging in community. Of course, people must meet what is sometimes termed a "volunteer threshold" obtain these benefits. Fortunately, the minimum amount of community engagement to achieve health benefits is not substantial. One or two hours per week of such activity is considered sufficient—though more engagement provides greater benefits. Further, volunteering must be done for the right reasons. One study in the journal Health Psychology suggested that volunteering "because you have to", as opposed to "it feels like the correct thing to do", is not associated with the same level of benefit. Therefore, the goal is to find something you enjoy doing or doing for others. It is important to also note that volunteering is not the only way to access the health benefits of community. Activities like singing in a choir, playing on a recreational sports team, and belonging to a hobby group are additional ways for people to feel like they are part of something, and these activities are associated with benefits. However, most of these fall short of the quality of indigenous communities because they lack several of the Necessary Features of Actual Community. That is not to write that we should not be involved in such groups—only that real community offers substantially more benefit if it can be located or created.

SURVIVAL OF THE THOSE WITH THE MOST COOPERATIVE CONNECTIONS

Nature is often depicted as a savage place where brutal acts are the norm and each organism vies against others for the acquisition of necessary resources. We are so occupied by the idea of struggle and competition among and between species that the concept posited by Charles Darwin—survival of the fittest, where only the largest, strongest, and fastest survive to reproduce and pass on their successful genes—is rarely questioned. This particular interpretation of what we observe in nature (competition) appears completely logical. Of course, this viewpoint hails from biologists and other scientists who grew up and reside within a civilization that is highly competitive and has abandoned many aspects of human life that were almost universally present prior to the adoption of agriculture. Is it possible that our current worldview, a product of high rivalry and antagonism between nations and individuals and a common feature of athletics, market place activity, and scholastic success, is clouding our view (at least to some extent) as to what is actually occurring outside of civilization?

What if instead of survival of the fittest (or at least in addition to this idea), we actually have a kind of cooperation acting on each landscape throughout the world and through time, so that those most likely to survive are the ones who cooperate the most? And each form of cooperation will look different (i.e., each species will have its unique way of collaborating with other life on the planet). In these ways, all wild life works together to contribute to the mega-organism we call earth. It could be said that each wild species has a role, a particular function, that it performs on its landscape. Some of these roles we have given titles, such as autotroph, herbivore, predator, and decomposer. Landscapes are less likely to experience severe disturbances when they have multiple species occupying each role; which is to write when an ecosystem has more biological diversity. Keeping in mind that (generally speaking) the most stable ecosystems are those that are more diverse—those with the most species interacting with one another—any force that reduces the number of cooperations is contributing to instability and a decline in health of an ecosystem.

Ecological titles (e.g., herbivore, predator, omnivore) generally look only at an organism's role at this moment in time, and rarely examine how living creatures cooperate with each through time to develop extraordinary traits. It is the speed and agility of North American doves and waterfowl that necessitated an ability of the peregrine falcon (*Falco peregrinus*) to stoop long distances through the air at astonishing quickness in order to capture them. It is the numerous predators of the ruffed grouse (*Bonasa umbellus*), including the various accipiters (i.e., hawks of forested areas), that has led to the remarkable mottled and striped plumage consisting of contrasting brown, gray, and light colors that functions as excellent camouflage (in fact, the birds are rarely seen before they flush into the air and fly away). It is the abundant tannins (which are antinutrients) found in the branchlets, winter buds, and leaves of various woody plants that have produced a unique trait in the moose (*Alces americanus*)—production of copious amounts of saliva with tannin-binding proteins to nullify some of the deleterious nutritional effects of these ubiquitous phytochemicals. While these are typically viewed as competition, these are also forms of cooperation. These interactions between different lifeforms leading to specialized traits are a form of coordinated change to become better adapted to their environment. After all, these traits would not have developed (i.e., there would be no need for them) without the interaction with other life.

There are many cases of cooperative connections between different species of wildlife that benefit all members involved (i.e., the interactions are mutually beneficial). There are also examples that, on the surface, appear to be an association that benefits only one member of the relationship but deeper study reveals otherwise. Acorn weevils (genus *Curculio*) lay eggs inside the immature fruits of several species of nut-bearing trees, including oaks (genus *Quercus*). As the nut matures, the eggs hatch and the weevil larvae, resembling a pale grub, consume the nut (which kills the fruit) and eventually bore a hole in the shell to exit. Therefore, the acorn weevil benefits from the fruit of the oak (the acorn), and that is the end of the story—no evidence of cooperation. But wait, not so fast. It turns out that careful examination of the situation reveals a different story. Research by Steele and colleagues in 1996 showed that gray squirrels (*Sciurus carolinensis*) have an ability to detect which acorns are infested with acorn weevil larvae and which are not. Examining their preferences for the acorns of three species of oak, they cache significantly more often those that are intact (i.e., uninfected) and disperse them further than those with weevil larva infections. The acorn weevil larvae increase the perishability of the acorn; therefore, it makes perfect sense that those free of infection are cached as they will last longer. However, the weevil larvae also increase the nutritional content of the acorn because this fruit contains abundant tannins that bind with proteins and make them unavailable to the squirrels. Further, the weevil larvae supply some minerals (e.g., phosphorous) that occur in low concentrations in acorns. Given that the study observed gray squirrels occasionally opening acorns and consuming only the weevil larva, the observations suggest that despite the fact the oak loses a proportion of acorns to weevils each year (damage from acorn weevils can result in a loss of upwards of 70% of the acorn crop in certain years), the acorns are more nutritious to the squirrels as a result. When one considers that other studies show that tree squirrels lose weight on a diet solely of acorns, it becomes clear that the weevils offer something to the squirrels (nutrition), who in turn offer something to the oaks (fruit dispersal), which benefits both the oaks and weevils by ultimately producing more oak trees. All three species benefit by the presence of the others. This is an excellent example of the kinds of cooperative connections that exist in nature.

One of the classic examples of cooperative relationships involves the gray wolves (*Canis lupus*) of Yellowstone National Park in (primarily) Wyoming. The wolves were eradicated from the park in 1926, initiating a series of unexpected changes. The elk (*Cervus canadensis*) were now without one of their primary predators (i.e., without one of their cooperative partners) and became very abundant. They began to over-browse woody vegetation along the stream shores, such as aspens, cottonwoods, and willows. Without the roots of these plants stabilizing the banks of the streams, the banks began to erode and collapse. This altered stream habitat for various species of fish because the absence of taller vegetation removed shade that kept streams cool, and also caused streams to widen and become more shallow (as their banks fell in). These trees were also preferred food for the American beaver (*Castor canadensis*), and as elk consumed them, including their new seedlings and sprouts, this aquatic rodent was unable to find enough food and their numbers dramatically declined in the park. Without wolves present, coyotes (*Canis latrans*) became more abundant. However, coyotes are too small to be regular predators of elk (though they sometimes take calves). Therefore, elk continued to over-populate the region and cause extensive damage to the plant resources. Further, without regular wolf kills, there were fewer elk carcasses for the animals that utilize carrion, such as the American badger (*Taxidea taxus*), bald eagle (*Haliaeetus leucocephalus*), common raven (*Corvus corax*), and red fox (*Vulpes vulpes*). With the return of the gray wolf to Yellowstone National Park, beginning in 1995, elk numbers were brought to a level where they did not cause extensive damage to the plant life. Further, these herbivores were less likely to remain in the open along stream courses (where they feed on the stream-side plants and cause erosion with their hooves). As a result, the vegetation has grown back and the stream banks are more stabilized, benefitting the fish and the beaver, the latter of whom now make wetlands with their dam building that creates a diversity of habitat for insects, amphibians, and their predators. This example illustrates the cooperation between the elk and gray wolves. While often viewed as competition when predators kill prey, this story exemplifies how their cooperative interaction ultimately protects riparian resources that benefit a broad range of wildlife in the region.

Wild humans (i.e., hunter-gatherers) also participated in cooperative connections with other wildlife. California Natives, such as the Miwok, gathered a species in the agave family called wavy-leaved soap-plant (*Chlorogalum pomeridianum*) for its edible bulbs, which were baked in earth ovens prior to consumption. Gathering the bulbs is lethal to the plant, so the Miwok needed to develop a cooperative strategy to prevent eradicating this important species of food plant. They removed the bulbs from the ground using a wooden digging stick. They would detach the lower part of the bulb, called the root crown, with their digging stick and replant this in the hole from where the bulb was removed. The root crown is capable of producing a new plant. Equally important was to time the collection of the bulbs when the fruits were present. In this way, the indigenous people could open the dry capsules and place the seeds in the freshly tilled earth, essentially planting this species for future harvest. Then, after a 3- to 5-year rest period, they returned to this location to repeat the harvest (see Kat Anderson 2005 for additional examples of Native American management practices). It is also worth mentioning that their digging in the soil would remove some plants that were growing near the harvested species, thereby opening space for this food species. The California Natives, like many indigenous people around the world, were able to turn a potentially destructive collection method into a process that benefitted them and increased the populations of wavy-leaved soap-plant. This is another example of a cooperative relationship that, on the surface, appears to be very one-sided arrangement. Beyond the illustration of the kinds of interactions that exist in nature, there are multiple important take-home messages from this example, two of which are: (1) what might appear on the surface to be a wanton act of collection actually represents a gathering system that includes numerous safeguards to protect plants from overharvest and (2) the simultaneous use and conservation of nature requires far more knowledge and skill than simply leaving nature alone (more on these in the final chapter).

Within hunter-gatherer groups, it is clear that cooperative connections are the norm, not the exception. Sharing of food harvests, for example, is an integral part of their lifeway and reinforces social relationships within the groups. The allocation of harvests to various members of the communities helps to insure that all members are protected from food shortages. Therefore, the act of sharing (i.e., cooperation in the feeding of all members of the community) increases the food security of the group as a whole. It may also contribute to the happiness observed in intact hunter-gatherer groups. Humans feel pleasure when they give to others. For example, a study examined the benefits of giving or receiving a small amount of money. Those who gave the money to charity had a region of the brain (called the reward center, which turns on when we feel pleasure) activated, whereas those who received the money did not. This is one of several studies that demonstrate emotional benefit to giving (which is to share one's "assets").

Harvest sharing contributes to social cohesion and increases acts of reciprocity. Because this form of food sharing is strongly tied to the definition of being a hunter-gatherer, it is part of the distinctiveness of indigenous communities; therefore, when harvest sharing ceases to occur, as often is the case when economic development disrupts indigenous lifeways, hunter-gatherers lose part of their cultural identity. Also of interest is that harvest sharing means that the entire group experiences bountiful periods as well as times of scarcity—the entire community is tied to the natural rhythm of that place, which further reinforces their relationship with their landscape. Figure 10.1 (left graphic) shows the harvest-sharing network in an Iñupiat village in extreme northwestern North America. Over 60 species of wild plant and animal foods were followed as they entered the village to identify the extent of food sharing. In the same figure (right graphic), the money that entered the village was also tracked. The cash-sharing network stands in stark contrast to the harvest-sharing network, where it is clear that certain aspects of social relationships have disintegrated. Despite the fact the observed community is considered to have strong interpersonal ties between the members, the cash is not widely shared among them.

Subsistence harvest-sharing network in an Inupiat village

Cash-sharing network in an Inupiat village

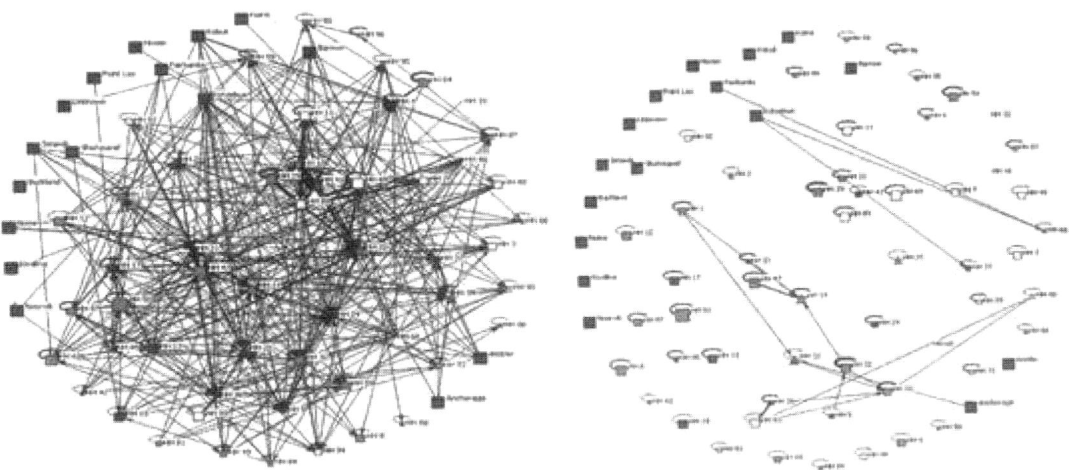

Figure 10.1. Comparison of food-sharing (which includes in this case fish, land animals, marine mammals, and plants) among individuals and to locations in an Iñupiat village with strong social ties and a comparison of cash-sharing in the same village, suggesting a deleterious effect of a market economy on community. Used with permission from: Haley, S., and J. Magdanz. 2008. The Impact of Resource Development on Social Ties: Theory and Methods for Assessment. *In* Earth Matters: Indigenous Peoples, the Extractive Industries, and Corporate Social Responsibility. C. O'Faircheallaigh and S. Ali (editors). Greenleaf Publishing, Sheffield, United Kingdom.

Given that cooperative connections are highly valuable to the survival (and even definition) of a community, it is interesting to note how the replacement of a indirect reciprocal gift economy with that of a cash economy leads to social dysfunction. Harvest sharing is based on community production, which creates strong social ties and cultivates trust between members of the community. Market economies, on the other hand, are based on the wage labor of an individual and utilize impersonal and often transient exchange relationships. As a result, cash economies erode social ties and diminish trust among members of the community. Part of the diminished trust is the result of the transient exchange relationships (i.e., business networking), where associations are forged for the benefit of the affiliates but are broken when one of the affiliates fails to provide benefit. Whereas communities work together to survive hardships, businesses create and sever bonds depending on their benefit to the business. This is the major difference between building a community and building networks—the former is focused on the entire network and long-term commitments, the latter focuses on the individual parts of the network and short-term commitments. In this way, cash economies mimic many other aspects of modern societies (i.e., they are egocentric and emphasize short-term thinking). It should also be noted that when indigenous cultures transition to a market economy (often as a result of outside pressure), individuals within the community report a decrease in feelings of social connectedness, a loss of overall common values, and a reduced sense of well-being.

Some people would dispute the need for community in the modern world, pointing out that they are comfortable (or even happy) living alone and may interact regularly with only few friends. Such people often immerse themselves in one or more solo hobbies or forms of entertainment that fill the time they would have normally (in healthy communities) spent interacting with other people and helping them perform the necessary duties of the group. Of course, no one today actually lives alone—such a belief can be held only by failing to critically examine details of their lifeway. People who spend much of their time in relative social isolation are still interacting with other people around the world. They are completely dependent on growers, builders, manufacturers, and thousands of other laborers who likely live in distant locations and are never met by the person living without community. The solo person, believing they are better off without a tight-knit group, has replaced strong social ties and direct interaction with the people who cooperate with them for weak economic relations and often no interaction with the people they rely on to grow their food, produce their clothing, and manufacture the goods and medicines they use. Essentially, the near majority of their life's interaction can be described as a network of superficial interactions with people that remain in their network only as a result of compulsory payments of labor (to the employer) and cash (to those who produce the items they need for survival and want for entertainment). People who prefer limited cooperative connections are often those who have been hurt by emotionally unhealthy people or are dealing with one or more disorders that cause them discomfort in social settings (e.g., Social Anxiety Disorder, Autism Spectrum Disorder, Asperger's Syndrome)—none of which are valid reasons for people (in general) to avoid social contact with others. To be very clear, a person who has experienced abuse of some kind or has a neurological issue cannot be used as evidence for humans to avoid contact with other humans. Their comfort avoiding socializing is, in some ways, similar to the alcoholic's comfort of drinking (i.e., we all recognize that the alcoholic needs assistance; likewise, those who prefer social isolation need our help). Asocial behavior is a symptom of an underlying problem that requires a holistic approach to generate more comfort interacting with other humans.

Survival of the fittest is not really an accurate description of what is occurring in nature but this common phrase has certainly influenced our worldview in really important ways. It allows domesticated humans to "write off" various events in the world that should have been prevented from occurring and, at the least, would have been mourned by people who have a deeper understanding of how connected life truly is. This phrase alters the way we view events in unhealthy ways. For example, when another indigenous language goes extinct, some people simply describe the situation as an unfortunate example of survival of the fittest (i.e., the indigenous culture did not survive the colonization by imperialists), never realizing that the language embodied a unique way of perceiving and relating to the world. The vanished language held part of the diversity of human awareness and its loss represents a further homogenization of the world. Uniformity of thought on a global scale is a serious impediment to solving the world's issues—especially when the world is moving more and more toward a nature-disconnected, industrial lifeway that favors temporary economic relations. These kinds of social and market interactions are in opposition to beneficial cooperative connections. Hopefully, it is clear at this point, that many of the ecological problems we face today are the result of separation from nature. Likewise, the dissolution of community is the separation from each other. In both cases, the total number of cooperative connections in the world is diminished. Nature can be described as a dynamic process of cooperative connections, and humans used to partake in such meaningful connections on a regular basis. Therefore, the ongoing loss of such relationships in the world can be viewed as a loss of human nature.

GENDER EQUALITY

Most modern societies today would be defined as patriarchal, where men generally have a greater authority within the family and within the society. Greater authority generally results in disparate representation in political offices, higher wages for the same job, and greater social privileges. For example, the 114th congress of the United States is 80% male—which is the most gender equal is has ever been (i.e., in the past, members of the House of Representatives and Congress were proportionally filled with even more males). In some countries today, women are not allowed to participate in political offices or can hold only minor positions and might not be able to vote. Regarding wages, there are a lot of misconceptions about this, but men in the United States do earn more than women for the same job. For the same job, women earn 91 cents for every dollar that men earn. The often used figure is that women earn 77 cents for dollar earned by men but this figure isn't controlled for a number of issues (e.g., actual hours worked, participation in unions, average income of different professions). That written, it still demonstrates a problem because many male roles are regarded with greater prestige than female roles. And this figure is much more dramatic if we were to examine some other countries where women are afforded few or no opportunities for education. One of the more striking examples of patriarchy regards household chores. Even though both genders may be working full time jobs, it is the female who is expected to do the bulk of the domestic labor (such as cooking, washing dishes and clothes, cleaning). These are viewed as traditionally feminine roles and men rarely share an even burden in this kind of work. What this means is that women do more unpaid work than men and men get to have more leisure time than women in most households.

Feminism, a movement with the purpose of achieving equality for women, campaigns on a premise of empowering women. On the surface, this seems like a laudable goal, one that all members of a given society should be involved in regardless of their gender. While feminism has brought more discussion to important women's issues, it suffers from one very significant shortcoming—it is attempting to create equality in a system where equality can never be achieved (for any gender). The problem is that feminism has failed to critically examine the system within which it operates. While feminism is a diverse movement with different goals and methods of reaching those goals, at least some forms of feminism would seek to put more women in elite places of power based on wealth, political influence, and religious authority. In this way, there would be a more even representation of men and women in elite positions. However, with more women in leading roles, this means that some women will sit above others of their gender (and of the other gender) on the hierarchical ladder of society. In doing this, it actually creates inequality because some women will have more wealth and social privilege than other women. Therefore, this movement creates stratified gender equality, a similar level of representation in the various social classes as men. This is not equality, it is merely men and women sharing the same level of social dysfunction.

While I am not intending that feminism is a movement that is without merit, I would argue it needs to examine carefully its intentions. If the goal is to achieve equal power as men through competing with them, then it is likely that women also will suffer the many ill consequences of this race for power. Historically, we see that feminism has had some unintended outcomes as a result of wanting equality with men—many of whom have pathologically adolescent egos as a result of being raised in a society that has forgotten how to nurture whole humans who understand service beyond self. For example, the Torches of Freedom campaign in the early 1900s was an effort to bring cigarette smoking to women, who did not participate in this activity at the same level as men. In fact, various US municipalities had laws prohibiting women from smoking. While initiated by men, this campaign was seen as a part of the women's liberation movement and a way to attain equal rights for women. Through smoking cigarettes, women acted to break social taboos and achieve equal social privilege. As a result of this grab for equal power, women began to suffer at the hands of chronic smoking, which is one of the leading preventable causes of death. More importantly, because women carry the fetus during pregnancy, smoking by females meant that a greater number of infants (of both sexes) would be born with a range of health insults as a result of exposure to cigarette smoke while in utero.

Of course, there are other examples of feminism leading to unintended consequences. The desire for women to avoid pain in childbirth has existed for a long time (long before industrial society came into being). However, it is with the rise of feminism that a relief from the discomfort of labor became a necessary woman's right. As a result, feminists popularized the use of a pain-relieving mixture called "twilight sleep" that consisted of morphine and scopolamine (the latter a psychoactive compound, toxic even in relatively low doses for neonates, derived from members of the nightshade family). This medicine produced analgesic and amnesic actions for the mother but, unfortunately, depressed the central nervous system of the infant, sometimes leading to infants who could not be resuscitated because they were not breathing normally (ultimately leading to the disuse of this pain relief method). Despite these outcomes, respite from pain in childbirth remained an important topic to some feminists. Treating the pain from labor sometimes led to other necessary medical interventions, increasing the frequency of poor maternal and neonatal health outcomes. While drugs for the reduction of labor (and the understanding of their appropriate dosages) have improved over the decades, there was substantial harm to many mothers and newborns in order to get us to the current point of knowledge.

The point of interest in this section is that few people are looking to the historical model of gender equality as a way to move forward or at the very least understand how it was accomplished (this is similar to modern human's avoidance of historical information concerning diets and other items of interest to health). Most hunter-gatherer groups that have been observed demonstrated high equality between the two genders. The model that was practiced could be described as "separate but equal", with the two genders generally performing different tasks, both of which were highly valued by the group as a whole. The two sexes often achieved a high level of skill in their respective tasks, performing them at a greater degree of competency than the other gender. Sometimes both males and females participated in a particular activity but then the methods used were frequently different. For example, males may have fished in deeper water using hooks and lines from dugout wooden canoes and females fished in shallower water using baskets to net fish. Despite the different roles in the tribe, it is clear that both genders were respected. There are a number of ways to demonstrate the validity of that statement. For example, in some groups, certain important groves of food trees were been passed to the next generation through the maternal line. Likewise, the decision among hunter-gatherers to move camp was made by the women who had a better understanding of local food and fuel resources needed by the people for everyday living. Keeping in mind that women were just as responsible for feeding the family as the men (if not more so in many groups, even though they often sought different kinds of the food than the men), women had a respected place in hunter-gatherer groups.

Work by anthropologists supports the contention that gender equality existed within hunter-gatherer groups, despite the prevailing public opinion that hunter-gatherer groups were male-dominated cultures. In a recent article by Mark Dyble and colleagues published in 2015, they discussed the social organization observed in wild humans in two widely separated locations (the Mbendjele BaYaka of the Democratic Republic of Congo and the Agta of the Philippines). In each case, people within the groups had a relatively lower number of kin than would be expected if one gender had a greater social standing than the other. This may seem significant; however, studies show that hunter-gatherers do have a preference for living with closely related family members. If we were to assume that one gender (such as males) experienced more power in social decision making than the other, then they would likely surround themselves with as many kin as possible, meaning women would have fewer kin in their groups than the men. In fact, what was noticed by the researchers is that there was a large number of unrelated people in the tribes. More to the point, no gender had more closely related kin than the other, demonstrating that both sexes had an equal role in the decision-making process of who the tribes would be composed of. This contrasts with traditional agricultural societies where men tended to have more kin within the groups than did the women. It turns out that equality in this kind of decision making has a number of advantages, including the ability to track kin from further away, which creates a broader network that humans can draw on in times of need. It also increases the likelihood of somewhat different methodologies, promoting a sharing of innovations.

Perhaps a relevant way to demonstrate the gender equality of men and women in hunter-gatherer groups (and the gender inequality in agricultural groups) would be to examine how children perceive the loss of the two genders when a male or female in their life has died. A pertinent study was done that compared two groups of children in central Africa: the Aka (hunter-gatherers) and the Ngandu (farmers). These two groups live nearby one another, making them an ideal study group to compare foragers with agriculturalists. As Bonnie Hewlett reported in 2009, these two groups of adolescents had some striking differences in how they perceived and dealt with the death of adult men vs. women in their groups. Aka children remembered a similar number of male and female deaths (Ngandu children remembered far more male deaths than female). Aka children generally reported similar levels of grief when a male or female died (Ngandu children were more likely to report greater grief upon the death of a male). Aka children remembered biological kin from both the maternal and paternal sides of the family (Ngandu children remembered deaths on primarily the paternal side of the family). Aka children connected the grief they experienced over the loss of an adult to the relationship they had with the individual (Ngandu children connected the grief they experienced over the loss of an adult to what that individual had provided for them). Aka children found that spending time with family and receiving physical comforting helped them best deal with the grief they experienced at the death of an adult (Ngandu children felt relief of their grief when they received material items that had belonged to the deceased or when the living adults gave them gifts). The results of this study support the contention that men and women are viewed and valued differently in agricultural societies (and that the accumulation of material possessions is given a different priority in each group).

It is quite clear that hunter-gatherers (the ancestors of all modern people) lived in egalitarian cultures that valued the input of both genders and experienced greater community health as a result. It is also clear that modern societies are quite patriarchal and despite efforts for equality have simply not achieved this goal. So, how do we move forward? How do we develop actual equality where both genders are valued for their contribution to the community? While feminism would state we should empower one gender, which essentially accomplishes the same level of egocentric pursuit in both genders (not a particularly admirable goal), egalitarianism accomplishes equality by depowering both genders. It states that all community roles are valuable and that no one deserves greater privilege. While someone's talents can be deeply appreciated, that skilled person (be it a healer, weaver, or hunter) is not allowed to sing their own praises (nor do they need to, because they are emotionally well and do not require constant attention). Arrogance and bragging are common features in modern society, whether it be among individuals, professionals, or politicians. Getting others' attention is a common activity in young children, and when this behavioral trait continues into adulthood, it is clear indication of a society's failure to create whole humans. Those seeking employment and politicians must boast of their talents to demonstrate why they are the ones who should be chosen for a particular job or political office (respectively) because they are part of a highly competitive society that does not cooperate for a common goal. Within such an economic and political system, it is doubtful to me that real equality can ever be achieved.

Compounding this problem is the fact that many female roles have been devalued by members of society (including by women themselves). This has occurred in two ways: the automation of jobs and the diminished prestige given to traditionally feminine roles. Food preparation, which includes much more than just cooking in a home that understands traditional nutrition, is a vitally important job that affects the health of the entire home. It involves grinding, soaking, sprouting, fermenting, drying, nixtamalizing, leaching, preserving, and a host of other tasks that make a huge impact on the nutritional availability of consumed foods. However, with the virtual automation of this task, epitomized by a microwave meal that requires only that someone be literate enough to follow simple directions for temperature and time, the skill required for this role (and the respect garnered) is next to nothing. Making clothing was a time-intensive task that required a very large skillset that was handed down through the generations to allow the fabrication of attire that would protect against the elements while allowing humans the full range of motion needed for wild living. The processing of hides into supple clothing and the weaving of plant fibers into fabrics are things few people in the modern world can now accomplish. Even in the most extreme environments of the world, women made the most amazing clothing, including footwear, without following preset patterns and using tools they made from natural features of their landscape. Often by simply eyeing the person whom the clothes were for, women created the functional garments, sometimes of intricate style, using methods that are now mostly forgotten. Today, clothing is purchased in a store and made of textiles created by machines. All anyone needs to know is a few measurements of their body or have a willingness to try on several sizes to find the correct fit. There is no skill anymore in providing clothes for your family. Hence, the respect for this duty has also diminished.

It is easy to continue finding examples of traditionally feminine jobs that have been automated and, as result, have lost the respect that was held for these roles in egalitarian communities. Consider the elaborate baskets that were made for a variety of purposes. There are women in some communities (such as Pomo of northern California) who could weave baskets with such skill that they were water tight. Now, we purchase containers of plastic, steel, and glass made in a factory. Even the washing of clothes and dishes is now automated by machines. If we compare this with usual male jobs in and around the home, we see that many of these are not automated. Carpentry, plumbing, wiring and other aspects of home repair still require skill and problem solving (sometimes necessitating complex solutions). Vehicle repairs, which may need substantial experience to even diagnose the problem, typically can't be accomplished by simply pushing a button. It is easy to understand why many traditionally male roles have retained some degree of esteem (that is not to write that one needs to value these jobs differently—all are necessary for a functioning home). I want to be clear and state that all roles in the modern home deserve gratitude for the time they require and the intention put forward but that does not mean that all jobs deserve respect for the skill they require.

But it goes further than this because many women I've spoken to don't want to "go backwards" and have to craft things by hand. And therein lie the problems. One, developing a talent around craftwork is seen as regressing by some women. The skill required for some of these projects is extraordinary. One only needs to visit a museum featuring indigenous baskets, ceramic vessels, and clothing to understand this view is uninformed (and if one tries to create these items by hand, it will become even clearer how difficult they are to manufacture). I humbly challenge someone unfamiliar with ancestral skills to create a pair of Yakut reindeer skin boots (eastern Russia), a large Diné ceramic vessel (southwestern United States), or a Natinixwe twined basket (California) using only tools constructed of natural materials (i.e., materials like bone, wood, stone, antler). To consider this a backward movement in their life compared with most modern jobs is the product of immersion in a society that often values total earnings of a profession above all else. And this is the second problem. Professions are not valued based on a suite of healthy criteria, such as how little damage they do to the world, how they foster equality, or how they help people live sustainably within their ecosystems. Rather, domesticated humans often accord the highest prestige to the highest earning professions, professions that, in many cases, can be quite harmful to the world and even promote inequality among people. To provide for your family through crafting with your own hands from raw materials sourced from your local area is today seen as a major setback (true for men and women). This speaks enormously about such a society—being able to do for yourself is going backwards, whereas forward progression is having someone else do your work (and in the progress you forget how the task is done).

There has been a strong movement to enforce equal pay for equal work. In other words, each gender should be paid the same for their employment (all things being equal). Of course this should be the case, but it misses a fundamental aspect of being human—that there are two genders—and such a model doesn't celebrate the differences (rather, it rolls everything into one bland, ungendered package called "human"). When either gender can do the job, there is no incentive for equality in hiring, wages, or benefits. The employer simply hires those they perceive as working harder or better or even those they prefer to be around (which could be men). The historical model was very different from this (and while some would argue that gender doesn't and has never existed, it is a natural phenomenon supported by many observations, including the fact men and women in traditional cultures had different gut floras and even navigated their landscapes using different systems). It understood that each gender had biological talents as a result of being male or female. Each gender took on largely different roles within the groups and specialized in their respective tasks, holding a special set of the information concerning biodiversity in their communities. Each was critically important to the other because men could not do (with the same proficiency) the work done by women and vice versa. Therefore, the indigenous model was essentially "equal respect for dissimilar jobs done at different proficiencies by the different genders", and such a model worked to create equality. While this is not as simple as a sound byte as "equal pay for equal work", it does have the distinction of being an actual method used around the world that truly generated both respect and equality for women.

It is often the case that the writing in the previous paragraph is interpreted as men are to hunt and women are to stay home with the children. However, this is not what I intended, and it is a massive oversimplification of what actually occurred in hunter-gatherer tribes. First, I encourage anyone who wants to hunt to do so, but if everyone in the community does this, the group won't last long because there are many other roles that need to be filled for a community to survive. And while child care did fall disproportionately to women for a number of reasons, including the ability to breastfeed and often the distances travelled during hunting precluded young people with short legs from participating, that shouldn't be taken as women get the lower prestige role (which is often the interpretation in a society where women want to emulate men in their pursuit of material gain). Isn't nurturing the next generation of providers, healers, educators, role models, protectors, and elders the most important role in any community? Keep in mind, research on hunter-gatherer groups shows that women were also responsible for other important tasks, such as feeding the members of the community—often to a greater extent than the men—and that they were not solely responsible for childcare, which was performed by a number of different people in the group (other relatives, older children, and elderly members of the village). Women did travel out of the village to perform various important tasks, sometimes with infants or children in tow and sometimes not. This is the amazing aspect of the feminine, to be able to accomplish critical work and nurture (in all senses of the word) the next generation along the way.

Returning to the question of how do we move forward as rewilded humans seeking equality, it will likely require people to initiate and build their own communities founded on the principles of egalitarianism, among which one of the most important is equality of all people (not just equal chances for either gender to ascend above others of their own sex). It will also require sharing of intent, and food, and land, and duties (though genders may do different duties, especially if the work calls to members of one sex more than the other). These features of community are almost impossible to create and/or maintain in a society so pervaded with hierarchy. But a group of people can establish these as tenets of their organization and allow members to experience true equality in at least some portion of their life. Another way to establish equality between the genders (though not one likely to be popular in an industrial society) is to remove certain automated technologies in the home. Seek a return to traditional cooking, with meals often beginning the day (or days) before in order for aging, sprouting, or fermenting to take place. Have someone in the home fabricate clothing from scratch (using plant fibers, animal fibers, or even hides). Rather than buying dishes and containers, learn to make them, such as ones made from clay, which can be beautiful, functional, and distinctive. And so on. All of this investment in time and experience will change the way the home chores are viewed (and benefit whoever is doing them, man or woman). Importantly, find ways to transcend the market economy and eliminate (as much as possible) your need for and use of money, even if only within your community. Money is usually saved (a euphemism for hoarding) and, when distributed, is not evenly shared between members of the group. The more that important tasks can be completed without money, the more the group will move away from inequality.

Egalitarianism is a difficult goal to achieve. Some people feel that they are more important, that they contribute more, or that they are entitled to more because of their expertise, wealth, heredity, or gender. Something that has been the norm their entire life is difficult to move beyond. Further, some men don't want to give up the power that affluent societies have given them. But equality has always been the norm for *Homo sapiens* until quite recently (when the nature divorcement and agricultural experiments began). Males and females contributed equally and received equal respect. There was no need to empower women, nor was there a need to focus on the feminine (at the expense of the masculine). In fact, some groups used male animals as a sign of feminine beauty and fertility without compromising the recognition of both genders. For example, the women of the Ju/wasi of the Kalahari considered the bull common eland (*Taurotragus oryx*) as a symbol of female fertility and figure this large antelope prominently in the menarchal ceremony of young women. The size of the bull common eland was associated with health and fertility because overly thin Ju/wasi women do not menstruate and, therefore, can't conceive. They chose an animal with importance to them that has large size and rounded curves to represent aspects of the feminine. While people in agricultural societies would consider the bull to be a quintessential masculine (and phallic) symbol, in cultures with healthy gender relations, men and women are free to take any symbol they wish without confusion or criticism.

THE NEED FOR CEREMONY

Humans, as social animals, have always needed tools to maintain social coherence. Ceremony, which is used for many different purposes, is one of those important tools that helps create bonds that mimic familial ties, even among unrelated people. Ceremonies are used to mark the passage of important milestones in people's lives, including birth, maturation, joining of partners, moving into new roles, and death. These ceremonies may be called rites of passage (or initiation rites), and some versions may include obstacles that a person or group of people must overcome to demonstrate personal growth from one stage of their life to another (in this way they mark achievement). Ceremonies are also used to establish specific moods and express gratitude. Ritualized events are found in all cultures around the world, though the modern versions found in many affluent societies, while still with some benefit, have often been modified in ways that their importance and meaning have been diminished.

Ceremonies contain important elements that do more than simply unite members of the community (though this is a key feature of a communal ritual). Ceremonies also can provide recognition for accomplishment, help provide guidance for people as they move into a new phase of life, and connect people to their landscapes. Of course, some are primarily celebratory and allow people the occasion to enjoy a gathering of fellow community members and, perhaps, distant friends and family, with music, food, and dance. While each version of ritual may vary from culture to culture, they often share common elements that help to give ceremony its power in building strong bonds. Such features include a theme that incorporates the intent of the ritual, formal tone (for at least some portion of the ritual) that helps to establish the significance of the ceremony, use of similar sets of actions when comparable ceremonies are performed (sometimes called invariance, which establishes a choreography and helps maintain tradition), a traditional manner of performing the ritual that connects present attendants to their ancestors who used some of the same procedures, and the use of symbolism (whether through objects or actions) to connect the ritual to important events, other beings, or the land. These five features (and others that could be discussed) are important for generating meaning, without which the event fails to have any significant effects on the participants.

Modern societies, while still possessing many rituals, have often sterilized their versions of ceremony so there is little mention of a connection to our ancestors, the landscape, or the energy that animates life. As such, they are more a celebration that focuses on enjoyment rather than significance. Many rites of passage are now transformed to become another opportunity to further material gain. The birthday custom here in the United States is an excellent example of a ceremony that has retained only part of its original significance and establishes, from an early age, that accumulating wealth is a valid manner of marking a person's journey through life. The "birthday party" is an extremely superficial way of honoring the maturation of the child or young adult. Without an acknowledgment, guidance, and expectation, today's young adults in affluent countries experience greater frequency of identity crises (something that is virtually absent in observed hunter-gatherer groups). Holidays, based on important events in the history of the society or influenced by the dominant religion of the country (e.g., Christmas, Easter), are often celebrated by people who make no reference to the original meaning of the ceremony. While some religious institutions do a better job at retaining important features of ceremony, many ceremonies are simply without the impact found in indigenous and traditional cultures. Considering that true rites of passage are found in healthy cultures where depression and greed are rare, and that the most powerful (read: influential) countries of the world have largely lost these rites, it stands to reason that a return to participation in this universal aspect of healthy community may have a place in healing (to a degree) some of the social pains so commonly witnessed today.

Many ceremonies can be broken into three parts, where there is an introduction or an opening formality where all of the participants of the ceremony are brought together (at least for the purpose of the ritual) as one community, even if they are actually of distant lands. The body of ceremony (the second portion) may contain any number of distinct parts where important aspects of the ritual are performed. This is usually where the main theme of the ceremony is articulated and actualized. The final portion, the ending, involves a clear and commemorating event that marks the completion of the ceremony, the potential disbanding of the participants (so they can return home), and acknowledgment of accomplishment of the ceremony, which may be acknowledging the achievement of an individual of focus in the ceremony or the entire community of participants. Realizing that ceremony benefits from theme, formality, invariance, symbolism, and (when possible) traditionalism, these allow people to adapt (or create) ceremonies to suit their community's needs.

I am of the opinion that the rite of passage is one of the most important ceremonies that we can participate in (followed closely by expression of gratitude). Initiation rites can be done very differently, to suit the needs of the individual, pair, or group of people that are undergoing this time-honored ritual. I have come to understand that rites of passage that are not to include a challenge work well when they include two elements: an acknowledgment by the community of what has been accomplished and an expression of the responsibilities for the next phase of life. The acknowledgment honors what the individual has achieved, creating the sense that they are recognized and valued by their community. The expression of responsibility outlines their role in the coming years of life. This is important for several reasons. For adolescents, it doesn't leave them to figure out how to navigate maturation (which could mean they find harmful associations and become involved in negative pursuits to prove their entry into adulthood). The community expresses the needs they have for the individual in general terms (this is not meant to dictate exactly how the individual is to spend the rest of their life). Further, the community recognizes that with the coming into a new level of maturation, the individual can benefit the community (which is an additional layer of respect added to the person by the group, increasing the person's feelings of self-worth, their perception of being needed, and identity within the community).

Many rites of passage seen in indigenous cultures include one or more challenges that must be accomplished to successfully transition to the next stage of life. A well-known rite of passage with a fierce test can be seen in the Sateré-Mawé of Brazil. The ceremony marks the transition of a male youth to an adult warrior and involves the use of a venomous insect. The Sateré-Mawé collect bullet ants (*Paraponera clavata*), a large ant of the neotropical zone with an intensely painful sting, to use in the rite of passage. The ants are sedated through use of an herbal concoction so that they may be inserted, abdomen first, between straps made of leaves that make up a woven mitten. Upon reviving, the bullet ants are trapped between the weaves and agitated as a result. Initiates will then don these ceremonial mittens with many tens of ants in each mitten, the ants stinging their hands with what is widely believed to be the most painful sting on the planet, creating excruciating pain and tremendous swelling. If the boy successfully wears the mitten for the predetermined time, they leave the territory of adolescence and enter the rank of male warrior. While this may seem extreme, overly severe, and incredibly intense, rituals such as these create an intensity around the experience that contributes to its serious tone and the value it has in marking the transition to adulthood.

Another example of an indigenous rite of passage that would be viewed as extreme by modern people is the initiatory rite formerly used by the Algonquian-speaking Native Americans of current-day Virginia. The rite of passage was called the Huskanawing ceremony, and involved a decoction called wysoccan, which included material from a species of thorn-apple (likely sacred thorn-apple, *Datura wrightii*), an entheogenic plant native to North America. This member of the nightshade family is rich in tropane alkaloids, especially scopolamine and hyoscyamine, which are intoxicating and psychoactive when ingested in sufficient amounts. Young men nearing the age of maturation were kept for an extended period of time in a small area and consumed beverages containing thorn-apple phytochemicals. As described by Schultes and colleagues in their work "Plants of the Gods", the young men experienced a deep intoxication that was intended to serve as an initiation rite for manhood where they would unlive their former lives as boys, enabling them to become men of their community.

The examples presented in the preceding two paragraphs are certainly extreme by many standards of modern society, though certain gangs and other bands operating at the fringe of society certainly have some initiation rites that would include pain, danger, and the potential of severe injury. Rites of passage do not necessarily require this kind of extremism to be valuable, though they still benefit from sufficient challenge. Friends of mine have used the tending of a fire all alone for 24 hours as an initiation into adulthood. One author discusses the use of a solo canoe trip as a rite of passage. It is clear that indigenous rites of passage included a strong emotional aspect as part of the ceremony. Often, these kinds of challenge-based initiations, within the typical outline of a ceremony, has three stages: separation of the individual or individuals participating in the rite of passage from the community, the transition to the new stage of life (marked by successful completion of the challenge), and reintegration into the community as a new person with new roles and responsibilities. The reintegration aspect, which assumes a community of people who can acknowledge the accomplishment and reinforce the transition by treating the successful initiate in a manner suitable to their new role, is critical for full impact of a rite of passage. Without the community, there are no people to celebrate the transition to the next life stage.

Giving thanks is one of the most healing activities that a human can participate in (in my opinion). It is one of the reasons why this has been a common theme near the end of most chapters throughout this book when listing ways a person can rewild their life. Gratitude changes the way a person looks at the world; it helps them transcend an entitled mentality common to many people of affluent countries to one that is more appreciative of the world's bounty. Essentially, it focuses the attention outward on those things people have to be grateful for rather than focusing on the individual. Those who truly are thankful for what they have often find ways to live more softly upon the planet and genuinely care about the condition they leave the world in for the people and other-than-human persons who are not yet born. While the United States has a holiday called Thanksgiving, in my experience, it rarely involves an actual expression of thanks. Whereas in many indigenous cultures, thanksgiving ceremonies and practices are normal ways of interacting with the earth. This is perhaps exemplified in the Haudenosaunee's Thanksgiving Address, which are traditional words of thanks intended to be a spiritual address to the powers of world, offered at the beginning of events to bring the participants together and set a thankful tone (a copy of this address can be found in the booklet entitled "Thanksgiving Address: Greetings to the Natural World" by Jake Swamp). While it may seem pointless or even corny to members of an industrial society to give thanks to the trees, sun, rivers, and animal life to kick off an event, personal experience (and that of other teachers, such as Michael Douglas of the Maine Primitive Skills School) suggests this results in better outcomes for classes and programs.

What many people may not know is that expressions of gratitude are associated with increases in well-being and health. Yes, being thankful has a selfish side because taking part in the giving of thanks benefits the person who does so. For example, in a study by Emmons and McCullough (published in 2003), they found that people who wrote down what they were thankful for experienced greater well-being than groups who described things that irritated them or merely journaled the neutral happenings in their life. The authors of the study suggest that a conscious focus on a person's blessings has emotional and interpersonal benefits. In a 2009 study titled "Gratitude influences sleep through the mechanism of pre-sleep cognitions", researchers found that people with high levels of gratitude had higher quality sleep and greater duration of sleep. Later studies have shown that expressing thanks also lessens feelings of anxiety and depression, and results in fewer physical problems. Another 2009 study showed that thankfulness increases activity in a region of the brain (called the ventral tegmental area) that produces dopamine, a neurotransmitter that helps the body modulate sleep and wakefulness, helping explain why (in part) being grateful assists sleep. Studies have shown that those who are more thankful tend to exercise more and experience less illness (i.e., gratitude influences other areas of their life). It is important to mention that people who receive gratefulness also experience emotional benefits, such as increased feelings of self-worth. Certainly, when someone is thanked, they are encouraged by this act to give back, which builds social ties and increases acts of reciprocity.

Thanksgiving can take many forms. In several studies (including some of those mentioned in the previous paragraph), gratitude was displayed through writing down items people were thankful for. Thanksgiving can be expressed during open ceremony, as part of prayer, or even as minor private acts, such as the offering of a small item when something is to be harvested. I personally utilize an Anishinaabe tradition of offering a small portion of wild rice grains that I have harvested from the wild to demonstrate my appreciation for that which I am about to harvest or participate in. Whether the act of gratitude is public or private, formality and invariance help to make the expression more meaningful, increasing the benefit to the person or persons expressing thanks. Whatever form you choose to use, I would encourage you to make it a regular part of your living and express gratitude for something important in your life at least every week (if not more frequently).

Ceremony is an important aspect of a healthy community and part of being a whole human. In the modern world, it is sometimes difficult to engage in traditional ceremonies that were practiced by nature-connected cultures because these rituals have been forgotten in many circles. However, there are people keeping important traditions alive, and I highly recommend seeking such people. For example, the Lakota sweat lodge ceremony, when offered by those trained by indigenous elders, is one of the most memorable and therapeutic rituals I have experienced. In any case, finding mentors for the learning of ceremony allows one to adapt these observances to fit the needs of the individual's or group's situation. Through ceremony, we are connected to our ancestors of many generations ago. In this way, they are sacred events—but if that word (sacred) causes you pause, then simply refer to ceremonies as important or special. Don't get hung up on the terminology being used. Ceremony is an act that has been performed by humans for far longer than this industrial lifeway we find ourselves immersed in (a lifeway that sometimes challenges the existence of sacred acts). When we practice ceremony, we are connecting with other people, other life, and/or our landscapes in a deeply meaningful way. A rekindling of these rituals can go a long way in helping heal the wounds generated by living in a nature-divorced society.

THE LOSS OF THE ELDER AND RISE OF THE YOUNGER

In indigenous and traditional communities, the elder was a vitally important role. Elders had accumulated a lifetime of experiences and held a vast amount of knowledge concerning living in that place. This knowledge went beyond how to gather this or craft that but included the traditions, the ceremonies, the history, the methods of problem resolution, and the core values of the community. The elders were focal points of the group, esteemed features that were repositories of traditional ecological knowledge and wisdom. As asserted by Amadou Hampâté Bâ in this adaptation of his 1960 quote:

"Whenever an elder dies, a library burns down."

To be without elders was similar to being without mothers or hunters or healers because they not only held important information but also were responsible for transmitting that information through various teaching models (e.g., storytelling, song, ritual, "informal" education). The role of elder was necessary to the healthy functioning of a community.

Human technology, the sum total of our skills and methods, which is embedded in and demonstrated by our crafts and devices, has generally progressed in a relatively slow manner with little change occurring over a generation. While certain tools and techniques were ultimately abandoned as new ones were developed, most of these technological advances did not cause rapid desertion of methodologies used over a person's lifetime. Therefore, people were able to keep pace with technological change. This also means that the older members of a community (i.e., the elders) were valuable because their life experiences were rich with an understanding of the technology being used by the next generation. As such, they could guide the process of learning the technology of that place (i.e., help the younger generation become fluent in the necessary ecological knowledge).

Today, the situation is quite different. Some technologies are changing so fast that within a single person's lifetime objects may have been invented, used extensively, and then become obsolete. For some items, they may still exist but have undergone so many renovations and overhauls that the original users of the invention may not even recognize the device any longer—and certainly don't know how to operate the new form of the technology. The elders, on the surface, have been transformed into olders. They are just more aged forms of young people. Olders are considered to be less valuable humans that are tucked away in homes and other locations where they are out of sight and out of mind. And in fairness to this title, many olders have spent their lives in wage slavery and the pursuit of material gain, never bothering to learn and engage in healthy community and healing practices. Compared with the elders of indigenous communities, they may have less to offer the young people, but that does not mean they are without value.

The youngers (i.e., the young people of the generation) are now in a position where they feel empowered. They have grown up in the current version of technology and have a greater understanding of how to use the innovations of the day. Even though the youngers are often without an understanding of how the technology is constructed or how it actually functions, these facets of technology are not prized in a consumer-based society where simply knowing how to use a given device is considered to be a demonstration of "expertise" by the user. To be clear, even though the younger cannot manufacture, repair, or even explain the inner workings of a particular item (e.g., mobile phone, computer, radio, car, wireless devices), the use of the technological object is really all that matters. Given this is where youngers place high value, the older is simply without value to their everyday living.

Further compounding on this issue is the fact that various media allow one to virtually travel around the world and study any region, or its people, its forms of industry, and its remaining biota. With vividly colored screens, youngers can see vibrant imagery of distant places and, from the confines of their bedroom, become a virtual expert in a distant country. Any topic that can be discussed, a younger can use the World Wide Web to research and extract pertinent bytes of information for an academic report or conversation with a fellow classmate. Of course, the younger has never visited that place and does not know the sounds of its music firsthand, the smell of its local cuisine, the texture of its ground under feet, or the emotional feel generated by being in that place. Many olders have this first-hand experience but storytelling has been replaced by a high definition screen. And while the latter form of learning has its merits, the recounting of personal tales is a form of learning that has been used by humans since they appeared on this planet. Storytelling has been used as a way to transmit information in a highly personalized manner that required creativity on the part of the speaker and the listener (i.e., it exercised the imaginative regions of the brain that are not used as much today). Further, it provided purpose for the elder and demonstrated one of their key values to the youngers.

All of the focus on screens of a computer, tablet, or smart phone, while seemingly increasing the ability to learn about our world, has actually resulted in a decline in first-hand experience by youngers (and people of any age). Studying a screen is learning in a way that is removed from the actual experience—it is removed from the actual person who captured the images and sounds. The information has been filtered through several versions of technological media and programming before reaching the eyes and ears of the one staring at a small screen. The media is not immersive in the way life is and, unlike a storyteller, it cannot adjust the tale on the fly to focus on this or that aspect of the story, to generate a greater emotional response, or provide human to human connection. The younger, without necessarily realizing it, focuses on a kind of learning that tricks them into believing they have had a richer life experience than they have actually lived. It is yet another way the younger feels they have risen above the older and have little use for the relics of society.

Are the olders without value (as treated by many members of our society)? Certainly not. Despite the fact they have been raised in a nature-divorced society that lacks many healthful aspects of community and instead praises competition and egocentric pursuit (even against members of their own town), the elderly people in our society still have much to share with the younger generations. They have lived through many decades and possess a large archive of historical events that can help youngers understand the course that humanity has taken. Just like the elders in hunter-gatherer bands, they may remember rare events that occur so infrequently that a young person might never have experienced them. As such, the older person may have solutions that can be useful—just like the indigenous elder who may remember a water source that remains during severe drought or the plants that can be eaten during food shortages. Olders have likely experienced a variety of hardships and sorrows during their lives. Their first-hand experience dealing with troubled times and overcoming grief (for those that learned methods of doing so) can be invaluable to healing youngers who are dealing with their own troubles. The elderly may have also witnessed many different ways of overcoming various problems and offer unique insights when dealing with difficulties (especially non-electronic kinds). Some of the olders in any affluent society still qualify as elders, and can be treasured resources in their place.

One of the main problems concerning olders in our society is that they no longer perform (fully) one of the important roles of the elder: transmission of information to the next generations. While certainly there is some sharing that occurs, elders (and parents) have primarily relegated teaching to the schools. It is in schools where youngers receive the bulk of their preparation for their adult lives. But schools do not teach a deep understanding of natural history, or imbue young people with a strong sense of place, or transfer customs and ceremonies that unite people and landscape. Nor do such institutions even believe that such things are valuable (as clearly indicated by the fact they are not part of the curricula). However, elders can transmit this kind of valuable information that can transform the current younger worldview to something more eco-centered (i.e., something more respectful of life). We desperately need a return of the elder. For this occur, we need the kind of upbringing and community that gives rise to true elders. Elders who can recite years of baseball statistics and talk of actors and actresses of times long gone are not what the world most needs at this moment. We need elders who have immersed themselves in more holistic understanding of nature, one that does not separate the secular and sacred. It is essential that we have elders who truly grasp that all things are connected and actions taken now influence (positively or negatively) humans and other-than-human persons who are not yet born. These are important aspects of living that transcend technology. No matter what the current music fad or the latest video game of interest, youngers will have every reason to admire elders when elders hold wisdom that restores empathy in people and rejuvenates the land. When we have had a resurgence of such elders, youngers will respect them, not because they are told to, but because they understand that the elders have their best intentions in mind.

FINDING YOUR GIFT

So many people today are simply wage slaves, working 40 or more hours a week at a job they dislike, earning money for some possessions and a brief respite on the weekend, only to repeat the entire process over again (and again and again). Over ⅓ of their waking hours (some more than ½) each week during their adult lives are spent performing work that is unpleasant and without gratification. A recent Gallup study (2013) revealed that 70% of Americans are negative about and disengaged from their jobs. Such people may never have the opportunity to express their gift, that talent that brings them alive and contributes in a meaningful way to their community (or the world). Spending so much time away from their passions, people lose an excitement for living, which ends up manifesting as apathy. This indifference becomes an emotional mire that holds people down and keeps them from ever acting on the behalf of others. If people do not relish life, they will not champion its protection. Helping people find their passion, whether it be a professional or leisure pursuit, is a way to awaken people from the doldrums of society.

One could state that meaningful engagement with the planet begins with one's self, and then extends to their community. For most people to find their gift, they must express their authentic self. In other words, they need to follow their passion (or passions) so that they can share that which may have been concealed or otherwise kept from the world. Many people simply find themselves in the wrong group of people to feel comfortable sharing what brings them alive. Some are fearful of taking a new road in life or are worried about failure. Others are genuinely confused and cannot, at this moment, determine what talent or message they can give to the world that would make an impact and provide purpose in their life. Whatever stands in your way, the first step to identifying your gift is to truly believe that you have something to offer your community. As stated by John Powell:

"You have a unique message to deliver, a unique song to sing, a unique act of love to bestow. This message, this song, and this act of love have been entrusted exclusively to the one and only you."

Time in reflection and real soul searching is a way to help people find what motivates them. Hectic lives with every waking moment filled with busy activity is a way to prevent you from finding your gift. Time alone, especially in natural areas, can be especially useful. The goal becomes finding what you love to do most. To be clear, if sitting indoors playing video games is what you love to do most, then I would politely note you have not had enough life experiences yet to search for your gift. Such a pursuit that is without merit to other people is not the kind of gift being described here. A strong feeling of self-worth and contribution accompanies most gifts because they benefit other life, whether that be people or other-than-human persons. Again, the goal is to be authentic—allowing yourself to be swayed by what you think people will feel about your passion will not allow you to realize your gift.

Sometimes our gift requires education or some form of training for us to actualize it. For example, someone who wishes to become a healer or an artist or a craftsperson may need years of study and practice under a mentor or one or more instructors to reach their full potential. It will be important to keep your vision alive during these times so that it is not forgotten in the business of life. Spend time each day moving toward your goal or at least nurturing the idea of your gift. Whether you use journaling, visualization, or discussions with friends, if you know your life's gift, keep it in the forefront of your awareness each day. Financial limitations can be significant obstacles for some chosen paths, though there are often ways to continue study even when monetary issues preclude enrollment in universities, vocational schools, and similar institutions. For what it is worth, I have witnessed people from poor economic backgrounds work through such hindrances and realize their gift due to hard work, creativity, and (sometimes) some providence along the way.

While there are a variety of tools to help find your gift, some facilitators favor the vision quest. This rite of passage has been used by various Native American groups (and other indigenous peoples) and is performed with the intent to help the questor find their purpose and how they can contribute to their community. Ceremonies vary but generally involve a community of people who help prepare a questor for time alone in a sacred location. The duration of the vision quest is often four days, during which the participant fasts and spends time in contemplation and prayer. The vision quest is more than just a search for purpose, as it is also a way to mark transition. Many people have found this rite of passage to clarify, provide direction, and empower. The vision quest is not something to take lightly and most reputable programs and mentors who use this ceremony actually use a training period to prepare questors for the challenge. While four days without food will seem extreme to most Americans, it is the extremeness of the ritual that that helps to catalyze thought and receipt of message. If you choose to partake in this ritual, do research the program that will guide you through this process because visions quests, while potentially of significant value, do entail some risk.

For those who are new to the rewilding path and wish to pursue answers about a lifeway that produces excitement and fulfillment without requiring the commitment of a vision quest, consider answering some of the following questions. What do you truly anticipate doing? What were your childhood passions (topics that brought you happiness before you learned to be guarded in public with your desires)? When you communicate with friends or write in a journal, what topic do you most enjoy expressing? If you asked others to describe what they feel brings you most alive, what would they answer? Seriously consider these questions when you can be alone in a place that calls to you (e.g., an outdoor location that you enjoy being in and brings you a sense of calm). And while you ask these questions, keep in mind that your gift (or gifts) should contribute in a meaningful way to your community. Your gift should make possible a world that embraces the next generation and allows them to experience the joy of realizing their gift. Any activity that makes it more difficult for later generations to find their passion is not a gift; it is an egocentric pursuit that lacks true significance. We are currently in a period of time where too much of what people in affluent countries spend their time with revolves around themselves—a lifestyle that is, unfortunately, considered completely appropriate. While finding entertainment is a perfectly acceptable thing to do, constant pursuit of such means personal growth is given a low priority. In order to become an elder (rather than an older) and help others find their gifts, we must have found our own and contributed that gift to our community.

An important part of finding your gift is to be cognizant of how contemporary society may have influenced your belief of how big your work must be. In the United States, success is often defined by material wealth, titles, prestige, and influence. Your gift need not have any of those criteria to be a valuable contribution to the world. The special ability you possess doesn't have to reach thousands or millions of people to be the proof of realizing your gift. Because we have been seeded throughout our education with grandiose visions of financial success (or similar pursuits), we frequently borrow such imprints when we consider our gift for the earth. This is not necessarily the case for any single person's talent. We have no ability to see into the future and comprehend how being a nurturing parent may ultimately change the course of events in some distant time and place. Your gift may touch only one or a few people in your lifetime—and this does not take away from its value to all living beings. I encourage you to not be seduced by contemporary society's ideals while exploring your special talent.

I urge you to approach each day with anticipation of finding that talent or skill that brings you alive and will let you have periods of genuine exuberance in this life. It is worth committing effort to. While others can help you to find your gift, and some can even stand in the way, ultimately it is up to you to realize your own path. No one else can speak the words waiting to be uttered by your lips as well as you can.

THE NEOABORIGINAL STRATEGY FOR ENGAGING IN AND BUILDING COMMUNITY

What we do as adults has a strong influence on our children. When the adults of a community are emotionally healthy, the children often follow suit. This assertion is reflected in the writing of Elizabeth Thomas, who studied the Ju/wasi, hunter-gatherers of the Kalahari Desert. As she noted in her book "The Old Way", the children rarely cried because they had little to cry about. Yelling, scolding, slapping, and such methods of punishment were rarely observed. In fact, most children never heard discouraging words until they approached adolescence. Even when reprimanded, the scolding came in a soft voice. The Ju/wasi children were free from frustration and anxiety, and, as a result, were sunny and cooperative. The lack of psychological stress helped to create intelligent, likeable, and confident children.

Clearly, these observations are the result of a suite of factors, one of which is the quality of the communal experience that the children are raised in (as well as healthy parenting practices that will be the topic of another book). Community is the most often neglected and hardest aspect of a rewilded lifestyle to realize. It will require substantial work for most people to locate or create community. I cannot endorse this enough, even if the healthy community can be experienced only on an infrequent basis. Being in the midst of people who value your presence, support your work, and understand that humans and nature are part of a whole is a powerful tool for emotional well-being.

Successful human communities have always shared resources (at least to a degree). They have engaged in indirect reciprocal gift economies that have helped all members of the group. This practice, exemplified by harvest sharing, increased the food security experienced by members of the tribe. But sharing was more than just a manner of feeding those individuals who were not successful in locating or acquiring food, it defined hunter-gatherers and was a measure of a person's worth. Unlike modern society, which values the accumulation of wealth by an individual, traditional communities valued generosity and reciprocity. As noted by Thomas Mayor in his article "Hunter-gatherers: The Original Libertarians":

"Hunter-gatherers appear to place a high value on esteem, and ethnographers frequently cite "generosity" as the chief means of acquiring esteem. This theme recurs in the ethnographic literature for virtually all known foraging societies. The superficial reader of this literature, however, might easily be misled into thinking that "generosity" applies only to the giving of a "gift," not to the repayment of the gift at a later date. Yet both actions are equally important and largely indistinguishable because typically a long chain of exchanges extends over a period of time. Thus, observed "givers" of food in fact may be living up to a prior bargain by repaying a loan or by making good on a commitment to provide hunger insurance."

Humans have a deep need to socialize with (i.e., bond to) other people in a healthy environment. Our emotional well-being is based on experiencing love, being part of a group with a common intent, feeling a degree of self-worth through contributing in a meaningful way, and knowing we will be aided by our community in times of need. We need to start committing the same level of effort to surrounding ourselves with supportive community members in the way we might prioritize healthful food or movement in our life. Most of us cannot have the kind of community that was experienced by hunter-gatherers. This means, like with the wild diet, we must find ways to emulate it in the modern world so that we can still reap the health benefits of a rewilded community and use that community as a way to further connect with our landscapes. Remember, social pain is real. The brain processes breakup from partners, quarrels with friends, social rejection, and failure to experience self-worth similar to the way it processes physical pain. How can we be healthy as humans if we frequently experience pain?

Following are ten ways you can move closer to experiencing real community in your life.

1. Start the process by identifying the **Necessary Features of Actual Community** that are present and those that are missing in your life. This will help you prioritize what actions you must take to improve your communal experience.

2. **Seek out community** that is accepting of your person. A healthy community brings out the best in people. In industrialized countries, such communities can be hard to locate. I suggest beginning with primitive living skills groups because these people often realize that humans can't live alone and need to be supported by members of a tribe. There are many primitive living skills gatherings that bring together like-minded people and may be able to offer assistance for your search.

3. If you cannot find a healthy group of people to interact with, then **create community in your place**. Many will feel this task is impossible, but it can be a successful way to engage in community. Using meet-up groups and other arrangements, people can start communal gatherings on an infrequent basis to establish norms and discover what works for the group. Don't sell yourself short, necessity can be a powerful motivator for creating the things you need in life to generate health.

4. Foster a **reciprocal gift economy** with your community. If you do not have a functioning community, then do so with friends and family that are dear to you. In doing so, attempt to disengage from the market economy during this resource sharing as much as possible. Sharing with others creates powerful, positive feelings that can go a long way toward creating happiness in the midst of a dysfunctional society.

5. **Participate in healthy cooperative connections**. Volunteering and being involved in your community are ways to initiate this process. But cooperative connections are not held only between people but between all life and even landscape features (e.g., mountains, rivers, lakes, plateaus, gorges). Find ways to benefit those wild foods, wildcrafted medicines, and natural places you seek rejuvenation. After all, if they are lost to industry, they will not be able to help you along your rewilding journey.

6. **Practice gender equality**. Through practicing true equality for all people, gender equality will come naturally. All roles have value to the community, and both genders contribute part of what it means to be human in the world. If gender equality is difficult to commence in your group, find ways to highlight the roles of the suppressed gender until the community matures and can see the value of all people.

7. **Engage in ceremony**, including rites of passage and expressions of thankfulness. Ceremony is a useful tool for creating strong social bonds. Further, initiations can help mark the transition to new roles and provide healthy acknowledgment for the maturation of the individual. Ceremony needn't always be elaborate. Begin small with minor rituals (e.g., smudging) until your comfort with this aspect of being human develops.

8. **Revere your elders** and find ways to include them in your community. If you are surrounded by olders, you can make a significant beneficial impact in their life by seeking their input and helping them feel valued in their later years. True elders are invaluable and have much to offer a rewilded group of people.

9. **Find and express your gift(s)**. Do not let your life pass you by without experiencing the satisfaction and joy of helping others in the unique way that you can. We all have a gift to share with our community, a gift that supports life and enables the next generation to also express their gifts.

10. **Express gratitude for your community** (whatever it may be at the moment). We all have, at the very least, some compassionate and helpful friends and family who make a huge impact in our life. Celebrate these people for they help shape us. Our community provides us with an outlet for sharing our gifts. Without them, we never become who we were intended to be.

11. Green choices: walking softly in the home and marketplace

We are a consumer-based society. People purchase the things that they need because they are largely unable to craft them for themselves. The products that enter the home come from distant locations that we likely will never visit (or witness the ecological injury as a result of the resource extraction and/or manufacturing). Green choices, purchasing in a manner that limits ecological harm, provide people living in urban areas with a way to contribute to the rewilding movement. While some rewilding authors would deride such a chapter as you are about to read, people become conscientious consumers before they become non-consumers. It is extremely difficult for a person who has a new awareness of the outcomes of industry to go from purchasing goods without any thought of the consequences of such products to purchasing nothing at all. It is also a completely unrealistic expectation given that the learning of ancestral skills takes years (and, ultimately, a functioning community). Usually, people who commit time to studying this topic become careful consumers initially and, if they follow through to the logical conclusions that such study reveals, begin to gather and craft more from their local landscapes (when possible). However, city dwellers will have limited ability to participate in such activities. But they can make a significant difference in their shopping habits. One million people who decide to purchase responsibly will make a bigger impact (in the short term) than 100 people who return to a relatively eco-centered lifeway. Consider that the Facebook page "rewild.com", an online group that promotes a return to ancestral living, has 2071 members at the time of this writing. Compare that with the facebook page for Walmart, which has 32,677,835 likes. These numbers make it clear that leaving urban residents out of this movement is a mistake. Conscientious consumerism is capable of leaving some forests standing, keeping some mountains from being turned into rubble, and some rivers still capable of supporting life. Green choices are an important part of the total strategy for protecting the earth and the humans who live upon it.

GREEN PURCHASING

Let's be completely honest and upfront about our purchasing. As most companies currently practice, the best we can do with green purchasing is to slow the damage being committed. When we are dealing with 7.3 billion people (a number representing far too many to live on this planet in a sustainable manner), combined with many companies acting in an irresponsible manner, altering our purchasing can only buy us more time. While more time to evolve our practices is a laudable goal, at some point we need industry that doesn't result in ecocide. Think of it in this way (as the famous example goes), pretend for a moment you live near the center of the United States, in the state of Kansas. You need to drive north to Canada. After a full day of driving, you realize you've been traveling south toward Mexico. Understand that no matter how much you slow down, you will never reach Canada. At some point, you need to turn around so that you can drive north. This is exactly what we need our industries to do. Using 10% less water or packaging in way that uses 20% less material (i.e., slowing down in our analogy) isn't the ultimate solution. Consider the example of a hybrid vehicle that is 15% more fuel efficient than a comparably sized car with a gasoline engine. People really celebrate this reduction in fuel use without stopping to consider that a hybrid car still does something that the solely gasoline-powered vehicle does—it pollutes. It just pollutes less. Therefore, this reduction in fuel doesn't imply that hybrid cars are "good", they are simply "less bad". Our industries (and the people who rely on industry, which are you and I) need to stop focusing on slowing damage and commit to halting damaging practices altogether. In order for this to happen, there will need to be massive reforms in how we go about business in the United States. Not until people demand that virtually no pollution be produced will it ever become a reality. In the meantime, those of us willing to make changes can buy the world more time. That is what this chapter is about.

Before we launch into the concepts behind green purchasing, let's discuss the ultimate buzzword: sustainable. This all-too-often-used word in marketing refers to a manner of interacting with the world in a way that such actions can be maintained indefinitely. Therefore, any trees that are felled for products should occur at or below the regrowth rate of the forest. As such, sustainable activity should preserve the biological integrity of natural systems (forever). The problem is, as noted in chapter 2, one cannot use the word "sustainable" without defining what they are sustaining. As Miles Olson wrote in "Unlearn, Rewild" [9]:

"The popular concept of sustainability paints a picture something like this: Humans are burning too much fossil fuel. There is nothing fundamentally wrong with how we live, or how we interact with this Earth, there are just some glitches in the system. Acidifying oceans, ozone holes and, most importantly, global warming. If we can only make a few simple changes—switch to green energy, organic farming, cloth bags instead of plastic, phase out fossil fuels—the Earth won't burn and industrial civilization will be able to continue indefinitely. I don't want to argue too much right here over whether it is possible for this culture to become sustainable. I think it is more important that we consider if it is even desirable! In the sustainability movement, there is no discussion on what it is we want to make sustainable …"

For example, sustaining a growing population isn't actually sustainable because the burgeoning populace will continue to use ever greater amounts of natural resources and, eventually, reach numbers that cannot be maintained without catastrophic exhaustion of the world's natural wealth—the very thing people need for life—and the resulting mass starvation that comes with reaching a landscape's carrying capacity. Considering that we are witnessing (and part of) the earth's sixth major extinction, demonstrating a loss of global biodiversity, we, as a species, are certainly not operating in a sustainable manner. The upside to this horrific story of modern-day resource use is that it can be turned around. We can act in a truly sustainable, or better, rejuvenative manner. It will require us to become conscientious consumers and not let a very sick society dictate our manner of purchasing.

One of the most important things we must keep in mind is whether or not we, the consumers, pay the full price of the product that is being bought. By this, I am not referring to acquiring goods on sale. Instead, I am introducing the topic of externalized costs. When companies practice cost externalizing, they are able to offer particular products at a cheaper price because they pay only the costs of manufacturing and bringing the products to market. Any negative consequences that are imparted to the world (society and/or environment) are not part of the market price the consumer pays. Very often with modern industry there are serious health consequences to local residents (and sometimes distant peoples as well) who are forced to pay the costs of medical treatment out of their own pockets (i.e., the company responsible for the health impacts does not pay for the charges resulting from hospitalization, medicine, lost work, and shortened life span). Corporations that act in this manner are self-centered and are often owned and/or managed by people who lack empathy and long-term vision. And while it is astonishing to me that people allow companies to externalize costs, especially when they do not use or benefit from the industry that is costing them part of their income, it is a very common practice in the industrial age.

---

[9] Miles Olson. 2012. Unlearn, Rewild. New Society Publishers, British Columbia, Canada.

Let's consider an example to make clear how cost externalizing is a wonderful practice for the business but very harmful to everyone else. If we look carefully at the coal industry in the United States, one can better understand this concept. Coal is responsible for 50% of the power generation in the US but it produces 81% of the carbon dioxide (CO_2) emissions, which contribute to climate change and extreme weather events. Coal mining and combustion releases much more than just CO_2, it also releases particulates, sulfur dioxide (SO_2), and a suite of toxic and carcinogenic substances, some of which include arsenic, beryllium, cadmium, chromium, lead, and mercury. All of these pollute the air, water, and ground, leading to health issues for people who live both near and downwind from coal-fired power plants. In the US, it is estimated that 70% of the railway traffic is dedicated to shipping coal around the country and railways are associated with accidents and deaths (which the coal industry does not compensate people for). Mountaintop removal is widespread in some southeastern states (e.g., Kentucky, Virginia, West Virginia). It is estimated that 500 sites have been completely altered, affecting 1.4 million acres, with rubble from the mining cast down into the valleys below. In Kentucky alone, nearly 300 mountaintop removal sites have polluted nearly 4000 kilometers (2500 miles) of streams. The extensive deforestation that accompanies mountaintop removal affects the world's ability to store carbon dioxide emissions (resulting in more greenhouse gases in the atmosphere), further exacerbating climate change. The resulting ecological catastrophe ultimately reduces property values for those living near these sites, diminishes outdoor recreation opportunities, decreases the opportunity to grow clean food (due to water contamination), and releases methane (another greenhouse gas). It was estimated by Epstein et al. in 2011 that the use of coal and its waste stream cost the residents of the United States 345,308,920,080 dollars (yes, that is more than ⅓ of a trillion dollars) in economic, health, environmental, and other impacts during the 2008 calendar year. If these costs were internalized (i.e., paid by the industry that generates them), the cost per kilowatt hour for electricity generated from coal would rise from 10.54 cents to 28.38 cents. This represents a 169% increase in the price to have those who purchase coal power pay the entire cost of this product. While this might not sound like a good idea, it would generate a massive movement to find less harmful energy sources. Keep in mind that it was not that long ago that coal mining companies were forced by federal regulations to pay for the costs of workers succumbing to black lung (pneumoconiosis). If it were not for this practice being mandatory, the coal industry would still externalize this health cost as well.

There are literally thousands of examples of cost externalizing by modern industry. Excessive fertilizer containing nitrogen and phosphorus added to agricultural fields in the Mississippi River drainage flows into the Gulf of Mexico, feeding large populations of algae. As the algae plants die and sink to the bottom, they are decomposed by bacteria that use up the available oxygen and create a large dead zone. This kills many kinds of invertebrates (e.g., worms, shellfish), which are the food for some species of fish. These dead zones impact life, and impact the people who work in the fishing industry. The industrial farmers in the Midwest do not pay for the damages they cause (though they would likely be very upset if the fishing industry did something to remove thousands of square kilometers of agricultural land from production). These practices will continue until farmers are forced to pay the full cost of the products they produce (which currently do not include any compensation for the harm they cause to other people and their livelihood). Externalizing costs is an unfair and selfish practice, something that can occur only when people consider it acceptable to compete against other people who live in the same country. It matters in the marketplace because people will purchase goods that are completely un-necessary if they are inexpensive in the short-term to them. People will also wastefully use electricity and fossil fuels if they are cheap. When people pay the full cost of these items, they use them in a more sensible manner, and they use less, reducing their harm to other people and the ecosystem.

Another very important concept for us to consider is the quality of the manufacturing, which in turn affects two very important items: how long the product will last and our decision making when the product requires repair. Clearly, cheaply made products that use less material, inferior materials, poor craftsmanship, and little or no product quality control will likely break, wear out, or fail to continue functioning sooner than similar goods designed by reputable companies that seek to produce a long-lasting product. Given that many goods cannot be recycled, this means that inferior goods enter the massive waste stream sooner (and more frequently). Because the United States and many other affluent countries utilize a cradle to grave system of technology (i.e., one where the good is created and then it is discarded without reusing its component materials), it is important that goods not enter the waste stream (for generations, if possible). An excellent example of inferior products can be found when examining frying pans. It is possible to purchase an inexpensive, lightweight aluminum frying pan with a non-stick coating for $14.35, whereas a comparably sized, quality cast iron skillet costs $37.00 dollars (these prices found by comparing online products offered by Walmart website and Lodge Cast Iron). Using price as the primary criterion to choose which product will be purchased, most people will choose the lightweight frying pan (as purchase surveys demonstrate). As well, the convenience factor of easy cleaning will weigh heavily in this decision-making process (even though properly used cast iron cookware is easy to clean). Of course, the anticipated lifespan of a cheaply constructed aluminum pan isn't measured in generations but in years. One estimate provided by a major company is that non-stick cookware can be used for 3–5 years of moderate usage before it should be discarded (according to Amanda Schaffer in 2007). Therefore, over the lifetime of a person, many such inferior pans will be purchased and thrown away, ultimately costing far more money (in the long run) to the consumer, and this is not mentioning the health hazards of the non-stick coating (look into perfluorooctanoic acid used in making Teflon). On the other hand, I'm using cast iron pans that are in their fifth generation of use (if we count my daughter in this calculation). It is very clear which kind of pan (aluminum non-stick or cast iron) causes more environmental damage, feeds the waste stream further, and costs more money to the consumer (over time).

The other important consideration for cheaply produced goods is the usual outcome when something breaks or malfunctions on the product. Rather than having it repaired, it is simply discarded and another similar product is purchased. This shopping behavior uses more of the world's resources and feeds additional material into the waste stream. A more expensive and highly valued product of the same kind will be repaired rather than discarded more of the time, possibly requiring only a small part to return the good to proper working order. But there are other facets of this topic to consider as well, and an example here will prove informative. I have a steel cart that has been used for years for various chores (e.g., moving materials around, hauling fuel wood to the home). The four tires on this cart eventually cracked apart and required replacement (i.e., they could not be repaired). The price to replace the four tires with on this cart was $74.00 (from the manufacturer). The price to purchase a new steel cart: $75.35 (on the Amazon website because the manufacturer does not sell them directly), which would include four new tires, the body of the cart, and the handle. The seemingly obvious thing to do here is to buy a new cart. Or is it? While my cart was banged up from use, all of the visible wear was merely cosmetic. The structure of the cart was sound. Therefore, to reduce the waste stream as much as possible and prevent the need for additional mining of ore (beyond the four rims for the tires), I purchased only the tires. Yes, I did not end up with a shiny new steel cart but, then, I didn't need a new cart, I needed only new tires. This is an example of purchasing to reduce resource use, something that inexpensive items made of inferior material typically work counter to.

Most people living in affluent countries spend very little time researching how the manufacturing and disposal of the items they use affect the world. This isn't meant to be a judgmental comment condemning people for lazy shopping practices. Most people have assumed that their governments would simply not allow harmful practices to occur. Please let this be the wake up call to an understanding that extremely wealthy people and corporations are allowed to pollute and cause extensive injury to natural systems for various reasons. Two very important ones for this include (1) the fact that they provide employment to people and, therefore, are considered necessary (and their pollution a necessary evil), and (2) their actions are defended by politicians who receive financial support from them (which is both a form of legal bribery and an obvious conflict of interest). Walking a rewilding path is much about generating awareness and taking responsibility for our own actions (rather than merely waiting for governments to force action through legislation). It is up to us to research and question companies we receive products from and discover their environmental and social practices. There is no better way to voice your opinion of a company's track record than by voting with your dollars. If a large proportion of people were to boycott purchasing from a company because of poor practices, the company would change (and will do so promptly) to regain consumer attention—and the change would occur much faster than merely following a regulatory channel of halting harmful practices.

However, before we condemn big business and consider it the root of all evil in the world, remember that big business can remain big only because we purchase from them (and frequently). We have a responsibility in the harm being caused to the world and to the less privileged people living where the resources are extracted, manufactured, and disposed of. Therefore, we need to change our purchasing habits. The following ten items are **Green Purchasing Criteria** for manufactured goods that can assist with evolving our market behaviors. Note that some of these questions apply equally well to food and medicine. These are the kinds of questions I ask before making a purchase of a good sold in the American (or global) marketplace.

1. **Do I really need the product**? This is the most important question that anyone in an affluent society can ask themselves. Often the answer is no. However, societal pressure encourages people to purchase more and more because material wealth is a fundamental way people demonstrate their success and arrange themselves on the ladder of social hierarchy. It also encourages people to stay current, upgrading to new technological devices when the device in hand works perfectly well. It is worth noting here that the more "success" one experiences, the more likely one is to possess more homes and cars and "things", all of which requires resource extraction and causes pollution during their manufacture and shipment. Therefore, the usual American measure of success is highly correlated with how much harm one causes to the world. Let your deeds define your success, not the total amount of belongings.

2. **Can the product be reused, recycled, or composted when it has reached the end of its use**? Many products are now designed from a cradle-to-grave viewpoint, where they are used and then the items are discarded because they, or a substantial portion of them, cannot be used for anything when the life of the product has ended. The mountains of home goods that can be found at some disposal sites attest to our deranged view of product life cycles that stand in stark contrast to natural systems—where everything is ultimately consumed by some organism and re-

enters the environment as food or foundational material for the next generation. We need goods designed with a cradle-to-cradle mindset, meaning they are designed for 100% reuse, recycling, or composting (i.e., none of the component parts enter the landfill). It is only through designing goods with cradle-to-cradle approaches that we cease the absurd amount of waste we are currently generating. We need also to consider the packaging that surrounds the product when we consider the lifecycle of the materials.

3. **What is the longevity of the product**? This is a huge consideration for limiting harm to ecosystems. Modern manufacturing is, in most cases, highly injurious to natural systems. Therefore, if we are going to purchase an item that had a tax on life, let us select items that last as long as possible so that the tax need not be exacted over and over again in our lifetime. Disposable goods, when durable versions exist, in most cases are simply the wrong choice. Cheap items that break and malfunction after limited use just cost the buyer more money (in the long run). Durable products, or those that can be reused over and over (rather than merely recycled) are the best options for limiting harm.

4. **Where does the product come from**? Locally produced products travel less distance and contribute less pollution due to their transport. However, the product's location of origin has additional considerations beyond how far it has travelled. Some countries have extremely lax environmental regulations and offer few or no employee protections from chronic workplace harm or compensation due to injury. It often costs more for the same product made in the United States than in China; however, the former country at least has some protections in place to shield the environment from exceedingly ruinous discharges and considers workplace safety an important human right. And within the United States, some companies are more committed than others to lessening ecological harm and producing near zero waste. Consider also that some small-scale and local growers and manufacturers may not be the most efficient when it comes to total energy use (and, therefore, the calculated carbon footprint) because they do not have the economy of scale working in their favor as with some larger companies. However, such local producers also contribute to community resiliency through decentralizing food production and manufacturing of necessary products. Therefore, total distance of travel should not necessarily be the only concern with regard to the location of origin of a particular product.

5. **Does the product use less power or none at all**? Manufactured goods that consume less energy during their use can help reduce our overall impact. Electricity is anything but free. It removes mountaintops and rains toxic metals onto landscapes (coal), clears forests and releases CO_2 (biomass), impounds rivers, floods biologically rich land, and prevents animal migrations (dams), and requires the production of specialized equipment that necessitates mining, industrial manufacture, and carbon emissions (solar, wind). Petroleum-powered engines obviously pollute as well. This is not to write that we should avoid all powered machines and devices, only that we need to consider how each of these technologies produces its own specific consequences. We have options. We can prioritize fuel economy (for example) over the size of the tires and loudness of the exhaust on a car. We can choose hand-powered household devices, items that use no electricity over their lifetime, help build self-reliance during power outages, and provide people with movement.

6. **What materials are the product manufactured from**? It is important to consider that many products can be made from a variety of materials, from natural items that are biodegradable and non-polluting to various polymers that ultimately end up in our oceans or in the ground, where they eventually break down over the course of thousands of years and may enter the groundwater

of unborn people many generations from now. Material selection also contributes to the durability of the product (number 3 in this list), and in many cases it makes more sense to select an item made from metal or wood than from plastic (when the choice exists). Products made from renewable resources are advantageous so long as the rate of resource extraction does not outstrip the rate of resource regeneration. Manufacturing from recycled components does place less strain on natural resources (some of which exist in finite amounts) and reduce the creation of waste, but in many cases this is not as green as we are led to believe (see the next section: Is Recycling Best?). And let us not forget that some materials are not safe for us to be exposed to for years or decades because they themselves are toxic, carcinogenic, or endocrine disrupting, or breakdown into molecules that are. Again, this also applies to the packaging the product comes in.

7. **What are the social and ecological practices of the company who manufactured the product**? People generally examine only the qualities of the product and rarely hold manufacturing companies accountable for their pollution, human rights violations, and impact to (i.e., acculturation of) indigenous populations. Corporate responsibility is a huge consideration and we should be supporting those companies that are leading the way in this arena. A company that builds innovative products while simultaneously polluting an entire watershed isn't doing the world any favors—this is comparable to providing gifts of medicine to one village and piling all the medical waste in another. Manufacturers that move out of the country to find places with laxer environmental regulations need to be boycotted (period). Companies need to take care of their workers because it is these people who ultimately allow companies to be successful. And remember, indigenous people living a traditional or somewhat traditional lifeway do not need our help. Modernizing their lives ultimately erodes their connection to the land, brings on the diseases of civilization, and eliminates the social and gender equality they may be experiencing. It is difficult for people of affluent countries to understand the harms we bring to people because we are largely unaware of them (though, if you have read this far, you should be starting to become acutely aware of them).

These seven items that make up the Green Purchasing Criteria are not meant to be a comprehensive list of all factors for consideration of every product in the world. In other words, each product has its own list of concerns that relates to the area, the ecosystem, the people, and corporations involved in the manufacturing, use, and (hopefully) rebirth of that product. This may seem like a lot of work to do before buying a product—and it is if you are accustomed to passive purchasing that does not consider anything except the price and how well the product appeals to your fancy. Of course, what is appealing is much the result of social conditioning and may have little or nothing to do with criteria we have just discussed. Much of this information can be found today in a variety of sources; it takes only a willingness on your part to transition to being a conscientious consumer. Finally, this list of criteria does not ask an obvious question: can I make the product myself from local, natural, non-toxic, renewable resources? This question is the topic of chapter 12.

IS RECYCLING BEST?

The answer to this question is "it depends", with various factors coming into play, such as the specific material we are discussing and what our end goals are (e.g., reduce energy use, reduce water use, reduce the need to procure virgin material). But, in general, despite the public perception of it, recycling is far from best. In fact, it can be seen to drive the single-use mentality so loved by members of affluent countries, serving to appease the guilt that would result from throwing away disposable items. We need to develop an awareness of what happens after recyclable items are placed in their collection bins. However, the problems with recycling don't fall entirely to the consumer. There is also the manufacturer of these goods, who relies on the "green message" of recycling to continue producing single-use products.

When you place a recyclable item into the appropriate bin, it usually gets transported to a facility (such as a transfer station) where it will be picked up by employees of a company who handle recycling. This requires energy (usually in the form of gasoline) to transport the product. After it is sorted, packed, and transported again, it arrives at a facility where the used goods will be turned into a raw material. This transport requires more energy, usually in the form of diesel or gasoline. The raw material is either converted into a new product or transported another time to a manufacturing facility where it will be formed into new goods. The creation of new products in an industrial facility uses more energy (in the form of electricity or fossil fuels) and generates pollution, some of which is carcinogenic. The finished good is then transported to a central distribution center or a market of some kind, using yet more energy (diesel or gasoline). The consumer then drives somewhere to purchase the product or orders it online, which requires further energy (more diesel or gasoline). Clearly, the recycling process is highly energy intensive and polluting. You may be thinking that this is better than extracting raw materials, which may be finite in nature or subject to overharvest in a non-renewable manner. While that is usually true, it misses the point that if we simply reused the container, switched to using durable goods, and moved away from a disposable mindset, the environmental cost of recycling would be reduced to the environmental cost of reusing the object, which can range from nothing to merely cleaning the item.

Aside from the problem that recycling is energy intensive and polluting, is the issue that some products we believe are recycled are actually downcycled. Recycling, using a strict definition, means that a product is converted back into a similar or more valuable product after its use. Further, this could occur indefinitely. Examples of this are a glass bottle or an aluminum can. However, some products cannot be formed back into their original items, and then can be used only to make products of lesser material quality. Certain plastics, such as those with a resin identification code of 2 (High Density Polyethylene) can be used only to make containers for food one time, after which they are made into other products (often by combining other polymers and chemicals with them). These include objects like plastic chairs and tables. Those items are frequently not recyclable, especially once they get the resin identification code of 7 (other). At this point, they enter the waste stream and become an inhabitant of landfills. So, all of those plastic milk and juice bottles that you believe are being recycled are actually being downcycled, having only one more use as a different product before they are disposed of.

Of course, all of this is moot if items you believe are being recycled aren't actually reprocessed into another product. This occurs more frequently than most realize. One problem is that recycled materials must vie with virgin raw materials for quality and purity. So cardboard that is heavily stained with food items, mixed pieces of glass of different color, and certain types of plastics that are difficult to recycle are simply transferred to landfills. Further, some objects are made of several kinds of materials and create difficulties for recycling. A good example is the Tetra-pak, a primarily cardboard container used to hold coconut water, milk, and other beverages. Such a container is made up of three different materials (paper, aluminum, and plastic), and only a small proportion of recycling facilities can actually separate the materials. Therefore, most such containers end up in landfills. Even when items are being recycled, there is a waste, referred to as residual, that cannot be recycled. This residual ends up in landfills.

Finally, let us not forget that recycling creates pollution and exposes people to contamination, some of which is very toxic. Many items that are recycled had various poisonous items in them, such as paint, solvents, sprays, sealants, and so forth. These chemicals can contaminate the next container in the recycling chain. If the container is used for packaging food, the consumer may be exposed to such. During the recycling of paper products, inks, chemicals, and heavy metals may end up leaching into the ground. Recycling of plastics is anything but green, with some plastics yielding chlorine, dioxins, phthalates, and heavy metals when they are reformed into new products. And it is well known that some recycling facilities are among the worst sources of air pollution emissions.

There is a familiar slogan in the United States that goes "reduce, reuse, recycle", a saying that is designed to help people remember ways to limit our use of raw materials. But it needs additional words that begin with the letter "r", such as reconsider, repair, and re-integrate to make it more useful. Reconsider is to remind us that the item or items may well be unnecessary and that other options exist. Repair is a clear prompt to find ways to continue the use of an item that may have suffered damage or has become worn but is still serviceable with some mending or restoration. Re-integrate is a memory aid for composting biodegradable items and integrating them back into the soil where they can be used to grow things of use (rather than sending such items to landfills). Collectively, the mantra could be "reconsider, reduce, reuse, repair, re-integrate, recycle", with recycle last in the list because it is the least environmentally appropriate action short of simply disposing of the item in a landfill. Recycling is not the solution we have been led to believe it is. It is a policy that assuages our guilt and allows large companies to continue producing single-use products without backlash from an aware and eco-minded segment of society. It may strike people as a surprise to learn that many beverages, including soda and beer, used to be served using refillable containers. It is happening today with some bulk items like laundry detergent and dish cleaners. It is entirely possible for us to return to this practice in a larger scale and make it safe for the consumer. It requires only an awareness that recycling, though better than discarding, is far worse than reusing, and the will of the consumers to shift away from selfish acts, thereby protecting landscapes that yet unborn children will need for healthy living.

WHAT CLOTHES YOUR BODY?

We rarely take the time to learn the full history of the products we use. There are any number of reasons for this. For some, it is apathy for this kind of accounting, simply not wanting to take the time to learn how to protect landscapes and people. Others believe that corporations and governments are responsible and will adhere to a set of regulations that safeguard against environmental damage. There are even individuals who disbelieve that people are capable of harming the earth and, in turn, affecting human health. All of this overlays the fact that some goods are deemed so necessary that regardless of the harm generated we must continue to produce and use them. This is true of our clothing. Garments are necessary for protecting people from the elements, which can include low temperatures, precipitation, intense or long-duration sunlight, biting insects, and vegetation armed with spines and prickles. Clothing is also useful for guarding against work conditions that involve sharp, abrasive, or otherwise injurious objects. In the modern world, they are further considered necessary for vanity and demonstrating social status. Unfortunately, as with most items produced in the industrial world, modern clothing represents a serious source of pollution and exposure to toxins. Of course, options exist for essentially everything we grow, manufacture, gather, or produce, meaning that our clothing doesn't have to be yet another way we divorce ourselves from nature.

One of the most ubiquitous fabrics that clothing is made from is the fibers of the cotton plant, including upland cotton (*Gossypium hirsutum*), which accounts for most of the worlds cultivated cotton, Egyptian cotton (*Gossypium barbardense*), Asiatic cotton (*Gossypium arboreum*), and others. These fibers, which surround and protect the seeds, constitute roughly half of the fabrics manufactured in the world and about 39% of clothing. Conventionally grown cotton is among the worst agricultural commodities because of the amount of chemicals that is used to grow this particular cultigen. For every kilogram of conventionally raised cotton fiber, it takes ⅓ of a kilogram of chemical fertilizers and pesticides to grow it. In fact, cotton is the most heavily sprayed crop in the world. While only 2.4% of the world's crop land is planted in cotton, this plant accounts for 24% of the world's insecticide use and 11% of the world's pesticide use. The collateral damage is immense and many studies have documented wildlife illness and death attributable to the chemicals used to grow this plant, especially to birds and fish. In one case from 1995, more than 240,000 fish were killed along a 25 km (15 mile) stretch of river in Alabama by the runoff of legally applied pesticides to cotton crops. And because the pesticides don't stay on the field, as the previous example illustrates and as documented in the Mississippi Embayment area by Thurman et al. in 1998, chemicals sprayed on cotton have been detected in human breast milk. Given that seven of the 15 commonly used cotton pesticides in the United States are labeled as possible, probable, likely, or known carcinogens, this means that cotton workers and those living near cotton fields (especially) are exposed to hazardous chemicals. Therefore, even if someone were not to care about their own health, the purchase of conventionally raised cotton supports an industry that harms people and other-than-human persons.

Approximately 58% of clothes today are made from synthetic materials, including polyester, nylon, acrylic, spandex, and rayon. These fabrics are made using petroleum and (sometimes) coal, along with a suite of other chemicals, in a process that links single molecules together to form long polymers that can formed into threads for making garments. They are frequently treated with various human-made compounds, including petrochemical dyes for coloring, formaldehyde to prevent shrinkage, perfluorinated chemicals to prevent wrinkles and function as flame retardants, and alkylphenols as surfactants. These chemicals, while harmful to the people who wear them, are even worse for the people who work in the facilities that manufacture and apply them. A responsible consumer would avoid the purchase of these fabrics because they are responsible for significant amounts of environmental pollution, including chemicals that last an extremely long time in the environment. The fact that these chemicals collectively produce irritation, allergic reaction, endocrine disruption, and cancer should be enough to get us to reconsider these as a textile sources. Unfortunately, we are only recently becoming aware of additional harms from synthetic clothing.

Like any clothing, synthetic garments, including polyester and acrylic types, get worn and lose some of their fibers. These fibers can be seen in the lint filter of many dryers. But they are also lost in large numbers in the washing cycle. These tiny fragments of synthetic fibers enter the waterways in many municipal systems and ultimately find their way into lakes, rivers, and oceans, where they are consumed by tiny and filter feeding organisms, such as various kinds of zooplankton, fish, and shellfish. While this might not sound particularly problematic, there are a few problems here that make this a serious issue. First, as Browne and colleagues published in 2011 in the journal Environmental Science and Technology, the microplastic particles are found throughout the world, on all six continents inhabited by people, and were distributed from the equator to the poles. Not one sample was devoid of the particles. Second, they are abundantly

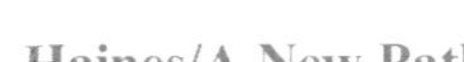

produced, with a single washing of synthetic clothing producing in excess of 1900 tiny fibers and particles. Third, the microplastic particles absorb fat-soluble toxins, like dioxins, polychlorinated biphenyls (PCBs), and polybrominated biphenyl ethers (PBBEs), which exert endocrine-disrupting effects on the organisms that consume them (in addition to the chemicals that they already carry). And, of course, we eat some of these organisms, meaning our pollution finds its way back into our bodies through this circuitous route. In other words, these microplastics, which are ubiquitous in many waters that would be considered relatively pristine, absorb certain kinds of environmental pollution and provide higher doses to the organisms that unknowingly consume these particles.

Animals, such as zooplankton, mistake microplastics for food and occasionally ingest the particles. The chemicals are then transferred to their body. For example, Chua et al. (2014) showed that PBBEs are relocated from the microplastics to the body tissue of a species of marine amphipod (*Allorchestes compressa*). Another study showed that fish who ingest plastic microparticles experienced a transfer of hazardous chemicals to their bodies and suffered liver pathology as a result (Rochman et al. 2013). These studies have documented that the plastic particles and the chemicals they carry are contaminating the lower trophic levels of the food chain, which are then passed from the small organisms to larger ones as they are consumed by their natural predators. Therefore, the larger aquatic and marine animals bioaccumulate toxins and suffer reduced health and vitality. In a recent study led by the Zoological Society of London, harbor porpoises (*Phocoena phocoena*) in the United Kingdom were found to be experiencing severe reproductive issues that were likely caused by exposure to PCBs. The researchers found that nearly 20% of the female porpoises showed reproductive failure (e.g., stillbirth, fetal death, miscarriage). A further 17% of the porpoises were revealed to have infections or tumors of their reproductive organs. While PCBs have not been used in that part of the world for more than 30 years, the microplastics are transferring these persistent toxins in the environment to living organisms. (The example of the porpoise was used here intentionally because of the hierarchy of life so commonly observed by modern humans—while zooplankton and small fish are not afforded much thought or compassion, the larger, charismatic animals are.)

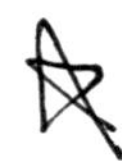

While all clothing produces lint and sheds fibers, fabrics made from organically raised cotton, flax, hemp, and wool produce fibers that are biodegradable and do not pose harm to our waters and the other-than-human persons that live there (unless they are treated or washed with conventional products; see the next section). Likewise, fabrics that are rarely used for clothing in the United States, such as buckskin (made from the tanned hides of various species of deer), produce a chemical-free garment that does not harm the people who wear them or the landscape they reside in. Synthetic fabrics are well known for their insulating qualities (even when wet) and ability to wick moisture from the skin to the next layer of clothing. However, this can also be accomplished by some natural fibers, including wool. While some feel that wool is too uncomfortable to wear, Merino wool can be worn next the skin without irritation and also provides insulation (even when wet) and wicking properties. Microplastic pollution is a serious issue, and the only way to deal with this is to have a return to natural fabrics produced in the least harmful manner possible (i.e., through avoiding industrial farming methods). At the very least, people should consider replacing synthetic garments that contact their skin with clothes made from natural fibers. Clothing choices in affluent countries are guided as much or more by popularity and perceived social status influences than by practical considerations. The ecological health effects of clothing have almost no influence on purchasing. We need to change this. We need to make natural fabrics "cool" again. We need people to consider the health of the world in their consumer habits. We've already polluted the world's oceans with plastic debris (both large and small), but we can stop the problem from continuing to get worse, which serves our own health interests at the same time.

WHILE IN THE HOME…

Keeping in mind that the average American spends 90% of their time indoors, what we do in that setting has substantial effects on our health. From the building materials we use, to the hygiene and cosmetic products, to the way we wash our dishes and clothing, the choices we make as a consumer contribute to a body burden of toxins within humans that also make their way into natural systems around and downstream of our buildings. Even the way we choose to light and heat our homes, which is exacerbated by the size of our homes because larger homes require more energy to illuminate and warm the space, has substantial impacts to air quality when we consider there are millions of homes and apartments contributing to the problem in this country alone. The goal of this chapter is to generate awareness of the problems we create when we go with the flow of American life and do not consider the materials we use and come into contact with. It is important to keep in mind here that the objective of most companies is not to generate health in your person or limit environmental pollution. Their goal is profit, and they incorporate human and ecological health only as much as they are required by regulatory agencies. We change this "do just enough" industry approach through choosing different products with our money (i.e., we choose companies that go further to limit harm). If we stop purchasing goods that detract from healthful living, these products will disappear and be replaced by more healthful versions—it requires only that consumers care enough to choose more eco-friendly products or make their own with non-toxic, natural ingredients. No company will make products that can't be sold. Not one. With this in mind, let's discuss some home topics that affect human and landscape health.

First, let us begin this discussion with mention of the building materials we use. I personally find it shocking how much of our homes, which are meant to protect us, produce toxic exposures, especially through degrading the quality of air inside our homes. While there are regulations in place to attempt to maintain some semblance of outdoor air quality (the Clean Air Acts of 1963, 1970, 1977, and 1990), there is nothing protecting indoor air quality other than you (and what you decide to purchase). According the US Environmental Protection Agency (EPA), our indoor air is usually 2- to 5-times worse than the air outside our homes (and some homes were found to have indoor air quality 100 times worse than the outside air). Why would this be? Because we have chosen to use chemical and synthetic products that off-gas, which is the release of gas molecules that were trapped or absorbed within a material, into the rooms we inhabit. This process supplies toxic, volatile chemicals into the air that we take into our body through breathing. These volatile compounds have a range of health effects, from asthma, to endocrine disruption, to cancer. For example, a 2012 report by the architectural firm Perkins+Will listed 374 known asthma-producing compounds in the constructed environment, a proportion of which were the building materials themselves (other items included on the list were cleaning and personal-care products).

We construct many wooden homes now with particle board or plywood, which uses a formaldehyde-containing resin to hold the wood particles together. Unfortunately, the formaldehyde does not all remain within the adhesive, making this building material the number one source of formaldehyde in indoor air. This chemical is an irritant, asthmagen, and a known carcinogen. It is also a sensitizer, which means that it makes a person more sensitive to other harmful chemicals found in the person's environment that they may otherwise have some resilience to. We put up walls made of drywall (also called sheet rock), which can be a source of sulfur if it was sourced from the wrong location (China), leading to irritation, asthma, and coughing. We paint the drywall with products containing volatile organic compounds (VOCs) that off-gas for long periods of time (not just while they dry). We cover our floors with carpets made of synthetic fibers that off-gas, which are treated with chemicals to be stain resistant, and need chemical adhesives to hold the floor covering in place, which further contributes to the VOCs in the air. These volatile compounds are responsible for an array of health issues, including headaches, dizziness, asthma, irritation, and (over longer periods) cancer. The sealing caulks and solvents we use further contribute to VOCs, as does the furniture and other things we choose to place in the home (such as vinyl shower curtains). And these are just the building materials and furnishings—the hygiene and cleaning products commonly purchased in the United States also contribute to the VOCs in our home. When the cumulative effects are totaled, it is easy to understand why the indoor air quality of American homes is so poor. It is a sad story because almost all of these sources of indoor air pollution can be avoided by simply choosing different building materials and furnishings (e.g., wooden boards over particle board, wood flooring and wool or cotton area rugs over synthetic carpets, cloth shower curtains over vinyl ones). And the topic rarely considered is that these materials become sources of environmental pollution when homes are remodeled and their building materials and furnishings, like plastic siding and carpets, are replaced.

After we build our homes with materials that do not support our health, we then keep them clean with an assortment of human-made chemicals. It is important that everyone understand that the industrial chemicals in this country are treated as innocent until proven guilty. The Toxic Substances Control Act of 1976 outlines that the EPA can't require any chemical-producing company to demonstrate the safety of their products unless the EPA itself can demonstrate the product poses a risk to health. This approach requires more resources than that agency possesses because of the large number of new applications each year (about 1500 according to one estimate). This means that you and your family become the test subjects, which you consented to through purchase of the product (and you also provided consent for your children, who have greater sensitivity than you do). But it is actually worse than you realize because the American government doesn't require companies to list all the chemicals found within cleaning products. For example, some carpet cleaners use perchloroethylene, which is known to damage the liver, kidneys, and nervous system and is a known human carcinogen. Another one, which we have already mentioned, is formaldehyde, which is an ingredient in some cleaning products. Manufacturers use a bit of deceit and may list this chemical under one of its synonyms, such as methanal, formalin, or methylaldehyde—names that don't generate the same concern for those few who understand that formaldehyde is not something to have within the home. Trichloroethanes are used in some cleaners because they are good solvents for items like adhesives, ink, and paint. The products that contain trichloroethanes rarely mention their entire range of health effects: damage to the liver and kidneys, respiratory irritation, depression of the central nervous system, and carcinogenesis. Nor do they mention the occupational exposure and loss of health of those who work in facilities where chemicals like these are produced. Certainly, nowhere on the packaging of products that contain these chemicals (and many others) is there a description of the contaminated sites around the country that resulted from spills or leaks during manufacturing and/or transport. And definitely, the chemical manufacturers don't discuss the ultimate fate of these compounds as they are washed down the drain and enter the environment, the same one that we grow and harvest our food from.

After we have built and furnished our homes with industrial chemicals, we use products with more industrial chemicals to clean them. And then, we use even more human-created substances to clean ourselves and the clothing we put in contact with our skin. For example, we put sodium lauryl sulfate (SLS) in our laundry detergents, shampoos, toothpastes, liquid soaps, body washes, and some makeup foundations, even though there are thousands of papers (literally) documenting its harm through irritation, organ toxicity, endocrine disruption, developmental issues, and cancer. We seem not to recognize the idea of cumulative exposure. Our product regulations ensure that we do not experience toxic exposures from THAT one product, but we use all THOSE products that also contain SLS. This means that some of us do, in fact, come into contact with enough of this chemical to impact our health. Given that there are similar products that function well and do not contain SLS, it is curious why this chemical would be used at all—a question I don't have a good answer to. I don't know why we need to put phthalates, which are linked with the occurrence of asthma, certain cancers, diabetes, obesity, low intelligence, autism spectrum disorder, and depressed fertility, in hygiene products at all. I also don't understand why we are still putting plastic microbeads in some soaps when we know these enter the environment and contribute to the plastic pollution that is becoming a global phenomenon. I can only speculate, but it seems clear that the increased incidence of health conditions is not acting as the harbinger of change that might be expected among a society that is paying attention to what is occurring around it and responding appropriately.

One reason for all this may be that we are interested in convenience and comfort enough that we are willing to experience, in trade, some health impacts. The clothes dryer is a good supporting example of this paragraph's opening statement. Residents of affluent countries use tremendous amounts of energy each year to dry their clothes inside a heated, rotating drum when clothing will dry on a line (outdoors or indoors) with no cost to air quality. Millions of tons of carbon dioxide enter the atmosphere each year to power clothes dryers. Humans have dried clothing for millennia without issue, but today a home is incomplete without a dryer. We have even gone so far as to outlaw hanging clothes on a line outdoors in some communities because it is considered unsightly. We should be providing recognition to people who take the extra few minutes to hang up clothes on the line because, simply put, this is one of the easiest and most inexpensive ways people can help protect air quality. However, online forums are filled with comments indicating people do not have time to hang up their clothes, even though it adds only a few minutes to the task. Others report that line-dried clothes are too stiff and scratchy and that lint and hair aren't removed from the clothing. And while solutions for this are easy, such as a compromise that uses the dryer ten minutes to tumble the clothes and remove some extraneous fibers and then finishes the drying process on the line, such answers require another minute or two on top of the few minutes needed already to line dry clothes. And many Americans simply don't want to spend that amount of time to limit air pollution (even though the pollution affects everyone). But we go further, adding dryer sheets to the load of clothing, which work to soften clothing by imparting chemicals onto the fabric that essentially lubricates the fibers. It turns out they contain a suite of harmful chemicals, like benzyl alcohol, chloroform, ethyl acetate, and pentane. Despite the fact there are several options for getting softer clothing without dryer sheets (and fabric softeners), these products will continue to be used until convenience isn't the overriding criterion. And until that time, we will continue to have daily exposures to toxic chemicals in the home.

At this point, some readers may be thinking this is all very alarmist. After all, many people live in modern homes and use conventional cleaning products and they are still living. In fact, human bodies are designed to deal with some level of toxic exposure without suffering any significant harm. And here is my response (which continues into the next paragraph). We are currently generating about 9,500,000,000 kilograms (over 21 billion pounds) of industrial chemicals that are released into our environment each year (according to data from the United Nations Environmental Program, the US Environmental Protection Agency, and other similar programs). Of these, about 20% are recognized carcinogens, meaning that about 65 kilograms (143 pounds) of cancer-causing chemicals are released each second. Since World War II, humans have generated 80,000 new chemicals that have been broadly dispersed into the environment. Today, breast milk has been shown to be contaminated with a host of chemicals, including flame retardants, dry-cleaning fluids, paint thinners, plastic components, chlorine derivatives, non-stick agents, deodorizers, gasoline byproducts, pesticides, fungicides, rocket fuel, and wood preservatives. That list doesn't include the suite of heavy metals that we also distribute into the environment. While this is not a call to shorten the duration of breastfeeding or completely cease this crucial interaction between mother and child, it is simply to point out that these chemicals are finding their way inside our bodies and causing health issues. Consider that a 2007 National Survey of Children's Health estimated that 22.3% of our youth possess one or more chronic conditions, including asthma, learning disabilities, attention deficit/hyperactivity disorder (and other mental health conditions), diabetes, cancer, and speech difficulty. A 2010 study in the Journal of the American Medical Association determined that the frequency of chronic health conditions among children increased 107% from 1994 to 2006. Isn't it clear that we are transforming human health (for the worse) with this lifeway? What is the point of living longer if you are also living sicker?

Americans (in this case) did, to some extent, consent to these exposures by purchasing these products and allowing various legislation to go forth that protects chemical manufacturers. The children of parents who buy such products did not—they cannot provide informed consent and relied on their parents, many of whom were very interested in convenience (e.g., a product that cleans really well with the least amount of physical effort). The wildlife near our homes also did not consent to these exposures, and many experience harm before humans do because of aspects of their biology (like amphibians who have highly permeable skin) or aspects of their ecology (they live in the river that we avoid because we know it is polluted). And what of people living in distant lands who use none of these products but still have exposures to harmful compounds? We projected into the environment, both intentionally and unintentionally, chemicals that persist for a long time and are transported by air and water currents and the movement of wildlife. As a result, almost nowhere on earth is completely free of industrial contamination. Even the people living without synthetic products, people who did not consent to the exposures, have these chemicals located in their tissues. All of this can be used as evidence for the extent of human domestication, a process that results in a sense of superiority (and even hubris) in those positioned to make important decisions for a society and a decline in the awareness and responsibility of the people who believe they must accept the decisions made by others.

The home is supposed to be a place of refuge and safety where human health is supported. Instead, the modern domicile is a location where people contribute to the body burden of industrial toxins that degrade the health of their families and reach out in the ecosystems (with their purchasing choices) and produce consequences there as well. The positive feature to focus on here is that consumer purchasing and habits can change. It can be our first steps on a rewilding path. It requires an awareness of the harms caused by the usual American choices in the marketplace and a desire to live in a more responsible manner. With those two guiding concepts (awareness and responsibility, both of which are important principles in rewilding), a country can make huge impacts by directing its purchasing dollars to less harmful products.

While this section is merely presented to generate awareness, interested persons will need more details to make their homes a safer place. I encourage everyone to read "What's Gotten into Us" by McKay Jenkins to learn more about our exposures. Likewise, books similar to "Green Goes with Everything" by Sloan Barnett will be of value. While that book isn't a rewilding reference, it does provide some background and a lot of practical tips for people looking to purchase safer cleaning, personal hygiene, cosmetic, and other home products. The author also describes how to make effective home cleaners with items as "toxic" as vinegar and citrus juice. Collectively, we can have a huge positive difference through small changes in our daily habits.

YOUR LAWN MAY BE GREEN, BUT IT ISN'T SO GREEN

The tidy, closely cropped, uniformly green area of turf grass around a home is a very common feature of United States and many affluent countries. Many home owners spend considerable amounts of time and earnings creating the perfect lawn. Frequent mowing, irrigation, weed pulling, and chemical application are common strategies for attaining the desired goal of homogenous green. Lawns are such a part of the American culture that they are seen as "beautiful" and a necessary feature of any home setting. Any lawn that does not receive constant upkeep is viewed negatively with the home owners of the offending tract receiving scorn and criticism from their neighbors. Open spaces around the domicile do have several nice features that help to garner greater enjoyment and safety for the residents, including better visibility, through flow of breezes, fire break, insect break, and open space for activity and games. However, many of these features of lawns can be enjoyed with other kinds of passive or active landscaping that do not have the tremendous environmental costs associated with highly manicured settings. Additionally, the lawn is an excellent example demonstrating the altered worldview and manner of landscape interaction found in domesticated humans, features that will serve as good discussion points to help us further understand how contemporary society has divorced itself from nature and disengaged from a wild (and healthy) ecology.

Let's look at what a lawn truly is. Most manicured areas of grasses are highly unnatural because they would not exist without (1) initial human planting of species that are usually native to other continents and (2) continued maintenance with fossil-fuel-powered machines and other products of industry (e.g., fertilizers, herbicides). Lawns are generally carved out of ecosystems comprised of many species at different stages of ecological succession to create a homogenous monocrop of one or few grass species (at least that is the goal). In other words, humans take natural communities of organisms with a large array of functions and values, capable of providing food, medicine, and raw materials for many species and convert them to something that has limited use for anyone except humans (who sometimes spend more time in upkeep of the lawn than actual time enjoying it). Lawns represent a place where the number of dynamic interconnections have been disturbed and reduced in number. They are a place where the tremendous structural diversity and infinite array of colors, shapes, and patterns have been changed to something with the geometrical complexity of an interior carpet.

The primary tool for maintaining the lawn is the lawn mower, which is 93% more polluting than the average car. For comparative purposes, it is approximately equal in fuel expenditure to use a lawn mower for one hour or drive the average car for four hours. As a result, lawn mowers are responsible for at least 5% of the air pollution in the United States (some estimates place this as high as 10%). The US EPA has estimated that 800 million gallons of gasoline are used each year to crop American lawns, emitting tons (literally) of pollution into the air. Let's not forget to mention the approximately 17 million gallons of gasoline that is spilled refueling lawn equipment. Lawn care frequently utilizes synthetic fertilizers that are applied in excess, resulting in runoff that enters watersheds. This ultimately feeds various species of algae that can fill waterways and deplete the area of oxygen when their plant bodies decay. Of course, water is also of major importance to lawn care, and in many parts of the country, lawns could not exist without extensive watering. In urban areas across the country, 30–60% of the total water used is for irrigating lawns. This amounts to nine billion gallons of water each day for landscape irrigation (the vast majority of which is lawn).

Waterways are also one of the recipients of an array of herbicides used to kill unwanted plants on American lawns. One study in the western United States found 23 different kinds of pesticides in the water, with five of them at concentrations sufficient to kill aquatic life. Another study by the US Geological Survey found that fish in 90% of the sampled streams contained at least one pesticide. If one critically examines the health concerns of the 30 commonly used chemicals to kill unwanted life on lawns, it will become quickly obvious that these chemicals should not be considered benign. Nearly ⅔ of the chemicals are linked to cancer, more than ⅔ to negative reproductive effects, more than ⅓ to endocrine disruption, approaching ½ to birth defects, and a full ½ to neurotoxicity (among other health insults that could be mentioned). These chemicals don't just enter watersheds, they are detected in groundwater and can leach into drinking water sources. They are toxic to many forms of life, not just aquatic organisms, including the bees that pollinate food crops and birds that consume insects considered to be a nuisance to humans. Exacerbating the issue are the amounts of chemicals used on lawns. The US EPA estimates that homeowners used up to ten times the amount of pesticides on their lawns as American farmers applied to food crops. If none of this bothers you, it should. Studies have shown that children who live in residences that have chemically treated lawns experience a 6.5 times higher rate of cancer than do people who do not treat their lawns. Not the best gift for anyone's children. And people using the lawns track those chemicals inside the home, so that everyone is exposed.

Lawns certainly would not be such a problem if there weren't so many of them. It is now estimated that over 16.5 million hectares (41 million acres) of the United States is lawn, with at least 5000 acres daily carved out of existing habitats to make new lawns. This means that lawns are the largest crop in the United States, covering 1.9% of the surface area of the country. The problem is that this particular "crop" does not produce food and it does not support animals similar to a forest, prairie, or marsh. The lawn became associated with status and hence it became popular in a stratified society looking to climb upward in rank, eminence, and prestige. Today, some people do not even know why they put so much effort into lawns. It is not necessarily that they are consciously trying to demonstrate their higher social rank. It is just a ubiquitous feature of our culture—you buy a home and maintain the lawn around it. There is little doubt that residents of the United States appear to be obsessed with lawns. It would very fortunate if they instead became obsessed with intact landscapes.

Allow me to be direct—lawns are mostly wasted space that reflects our desire to control the natural world. We take many aspects of natural diversity that support an array of cooperative connections and reduce them down to a well-ordered and closely cropped monochrome surface. Rather than a nearly infinite array of heights and branch angles that would occur in a forest or a multitude of flowers at different stages that would brighten the landscape in a prairie, our society considers lawns to be an improvement over the seeming disarray of nature. Perhaps, though, this apparent disarray appears as such because we spend too little time on wild landscapes to make sense of it. Much like the definition of human beauty changes between different cultures, the idea that a lawn is beautiful is completely a product of social upbringing. It is our domestication that leads us to believe that a reduction in the number of species occurring in an area, the conversion to a landscape that does not contain useful plants, and the loss of structural complexity that would have supported a greater array of niches and interactions is a sign of higher status. This belief is simply another example of nature divorcement. When one critically examines the lawn, it can be seen to be largely bereft of natural beauty. In nature, one of the fundamental aspects of beauty is diversity on many scales.

So what do we do about lawns? Get rid of them, or at least a significant portion of them. Let the borders grow up into whatever natural community would occur in your part of the world. Use the space to build "gardens" based on polyculture principles and perennial species. If you choose to design the landscape, plant native species for ornament, food, medicine, and landscape heterogeneity. Regain the structural diversity that may have existed there before by planting sun-tolerant species that produce shade for species underneath them that require less light (the more layers, the more life will return to your home). These gardens can be quite beautiful, satisfy local ordinances about unkempt residential spaces, and require little or no watering (if the correct species are chosen). Keep in mind that 96% of our songbirds require insects to feed their fledglings, even if they are primarily consumers of different foods (such as fruits) at other times of the year (note that there are other species similar to humans in that the developing young have different nutritional needs from the adults). Non-native plants are generally less palatable to native insects, which means that our native birds suffer when we choose species native to other continents. I want to state this again—when we consider other options beyond the lawn, we want to consider native plants as much as possible (whether we passively let them colonize the area or we actively plant them). If getting rid of the lawn isn't practical or possible in your situation, then manicure it less. This means mow it less often (remember, taller grass needs less water). Let other species colonize it and let those species flower sometimes before your mow (it will attract species such as butterflies that utilize the nectar from flowers). Forgo any and all uses of synthetic chemicals. Water it less or not at all. If you think that failure to irrigate means your lawn will die, this is untrue. It means only that the species that require lots of water may die (or become dormant during periods of water stress). Species that can survive on less water will eventually find your lawn and inhabit it. There are many options beyond the lawn, only a few of which I have mentioned here. The first step is to realize how limiting this kind of landscape is and how damaging its maintenance can be.

AMERICA'S BEVERAGE

Residents of the United States enjoy drinks made from coffee plants (*Coffea* species, primarily *C. arabica*), woody plants native to the African and Asian continents. The "beans" used to make coffee are the seeds gathered from the fruits. The beverages brewed from the roasted seeds have a characteristic flavor and are stimulating due to the presence of the alkaloid caffeine. Americans spend approximately 40 billion dollars each year on coffee. With the seeds of this plant being the second-most traded commodity in the world (after oil), it stands to reason that what kind of coffee we purchase can make a huge impact on the world, especially in the places where coffee plants are grown. Skeptical? Consider that 2.5 million acres have been cleared in Central America alone for monoculture of sun-grown coffee. As the World Wildlife Fund has noted, 37 of the 50 countries with the highest rates of deforestation are also countries that produce coffee. And most Americans, what do they have to say about this? Nothing—they discuss at great length which brands and methods produce the best flavored beverage but are largely unaware of the environmental costs. So, let's change this.

Wild coffee plants are species that grow in the shade of taller trees. As such, they are part of a forested community with both a diversity of species and a complex structure of different height plants. This contributes to a valuable environment that provides a variety of different settings and niches that harbors a greater array of animal species, including birds, insects, and amphibians. Cultivated coffee plants can be grown in this setting (i.e., in the shade of trees). However, what can be seen happening around the world is a transition to coffee plants grown in the open sun—after the trees that used to be there have been removed (and the subsequent death or exodus of the animals that used to live in that forest). Why is this done? Because monocrops of coffee plants grown closely together can produce greater yields and derive more income for the corporations that receive the greatest benefit from coffee farming. While the people living in the countries where coffee is cultivated do receive some income, they earn a tiny fraction of the profits generated and lose their forests (including the edible, medicinal, and useful plants that grew within them prior to the felling of the trees).

Of course, more than humans are impacted by this practice of sun-grown coffee (an agricultural method also known as "unshaded monoculture"). By the removal of the forests, all species that depended on trees and what grows in the shade of trees are affected. For example, many migratory birds in the United States visit Central and South America during the winter season. Those birds that require forests are finding less and less suitable habitat to overwinter in. The very winged animals that fill our soundscape with a symphony of vernal song and consume untold numbers of insects (some of which are considered pests) to feed their fledglings are unable to find appropriate habitat at the southern end of their ranges. One estimate places the number of bird species at 95% fewer in sun-grown coffee tracts compared with a better option—growing coffee plants in the shade of trees. According to the American Birding Association, shade-grown coffee plantations are second only to intact forests when it comes to providing valuable habitat for forest-dwelling birds. The reason for this is because shade-grown coffee plantations still provide functional habitat and abundant food resources, including fruits from wild trees, nectar from flowers, and insects living on the plants.

Shade-grown coffee has a number of additional advantages. It requires fewer (or no) chemicals because the leaf litter falling from the trees adds compost to the soil, and the resident birds can provide a pest control function. This latter trait of shade-grown coffee should not be underestimated. One study in Jamaica showed that when birds were excluded from coffee plants, those plants had a 70% greater infection rate of their fruits by a species of beetle called the coffee berry borer (*Hypothenemus hampei*), which damages the seeds of the coffee plant. Studies conducted on sun-grown coffee showed that synthetic fertilizers and chemical pesticides were used extensively, which not only polluted the landscape but also harmed the health of the workers who were exposed to these compounds. Shade-grown coffee also protects the topsoil far better than monocrop farming and limits erosion that is inherent to industrial agriculture. Further, there is substantially greater water retention in shade-grown plantations because of the abundance of plants, their roots, and the leaf litter. This results in less runoff and less leaching of nutrients out of the plantation (again, requiring less industrial inputs to replace lost nutrients to the soil). A final item worthy of mention is that shade-grown coffee plantations also serve as an important carbon sink because carbon that would end up in the atmosphere is stored in the tree's roots, trunks, and branches, as well as in the soil. In contrast, sun-grown coffee farms contribute to climate change (as does most industrial farming in the world).

Unfortunately for the consumer, simply looking for shade-grown coffee cultivated in an organic manner is not enough because there are different versions of shade growing, some of which are far more beneficial to the wildlife than others. There are four methods used by farmers to grow coffee in the shade of trees (listed from least to most forest altering): rustic, traditional polyculture, commercial polyculture, and shade. Rustic represents the most eco-conscientious way to grow coffee. Using this method, coffee plants are grown within an intact forest with only some clearing of the lowest level of wild plants to provide room for the cultivated species. This method has lower yields than more intensive methods but also leaves wild fruit and medicine trees, which can be foundations for local resources or additional income. Traditional polyculture uses shade from native and cultivated trees to produce coffee. The planted trees often include species with edible fruits, medicinal parts, or other uses (e.g., fuelwood). Similar to the preceding method, chemical fertilizers and pesticides are rarely used. Commercial polyculture represents a more intensive system of using shade trees. With this method, the trees are typically all planted and much more extensive clearing is done to make room for more coffee plants. Pruning and removal of epiphytes (i.e., those plants that grow upon other plants) is generally used to allow more light to reach the coffee plants. Further, this system generally uses some fertilizers and pesticides because the forest alteration is becoming too extensive to maintain a functional ecology of wild organisms. The final shade-grown method is shade monoculture. This method represents a significant impact to the landscape and clearly looks imposed on the landscape due to its lack of complexity (though it is still better, in many ways, than sun-grown coffee). Coffee plants are grown under a monoculture (or rarely two species) of planted trees. Due to extensive pruning and epiphyte removal, the coffee plantations have only two strata: coffee plants and trees (usually a species of shimbillo, genus *Inga*, in the legume family). Coffee plants are grown quite densely in this system, producing higher yields than other shaded methods, and chemical inputs are common. Even with these brief explanations, it should be clear to most people that rustic and traditional polyculture are the best methods for producing coffee with the least harm.

The discussion of America's beverage and its environmental harm doesn't stop with the discussion of cultivation methods. An important aspect of this conversation also centers on the container the brewed coffee is placed in. It is estimated that 130 billion paper cups are given away for beverages each year in the United States, with 52 billion cups specifically for coffee (see Grishchenko 2007). Americans produce more than 53% of the world's disposable cup waste. The switch to single-use products got under way in the early 1900s when tuberculosis and influenza concerns suggested sharing common implements (such as a ladle at a public water source) could promote the spread of infections. Americans, who are now the quintessential consumer society, initially resisted the switch to paper cups and similar disposable products. However, the country has now fully embraced a move to one-use goods and spends very little time thinking about how these kinds of merchandise affect the world. Paper cups have substantial pollution and resource consumption at all stages of their production, use, and disposal. While some studies have tried to convince people that paper food containers are an eco-friendly choice, such studies have omitted important aspects of the food container's life cycle (i.e., they have been incomplete and misleading). A 2006 study commissioned by Starbucks (one of the world's leading users of disposable cups) showed that a ceramic mug is by far the better choice. Such a beverage container reaches its "break-even point" in terms of environmental harm with a disposable cup at 70 uses, which is easily accomplished by ceramic mugs that can be used thousands of times over their life. Even considering the fact that a ceramic cup must be washed, it still reduces water use by 64% and water pollution by 99% compared with a paper cup over its lifecycle. Equally important is the fact that solid waste is reduced by 86% through reusing a durable beverage container.

Today, the environmental harm created by the coffee industry has burgeoned further with the popularity of home devices such as the Keurig K-cup. Such machines utilize a small, foil-covered plastic "pod" that contains coffee seed grounds and a paper filter that is inserted into an automated device that brews a single cup of coffee. Once the coffee has been brewed, the pod is removed from the machine and thrown away. There are several problems with the K-cup design, including the fact that the pods are difficult to recycle because they are constructed of a specialty composite plastic and contain several different materials that would need to be separated somehow. Each year, many billions of K-cups are purchased and thrown away, so many that if these pods were lined up end to end they would encircle the earth more than 12 times. In the distant future, when the plastic of the pod breaks down, it will leach into the water of a population of people many generations yet to be born and pollute the rivers, lakes, oceans, and drinking water they rely on. And while reusable pods made of stainless steel have been designed, they are unpopular because they need to be washed between each use and some companies have designed their K-cup machines to not function with anything except a single-use, plastic K-cup.

So, you may be thinking, what does coffee have to do with rewilding? This particular topic, among many that could be chosen, exemplifies the problems with domesticated humans and industrial living. It is a good example from which we can apply lessons to other market-related topics. At the beginning of this book I made the statement that modern humans are selfish and unaware. This was a pointed statement to begin a book with and probably seemed overly harsh and judgmental. However, we have discussed many topics throughout this book that support that statement. The fact is, we are so interested in convenience that we will allow the last forests to fall and the remaining clean soil and water to be fouled by pollution. To simply avoid the "hassle" of carrying a reusable cup with us and washing it between uses, we will ultimately damage some of the remaining wilderness areas left on the planet. Further, we feel so entitled to coffee that no matter the area of forest that falls to grow this plant or the amount of waste produced, these inconvenient details are simply considered necessary expenses that must be paid—even if they are paid by people living in distant lands who lost their forests or by people yet unborn who will deal with the pollution. How can this be described as anything but selfish or unaware? Of course, the tragic issues surrounding America's beverage (combined with other aspects of industry) is that humanity will have no place left to rewild to. Without open spaces where abundant cooperative connections exist, entire generations of people will fail to experience the physical, emotional, and spiritual benefits of immersing themselves in nature. It is imperative that humans cease using convenience as a primary criterion for designing goods. Most manufacturers won't do this of their own accord for fear of losing revenue. This is why we need unselfish consumerism, a form of purchasing that considers other life (present and future) in the decision making process. If we refuse to purchase coffee from anything but shade-grown plantations, this will be the only way it is grown. If we stop purchasing single-use cups and pods, manufacturers will stop making them. The solution is actually quite easy, it comes down to only whether or not humans will make the decision to inform themselves and act mindfully.

PRODUCING FOOD WITHOUT CRUELTY AND ECOLOGICAL HARM

Try to imagine a life where you are detached from your mother prematurely, rarely experience sunlight on your skin, seldom (or never) feel the earth beneath your feet, and are fed a biologically inappropriate diet that ultimately leads to sickness and disease. This is the life of many domesticated food animals in affluent countries (and, if one were to think about it, the life of many domesticated humans as well). But it is much worse than this for some animals.

Factory farming (or industrial farming) is a form of husbandry that sees animals living the entire lives within the confines of tiny cages, standing or sleeping in their own feces, and being provided a highly unnatural diet that consists even of dead animals, recycled newspaper, and their own manure fed back to them. Animal mutilation, including such practices as removing tails and beaks (in the latter case with a heated metal tool), to deal with issues that arise when animals are not provided sufficient space, is an excellent indication of how little empathy modern humans have for other life (including the lives that sustain them). That cruelty exists on some farms is not anything that requires debate—it is an unfortunate reality that reflects very poorly on the people who practice, condone, and promote this method of food production.

There is a slowly growing awareness regarding the destructive and unkind practices of factory farming that considers life (plants or animals) merely as industrial outputs. But, as with many topics, there is abundant opportunity to broadly generalize in an inaccurate manner and condemn those who raise animals in a compassionate manner that is in-line with the animal's nutritional, social, and environmental needs. We will here focus primarily on animals because it is with these organisms that we need to address some persistent myths that are promulgated by those who have not critically thought about the arguments they present. While this immediately reads as standing in odds with a particular group of people (to be named shortly), I am very respectful of their decision not to participate in this this form of barbarism. What we must contend with is whether or not raising animals is destructive to the landscape and whether or not raising animals is a cruel practice that needs to be stopped entirely.

To begin, I will apologize for appearing to single out one of the few groups of people (vegans) who have made a stance and are actually doing something constructive to combat industrial farming practices. But what is not constructive (though a very common practice among vegans) is to attack people who consume animal foods but do not participate or support in any way cruel animal husbandry. The typical argument used is to find the worst form of factory farming and apply their observations of this system to all animal-raising systems and chastise people who eat from the animal kingdom. This is analogous to someone claiming they refuse to eat plants because some crops are transgenically modified (i.e., GMO) to allow a greater amount of glyphosate herbicide to be applied to them. While this is true of some plants, it is not characteristic of all cultivated species (and certainly not representative of wild plants). To consider all people that practice omnivory as supporting factory farming is a gross mischaracterization that disrespects both the consumers and the producers of humanely raised animals. So, to be very clear, I am thankful and commending of vegans for refusing to participate in the factory farming of animals. This form of food production needs to be stopped (yesterday). However, I do not agree with their assertion that all animal husbandry is characterized by human cruelty on other-than-human persons.

Clearly, the question that needs to be asked is this: is any form of animal husbandry humane? Asked another way: can human tenders treat domesticated animals compassionately and utilize methods that support their physical and emotional health until their lives are taken? The answer to both of these questions is a yes but, at present, only a minority of farms actually succeed in doing so. However, this is not a reason to abandon animal husbandry but a motive to better rearing practices across the globe. To examine what it would take to practice conscientious farming, let us first look at what are the needs of an animal (and I'm not just referring to survival but, rather, a healthy life that has elements of what similar animals in the wild would experience). Animals require space outdoors to roam, forage, browse, wander, interact, explore, rest, and move. They are like us in that they require lots of movement for health. Animals require clean water and biologically appropriate food. Such food is in-line with their evolutionary needs (e.g., cows graze on grasses and forbs, they do not eat solely grain) and should produce health and vitality throughout the lives of the animals so that medical intervention is rarely needed. Further, it should be free of contamination (which is to write that it should be wild or organically grown). Animals need members of their own species to socialize with, and this includes breeding and all the behaviors associated with it. They require shelter from the elements, including shade during the summer sun and structures to protect them from precipitation and keep them warm during the winter (all depending on the location and the animal in question). Animals deserve our gratitude. They also deserve a longer life than most are given and a death free of pain and emotional trauma.

Many people focus on the death of farm animals, and rightly so given how little empathy these living beings have been shown and the deplorable methods that have been used on them. However, it is completely possible to arrange a farm such that the killing of animals is without stress and without suffering. Let us look closer at this situation. As written by Sheldon Frith, there are essentially three manners that an animal in the wild or on the farm can die: a death without intervention, a death via non-human predators, and a death by human intervention. The first would include such deaths as old age, disease, starvation, and infection. Death by old age is extremely rare in the wild because animals weakened by age are generally targeted and killed by their natural predators. Animals that die slowly of disease and starvation experience a pretty horrible end to their life filled with significant pain and suffering. Death by non-human predators often involves fear from a chase and some suffering. While some deaths can be quick, others are prolonged as predators overcome the animals by wounds, bleeding, suffocation, or venom. In fact, some wild animals are even partially eaten while they are still alive. A death by human intervention can be one of the least traumatic ways to die—assuming that the human tender is attempting to create a peaceful death. Areas where animals are killed can be arranged to avoid items that cause them fear, such as ramps, dark interiors, loud machinery, and the site of other animals being killed. There exist several methods of killing that are quiet, without dramatic movement that would cause anxiety, and kill instantly (such as an air-powered piston-type gun that targets the brain). In fact, when all items are considered, it is possible for a death by human intervention to produce the least terror and suffering. If we are accepting of wild predators using claws and teeth to tear open their prey species, we should be comfortable with an instantaneous death by human intervention (it is, in actuality, much more gentle). This is not to judge or condemn the methods of wild predators or suggest that all animals should come under human care, only that if suffering is important to us, human intervention that is guided by empathy and gratitude can be non-traumatic.

Another farming topic that is often in the spotlight is the age when animals are killed. Many animals are taken when very young. For example, some chickens that are raised for meat are killed at six weeks of age. Pigs vary at the age of death but some farms do kill piglets that are less than 3 months old. Some calves are killed literally when they are days old for veal. While it is certainly true that wild predators often take young animals borne that year, domesticated animals are in our care and deserve some length of life. By allowing farm animals to live a life outdoors on ample range, socializing with animals of their own kind, and even having an opportunity to breed and raise young of their own, they would potentially experience more of their life than if they were wild animals (where they may be killed by their natural predators within hours or days after birth). Again, it is possible for human-tended animals to have longer lives that are without hunger, pain, or stress (all things wild animals experience). This all suggests (if not demonstrates) that humans raising animals can be an ethical way of producing food. Of course, people will need to shift some of their dietary habits to accept older farm animals as food. These animals present meats that may be less tender and have a stronger flavor. Of course, this is easily remedied by proper preparation, including slow cooking methods and marinating. For example, I occasionally acquire mutton (which is the meat from a sheep that is more than two years old) from a friend who raises sheep on an island off the coast of Maine. These social animals live in small flocks in a relatively wild setting without fences (i.e., they are free to roam over the entire island). Their diet consists entirely of wild plants (grasses, forbs, and seaweeds) and they are protected from the harsh climate by their thick wool coats. The meat from these free-range, older animals has a stronger taste than that of lamb (which is the meat from a sheep that is less than one year old). However, properly prepared, it can be made very flavorful, and I have served it to many guests who have come back for a second helping. While the lamb is preferred by most, the mutton is a more ethical choice because it provides the animals with a longer opportunity to experience life that would be relatively similar to the wild progenitor of the sheep (*Ovis orientalis*—mouflon).

Some animal activists would argue that all domesticated animals should be set free, permitting the domesticated animals from the farms to live wild lives again. This would, on the surface, appear to be the most ethical way to treat our farm animals—allowing them to live without the shackles of domestication. First, if you subscribe to the "free the animals" idea and own a pet, you are being a hypocrite (while I am being blunt, I am not intending to be rude here). Of course, many would state that their pet is not being kept against its will. I would argue that farm animals raised in a conscientious environment are also not kept against their will (it is only the death that is without consent—which is true of all lives that are consumed by other life). But, to continue this discussion, what would happen to your family dog if you let it go in a large wilderness area? Or how about if all the cows living in northern areas with abundant snowfall were not provided hay and silage over the winter season? What would happen to you (a domesticated human) if you were taken to an extensive uninhabited region without your human tenders? The fact is, most domesticated animals have lost either some of the faculties needed for survival in wild environments (similar to most humans) or have been raised in areas that are outside of their ancestral range, a place where they would still be somewhat adapted to the local environmental conditions. Domesticated animals that are released into the wild would largely die of painful deaths from injury, starvation, dehydration, or predation. While it is true that some domesticated animals become feral and rewild themselves when they escape (e.g., feral pigs in the southern United States and elsewhere, chickens in Hawaii, horses in the southwestern United States), these are exceptions, not the rule. Further, those animals that escape into natural communities often cause great damage to the landscape for a host of reasons (for a good example, research the harm caused to the forests, streams, and oceans caused by feral pigs in Hawaii). While some readers may consider these last paragraphs as hostile to their life views, I intend no disrespect (sincerely). Sometimes awareness creates grief and even anger.

Another issue that is often raised concerning animal farms is the harm caused to the landscape by the animals themselves. This appears as a very valid reason to stop all animal husbandry, although raising plants for human food is also destructive but is never considered to be something that should be stopped altogether. In other words, most everyone agrees that it is logical and ethical for humans to feed themselves in some manner. I, and others, would simply argue that we should be using best practices (which, usually, we are not). Given that growing plants is, on average, less harmful than raising animals as currently practiced, it is considered the path forward for greater ecological sanctity (when it is merely "less bad"). However, the idea that animals harm the landscape is, again, accurate only when we examine the usual practices in the United States and elsewhere. We are frequently told that animal rearing injures the soil, depletes and pollutes the water resources, and even contributes to climate change, a serious issue that threatens much of the life on this planet in some way. I'm in complete agreement that those practices should be immediately halted. However, they are not inherent features of animal lives (wild or domesticated). Further, it has been shown that proper animal rearing can even heal a landscape from trauma it has experienced in the past.

If one wants to make the assertion that large numbers of animals always harm the landscape in some manner, we might look to wild populations of some species of herbivores, such as the American bison (*Bison bison*) on the North American continent or the blue wildebeest (*Connochaetes taurinus*) on the African continent. These are animals that currently or formerly existed in massive herds of many thousands of animals together in one location, and with millions of animals collectively on the continent. Such species would have exerted a tremendous influence on their respective lands. What we see, though, is that such animals, in a wild setting, are quite beneficial to their ecosystems. These animals (and many other similar ones that we could mention) are often in a state of continuous movement, due to the temporary abundance of plants they consume and pressures from their natural predators. In these ways, the animals do not remain in place for a long period of time where they can overgraze a range, cause erosion, and pollute water sources with their dung. When they are present in an area, their hooves push the seeds of various plants into the soil (allowing for better germination) and push plant material into the soil, which breaks down more rapidly and (along with their manure) helps nourish the soil. The intense but short duration grazing actually stimulates plant and soil micro-organism growth, which is a major source for carbon sequestering (i.e., it stores carbon that would be emitted into the atmosphere as carbon dioxide). In fact, productive grasslands can sequester more carbon than forests, so long as they are grazed (otherwise, the growth stalls and decay becomes a major carbon source). Further, fungi that act in a symbiotic manner with range land plants (e.g., mycorrhizal fungi), also benefit from grazers and can sequester additional carbon.

Any discussion of climate change and pasturing of animals must include the topic of methane (CH_4). Methane is produced through the fermentation of forage plants by bacteria that reside in the digestive system of ruminant animals and is released into the air primarily through belching by the animals. This gas is of concern because it is a potent greenhouse gas—many times more potent than CO_2. Of note is that some species of soil bacteria called methanotrophs (or methane-oxidizing bacteria) utilize the methane produced by the grazing animals as a food source. Nearly all discussions of methane center on the production by grazing animals and not the bacteria within the grasslands that make use of methane. Rangelands are systems that have production and consumption components, yet people highlight only the production aspect of the system. This is analogous to generating fear through discussing all the water entering a lake but failing to mention the lake has an outlet that drains the inflowing water. Research demonstrates that methanotrophs make use of significant portions of the methane produced by ruminant animals (and some measurements have found the grasslands system to be a net zero source of methane). Further, there are strategies documented to reduce methane emissions, which can be integrated into animal husbandry practices. The quality of the forage is a major determining factor, and when animals are rotated onto fresh pasture (as would happen in the wild), methane emissions decrease. However, the number one way to reduce methane emissions from grazing animals is to cease factory farming. It relies extensively on fossil fuels (the number one source of methane emissions in the world), transports foods at great distances, and ultimately produces massive amounts of food waste (another major source of methane—Nicolette Niman notes that almost 40% of the food produced in the US in thrown away). Properly managed grassland systems aren't the problem—they've always existed with very large herds of methane-producing animals—it is the industry that we currently use to generate and transport food.

It can be shown that many grasslands and areas that have been converted to grasslands do much better with herbivore activity that mimics ecological patterns. The problem, of course, is that most animal husbandry does not even attempt to emulate such practices, which is to write that they do not try to mimic the cooperative connections between similar wild animals and range lands. The animals are confined and kept on a piece of property continuously. Further, they are not kept together by predators but spread out over an area and slowly degrade that setting (depending on the number of animals present). And while their numbers would not be harmful if they moved on in a natural migration, the fact that they are confined to one place means they produce so much waste that it ends up being a source of pollution (when it should be a source of nourishment to the plants). Continuous grazing and no grazing have some of the same effects—the composting and regeneration that is facilitated by the temporary presence of animals does not occur. Soil micro-organisms can be harmed by agricultural chemicals, which are very common in today's industrial farming, including the methanotrophic bacteria that can utilize methane and prevent it from exerting a greenhouse-gas effect. There is no doubt that animal farming practices need to change in the United States. What is healthier for the environment (including the soil, air, and water) is healthier for both us and the animals we raise.

While we could go on and on dealing with the issues and myths of animal farming, there is one additional item that is necessary for us to discuss. The idea goes as such: it requires more land to produce a pound of animal food than it does to produce a pound of plant food, so we should focus on producing plant foods (and feed more people). Given certain assumptions, this idea is generally true because herbivores do not convert the plant foods they eat into more of their own tissues at a 100% efficiency rate. Therefore, much of the plant matter ingested is lost in the conversion to animal matter. While aspects of this argument have already been dealt with in chapter 3 (in the section titled "the vegan assertion"), here, we will present additional information that is counter to this belief. For this idea to be true, it would mean that all land used for raising animals could be used to grow grain (for example) to feed people. And that is simply not the case. Nicolette Niman estimates that 85% of the land in the United States used to graze cattle is unsuitable for crop cultivation (i.e., is non-arable land). Therefore, land used for cattle grazing, especially in the western portion of the country, is not being taken away from growing grain for human consumption. Equally important is the fact that grazing animals on ranges do not require the land to be tilled (or plowed), which means that the soil biology remains intact, preserving moisture, symbiotic fungi, methanotrophs, and the carbon sequestering properties of the system itself. Considering the tremendous declines in large herbivores (e.g., American bison) in parts of the North American continent, open expanses of land can experience the beneficial effects of herds of animals using domesticated cows that are managed in a fashion that mimics wild herbivore populations.

Now, it may seem strange that I'm defending the rearing of domesticated animals in a book about the rewilding of humanity. However, there are several reasons why this section is important to a book of this kind. One, there are far too many inaccurate statements that need to be addressed and serve only to confuse the entire issue. Two, omnivory is one of the pillars of a nutrient-dense diet. Therefore, animal foods are necessary for the proper development of a healthy and well-formed human. Three, many people do not have access to wild animal foods, and domesticated animals raised in a conscientious manner can serve as an important source of animal nutrition. Four, people should be able to feed themselves with a diet that is biologically appropriate (which is omnivory). Five, there are several herder-gatherer cultures around the world that combined animal husbandry with foraging and have experienced health and beautiful form. Six, animal rearing can be done in a fashion that keeps landscapes intact or at least more intact than conversion to annual mono-cropping of cultivated plants (which can be highly injurious to the land and causes substantial declines in local biodiversity). Given that herds of animals of a million strong in water-stressed environments did not destroy the landscape nor exacerbate climate change issues, the problem we face is the method of animal husbandry, not the raising of animals itself. We, the consumers of animal products, need to drive the change to animal farming based on ecological principles. This is our responsibility as residents of the earth, to nurture health, not just in ourselves, but in the coming generations of people. To do this, we will need to realize we are intimately connected to our landscapes and the health they experience. Therefore, we need to stop imposing industrial methods on the land and start emulating wild patterns.

THE NEOABORIGINAL STRATEGY FOR MAKING GREEN CONSUMER CHOICES

Humans have shifted in a relatively short period of time from being organisms who gathered and crafted the items they need for living to people who purchase goods. We transitioned from being an integral part of the ecosystem to consumers, who have the capability to shelter or degrade ecosystems with their purchasing choices. And while it is likely that no industrially produced goods can save this planet (because they all exert an ecological tax), we can make significant differences in the quality of our air, water, and soil by simply changing what companies we support with our purchasing dollars. It can be shown, through examining our collective purchasing history, that people in affluent countries prize many things above the protection of ecosystems, including price, convenience, comfort, and perceived social effect. It is possible, through education, role modeling, and polite social pressure, to change all this so that other factors are considered more important (or at least equally important). We don't get there by judging others because this creates a defensive and often confrontational tone. Further, no one, including me, is doing everything in a perfect manner (if there is such a thing).

In order to facilitate social evolution in the market place, we need to become informed and pass this information on to our children. It needs to be part of the curriculum the next generation learns in the home (i.e., this isn't going to be taught at school, at least not to the level required for substantive change). We have spent too many generations allowing our elected officials, who receive legal bribes (in the form of campaign contributions) that sway their voting patterns, to watch out for our health and that of our landscapes. This method, of allowing our personal sovereignty to slowly dissolve and letting others stand in charge of our health, clearly isn't working. And following the actions of our friends and family, most of whom have not spent time to become informed, is not a genuine solution for health either. Remember, we have all been raised in a country that promotes a lifeway of amassing wealth and physical goods at the expense of the environment. The more one earns, the greater the success they are said to experience. We have glorified those who have the most, and, perhaps without realizing it, we are concurrently admiring the people who produce the most waste and pollution. Making matters worse, these are generally the people we have placed in the role of elected representatives (most members of the Senate and the House of Representatives would be described as wealthy and experience privilege many other Americans do not). Therefore, change will not only require individuals to evolve but also our concept of "success" and who we decide will make decisions on our behalf. While some would state no one is their master, like it or not, people are making decisions that affect the ecological sanctity of the world we live in.

Taking clues from hunter-gatherers, we see that across cultures, amassing material goods were not considered the goal of life for the original humans. They led overall happy, contented lives with more leisure time than most people in industrialized countries experience, and never needed to import goods from other continents or worry about climbing a social ladder based on the clothing they chose to wear. They let their deeds demonstrate the qualities of their person, not the products they owned that were manufactured by other peoples in a distant land. However, we view these wild people as poor, impoverished, and underprivileged, never realizing that we are viewing their lives through a highly biased lens. As Marshal Sahlins notes in his article "The Original Affluent Society":

"Consumption is a double tragedy: what begins in inadequacy will end in deprivation. Bringing together an international division of labour, the market makes available a dazzling array of products: all these Good Things within a man's reach, but never all within his grasp. Worse, in this game of consumer free choice, every acquisition is simultaneously a deprivation of something else only marginally less desirable or perhaps more desirable. This sentence of 'life at hard labour' was passed uniquely on us. Scarcity is the judgment decreed by our economy. From our anxious vantage point we look back on hunters. Having equipped the hunter with bourgeois impulses and palaeolithic tools, we judge his situation hopeless in advance."

Of course, hunter-gatherers did not have such impulses (to amass material goods). Too many possessions were an encumbrance, especially because they impeded mobility (which directly related to the freedom of hunter-gatherers). As a result, they simply never got caught up in the continual pursuit of material acquisition, and as a result of this, lived the least destructive lives humans have ever lived. Marshal Sahlins points out that:

"Hunter-gatherers consume less energy per person yearly than any other group of human beings. Yet the original affluent society was none other than the hunter's, where all people's material wants were easily satisfied. To accept hunters as affluent is also to recognise the tragedy of modern times in the current human condition with people slaving to bridge the gap between unlimited wants and insufficient means."

At some point, we will need to state that enough is enough. We need to change our current paradigm of pursuing the fulfillment of unnecessary material wants. We will also need to stop focusing on small reductions in pollution, where we exalt products that produce 10% less waste. We will need to stop focusing on regulation to alter industry's path because regulation is an admission of failure—there would be no need to regulate emissions if those emissions were non-toxic. We are going to need to incorporate attributes of cultures that focus on long-term existence. Until that time, here are ten ways the neoaboriginal can modify their consumer habits.

1. **Become informed**. This is one of the most powerful tools for preventing ecological devastation and protecting future generations. Modern humans make far too many assumptions about their respective societies and the goods they produce and use. An aware human will make substantive changes to their daily living because they realize it benefits them, their local landscapes, and ecosystems they may never visit in their lifetime.

2. **Determine if you really need the product**. The purpose of a modern human's life is not to fill the largest home they can afford with physical goods. Members of affluent countries purchase so many unnecessary items, many of which are fragile or otherwise poorly constructed and end up in landfills within days or weeks. At some point, we are going to need to derive

happiness not from consuming the world's resources but through engaging with our human and wild communities.

3. Whatever you do choose to purchase, **acquire quality versions**. Seek out durable sorts that last as long as possible. This may mean you can't buy an entire home set immediately, and that is perfectly fine. Items that last generations do the world much less harm than a comparable item that lasts a decade.

4. **Reuse** as your first line of defense against single-use, disposable products. This requires a willingness to carry a mug, a bowl, and utensils with you as you travel for work, education, or pleasure, similar to the call to bring a cloth shopping bag along when you visit the supermarket. It's not a big request, and it robs companies that produce throw-away items of their revenue, which will force them to transition to more ecoconcientious goods.

5. When at all possible, direct purchases to goods that are **dispensable or concentrated**. Dispensable goods include some home cleaning products and foods, both of which can be distributed into reusable containers and bags brought from home. The next best option is concentrated goods, which require tiny amounts or are diluted at home. Dispensable and concentrated products produce, over the long run, many fewer containers that ultimately end up in landfills.

6. **Buy local** is a real strategy for promoting health in a community. It isn't merely a manner of reducing the long-distance transportation of goods. Acquiring products from local growers and manufacturers promotes community resiliency through financially supporting people who produce what you need for living. It is also easier for you to gain first-hand knowledge of their activity, making their production practices more transparent (and likely more in line with human and ecological health regulations).

7. **Transition away from synthetic ingredients** in your clothing, home construction, cleaning supplies, hygiene products, and so on. Even when used as directed, these chemicals are exerting an array of effects, especially on younger people and those who live near where these products are grown or manufactured. One strategy in the reformatting of our entire system of production and transition from cradle to grave to cradle to cradle technologies is to move toward natural, non-toxic, and biodegradable components. That way, when a shirt reaches the end of its life, it can become soil that nourishes the growth of food, medicine, or raw materials.

8. **Support conscientious and ecology-based animal husbandry** that places an appropriate number of animals on the landscape, uses rotational grazing, relies less on cultivated grains, and promotes a productive landscape through following ecological principles (rather than using agricultural chemical inputs). Animals raised in these conditions are healthier for us to eat and support the ecology of the range lands.

9. **Purchase products that are priced accurately**. Companies that sell inexpensive products because they externalize significant portions of the true costs of growing or manufacturing the good should not be supported. Frankly, these are selfish companies that do not have community interests in mind. Such practices, as epitomized by coal, factory farming, hydraulic fracturing ("fracking"), and oil sands extraction, are socially irresponsible because they cause significant harms that they do not pay for.

10. Have **gratitude** for the amazing array of choices available to people in affluent countries. The large selection of products is not a birthright or an entitlement; it is the result of fortune of birthplace or immigration. Because of our choices, we have the capacity to encourage less harmful manufacturing processes, and this is something that all people, urban and rural, can contribute to.

12. Primitive technologies: becoming self-reliant

Primitive technologies, or perhaps better referred to as ancestral lifeways, are the collection of techniques, methods, and material items used by hunter-gatherers for living in their location through the seasons. These were place-based technologies, using the natural materials found and procured around them, which were fashioned into tools, containers, hunting weapons, cordage, clothing, shelters, and so on. While the term "primitive" carries a negative connotation today, these are, in certain cases, complex skill sets requiring years to understand, implement, and transfer to the next generation. Therefore, here (and throughout this book) primitive refers to the archetypal (i.e., the original form). The advantages of these technologies are many, including that they allow true self-reliance, freedom from domestication (and any other forms of subjugation), and are truly sustainable practices when used in the context of Traditional Ecological Knowledge and Wisdom. But more than this, they are part of each and every person on this planet, having been practiced by the ancestors of every living human. Our physical form has been shaped by the ancestral technologies that were employed prior to appearance of agriculture. Further, our ability to form complex thoughts and even communicate through oral language has been molded by the crafting of tools that demanded a specialized set of techniques (grammar), detailed understanding of the process (vocabulary). and a specific order of steps (syntax). While contemporary humans have largely forgotten the very tools that allowed us to be successful in our natural environments, we are a species that is healthiest when we use our original skills, and our landscapes benefit as well.

THE ORIGINAL AFFLUENCE

Affluence in the modern world is tied to wealth. Through wealth, one is able to satisfy their needs and abate some of their wants through the purchase of goods and services. Wealth also has the potential to liberate a person from the continual financial burden of living in a society where costs, payments, taxes, mortgages, fees, and fines are found at every turn. But for many, wealth also produces additional problems because it generates greater and greater wants—the more money one has, the more possible it is to acquire luxury items, additional vehicles, vacation homes, and similar such items that produce additional prestige. This constant inability to satiate material desire is an erosive force for a person's sense of contentment. Financial affluence can never heal the wound created by insatiability, a wound that was formed early in life when every holiday and right-of-passage was taught to be a new opportunity for material gain. We have created a society filled with people who produce little of what they need and desire much. Further, this form of affluence, which is shaped by a person's social environment, is tied to a society that can experience deep troubles with its economic institutions. It is a kind of affluence that can disappear (when money loses its value and becomes nothing more than paper and coin), and there are situations where even wealthy people can be at risk of starvation.

The original affluence was much different. It resided within people. It was a practice of producing all the necessary items for living and wanting very little (in the way of material possessions). Rather than seeking the temporary decline in desire for material things produced through a new purchase, ancestral humans sought the wholeness of spirit found by connecting with their communities (social and ecological). Ture affluence is an ability to satisfy our wants. Hunter-gatherers possessed the most highly advanced form of affluence because they were able to satisfy their wants anywhere they travelled within their homeland. They did this without bringing along vast amounts of supplies or travelling with cutting-edge, lightweight, backpacking gear. They possessed an ecological skillset that allowed them to procure food and the other items necessary for living. This is perhaps best explained by Elizabeth Thomas in her book "The Old Way", where she was part of a team that entered the Kalahari region to live among the Ju/wasi. Her team required massive amounts of equipment. This included gear for sleeping and sitting (e.g., tents, cots, sleeping bags, folding chairs). They needed tools for orienteering (e.g., compass, maps). They were travelling in a vehicle; therefore, they needed to be able to deal with repairs and refueling (e.g., spare tires, inner tubes, tire patches, jacks, toolboxes, auto parts, winches, motor oil, gasoline). They needed to carry with them the items that would protect them from the elements (e.g., pants, sneakers, boots, underwear, shirts, socks). The list goes on and on (e.g., sewing kit, rifle, bullets, scissors, safety pins, reading glasses, soap, washcloths, toothpaste, water, utensils, cooking equipment, dry food, canned food, disinfectants, antivenom for snakebites, notebooks, pencils). The list included essentially everything they used. These items had to be carried with them because they could not create them from the landscape. In contrast, the Ju/wasi they spent time with carried very little—sticks, skins, eggshells, and grass.

Most people in the modern world consider hunter-gatherers as poor because, in large part, they have so few possessions. Clearly, this is examining wild people through a highly biased lens, a civilized lens where more possessions equal greater wealth. Given that hunter-gatherers spent less time at work than we do (3–6 hours, on average, spent each day toward food procurement), it is clear that they were not routinely experiencing scarcity (if they were hungry, they would have spent more time trying to locate food). While city builders would consider them to be in a state of dire poverty because of their few possessions, hunter-gatherers actually experienced greater nutrition than most people alive today. It is estimated that 1 in 8 people in the world are experiencing chronic hunger and malnutrition (with this figure reaching 1 in 5 on some continents; figures from The State of Food Security in the World, 2015). Given this, one could assert that, as a whole, human affluence has actually decreased. Poverty, and the resulting inability to secure nourishment, is a social position that was invented by society. The intrinsic inequality produced by society was not experienced by hunter-gatherers. If we define affluence as an ability to satisfy your wants, then indigenous people experienced a greater degree of affluence and more equal affluence than we do.

With the original affluence, humanity had so much, but we have lost most of it. We are convinced that our technological supremacy is a major step forward, unwilling to admit that it has resulted in a form of enslavement. Without an ability to do for ourselves, we are completely dependent on our income-producing activity and, when it is lost (as sometimes happens when we become unemployed), there is tremendous stress because we no longer can feed ourselves and may lose some of our possessions (which is a concurrent loss of prestige). The lure of industrial technology is very seductive. But an objective view would show it to be a trap. While a given task might be more easily accomplished with some machine, we must work more hours each day to pay for the machine, its maintenance, a way to transport it, and a building to house it in. But, the penalties of industrial technology are more than just lost free time. As Miles Olson noted[10]:

> "Every succeeding level of technology creates a further disconnect, with a simultaneous increase in power, control and efficiency—a troublesome combination. You can dig a hole much faster with a shovel than your hands, but you no longer feel the soil. You can cut a tree down much faster with a saw than stone tools, with a chainsaw than a hand saw, and with a feller-buncher than a chainsaw. In every stage the person doing the cutting becomes more removed from the process, more alienated from the individual tree that is being cut. You kill faster, feel less."

---

[10] Miles Olson. 2012. Unlearn, Rewild. New Society Publishers, British Columbia, Canada.

There is little doubt that each increment of technological sophistication is accompanied by an increment of separation from nature (and all that ensues from that increase in separation).

We (as a species) used to use our creative talents to construct beneficial and beautiful items from natural materials. Today, we have nearly lost that ability, to the degree that we often can't even mend clothing that has developed a tear. Instead, we shop. But while this may temporarily feed the need for creating, it falls short in its ability to satisfy our longings and promotes consumerism that harms the planet's life. It is entirely possible for people to recapture the gratification that comes from crafting for one's self. It goes beyond the joy of purchasing because it represents more than just a novel item; it fundamentally embodies self-reliance. The ability to create the things we need from our landscape is the ultimate freedom. The more we are capable of doing, the more freedom we experience. We can return to a previous level of technology, even if in only some aspects of our life. Such a move is not a step backward, but a journey forward into autonomy. It imparts a greater degree of connection to the life and other materials involved in the activity. Further, it means that we do not need to support industry in those realms within which we have gained an ancestral expertise. Humans are amazing creators of useful tools and attractive objects. It was the reason we were so successful at living in our place. We can enjoy that original affluence again. It requires a return to our roots and a retrieval of our traditions. Remember, as Gustav Mahler wrote (or some variation thereof):

"tradition is not the worship of ashes, but the preservation of fire."

BECOMING A STEWARD OF FIRE

While there are many unique aspects of the ecology of *Homo sapiens*, perhaps none is as striking and important as the ability to produce and control fire. While there are many species adapted to ecosystems that experience fire, no other animals can create it where none exists, maintain its combustion for long periods of time, and even intentionally transport embers from one place to another to rekindle the fire. There is nowhere on earth where and no time in the history of the human species when fire was not used for some very important purpose. The use of fire continues today, though, like many aspects of modern living, humans are separated from this natural element. It powers our vehicles, it generates electricity, and it shapes the products we use in daily living. But we do not kindle it, tend it, or extinguish it—this takes place remotely through the use of chemical reactions or electric currents, the pushing of buttons, and the turning of keys. We are separated from the fire, and most have lost the ability to steward this magnificent resource without the use of industrial technology. Fortunately, there are those who keep the skill of creating fire alive, who teach people how to caretake this transformative force. The story of fire, told briefly in chapter 3 (How Fire Has Shaped Us), is continued and expanded here.

First and foremost, fire is a tool. We primarily think of it as a way to warm our homes and cook our food. And while fire is certainly those things, it is so much more than these to wild humans. The heat of fire can shape materials into tools, such as wood for making a hunting bow with curved limbs. It can liquefy material for ease of mixing or application, such as resin and other mastics and water-proofing agents. It can soften material to allow better extraction, such as plant roots for use in a medicinal tea. It is capable of transforming materials into something new, such as clay to an earthenware pot. Fire can also be used to create smoke, for smudging shelters and living spaces to drive away insect pests. The fact that it can be used to keep a domicile within a livable temperature during extreme weather, detoxify foods through killing potential pathogens in and on the nourishments, and reduce or eliminate various toxins and antinutrients simply adds to its incredible value to humanity.

Fire was also an important social and cultural tool. It was the meeting place on cold evenings, where people gathered to share cooked foods, and where stories were told to the next generation. While replaced today by the television, fire kindled imagination and stimulated the use of creativity. This is in stark contrast to the television, which fills the head with already formed images and obviates the need to recreate stories from only the words, facial expressions, hand gestures, and tone of the story teller (i.e., we took the art of storytelling and gave it away to film makers). Fire was a rallying point that brought together the generations and provided safety from the elements, from large predators, and from the apparitions that walked at night. It was a center of the community and the flammable gases that were burned in their bright displays captured the attention of humans then, just as they are capable of doing today.

Around the world, indigenous and traditional people had time-proven methods of generating fire in a place. The methods usually involved the use of friction (though percussion methods were also used that relied on various chalcedony stones struck against marcasite to generate a spark). While it is often described as "rubbing two sticks together", the creation of fire by friction is more accurately described as spinning, sawing, or plowing one piece of plant material on a stationary piece of plant material. These movements generate heat from friction and also abrade away heated plant dust (called char), which collects in a notch or hole and gathers enough heat to ignite (i.e., pyrolysis). Once a glowing ember has been formed, the ember can be transferred to tinder (a dry, often fibrous, material that readily ignites with low heat) and coaxed into flame through the use of wind or, more commonly, human breath. There are innumerable variations on the friction fire theme, each one being adapted to the particular environment that the hunter-gatherers resided within. Some of those variations are described below.

One of the most widely used methods of friction fire around the world was and is the hand drill. This is also one of the simplest methods of creating an ember because it consists of only two parts: a long, slender, relatively straight spindle and a short section of branch or board called the hearth board (or sometimes the fire board). The spindle is spun between the palm of the hands as the hands slide down the spindle to create downward pressure. Once reaching the bottom of the spindle, the hands are reset near the top and continue to spin the spindle. To watch someone skilled with the hand drill is deceptive because it appears very easy to perform (though nearly everyone who tries is astonished at its difficulty to perform repeatedly, especially in different weather conditions). Most of those people who use this method carve a small notch in the socket where the spindle meets the fireboard to allow for an accumulation of the char (and the heat). The choice of plant materials is of paramount importance for friction fire methods because different materials ignite at different temperatures. This is especially true of the hand drill method, where it is the person's strength and technique that allows the spindle to spin on the hearth board at sufficient speed and pressure to generate enough friction to create an ember through pyrolysis. The spindle is frequently made from a stalk of an herbaceous plant with a pithy interior, though woody species were sometimes used as well. The hearth board is made from relatively soft woods, the pithy stalks of yuccas, the midrib of palm leaves, and similar materials. For example, the Tübatulabal people of southern California used the stalk of Douglas' false willow (*Baccharis glutinosa*) for the spindle and the root wood of Fremont's cottonwood (*Populus fremontii*) for the hearth board. In my part of the world (northeastern North America), I use several different combinations of plants, most often employing Canada fleabane (*Erigeron canadensis*) for the spindle and the wood of northern white cedar (*Thuja occidentalis*) for the hearth board. No doubt that this method was invented while drilling through materials to make a hole, where the resulting heat from friction accidentally created an ember and was eventually understood well enough to intentionally make fire when it was needed.

In some portions of the world, weather and other conditions required a greater ability to generate friction, especially through the use of a handhold that could be pressed down onto the twirling spindle to produce the necessary heat. Enter the bow drill, a more complicated friction fire device that can be used to produce an ember even in the regions of extreme cold and humidity. A small bow was used with enough slack in the bow string to wrap the cord around the spindle, providing a method of spinning the spindle much faster than the hands can accomplish through moving the bow back and forth by a push and pull motion. A handhold with a socket, made most often from bone, stone, or wood, held the spindle in place and applied the downward pressure to create friction against the hearth board as it spun. Sometimes, as in the northern North America cultures, the handhold was replaced by a mouthhold, which would then allow the hearth board (or the item being drilled) to be held off the ground and kept dry by the free hand (with the entire fire-making apparatus usually stabilized on the knee or some other surface). A wide range of materials (again) have been used for the bow drill. I prefer the woods of balsam fir (*Abies balsamea*), northern white cedar, and American linden (*Tilia americana*), in that order, for constructing the spindle and hearth boards of the bow drill.

There are many other versions of friction fire methods used around the world. The pump drill, which utilized a counterweight to keep a spindle spinning during the reset of the handle, was used by the Penobscot natives of Maine (and many other groups around the world). The fire saw (different variations), which used a piece of plant material such as a shaped stick or a piece of bamboo moved back and forth quickly over a stationary piece with a groove, was used in parts of southwest Asia and Australia. There were even flexible materials that were fashioned into a thong, such as species of climbing palm known as rattan, to saw back and forth on a stationary piece (the fire thong, as used in southeast Asia). Some of these devices were made beforehand, others were fashioned on the spot. Some were bulky (like some versions of the fire saw made from bamboo), others were compact and easily carried (like the strap drill of northern North America).

Much as with food, hunting weapons, and so on, friction fire methods were specific to each place because they used different techniques and different materials (i.e., different species of plants) to accomplish creating fire in their place. The use of friction fire methods is simply another way people connect to their landscapes and their ancestry. The stewardship of fire is an essential skill for wild living. It is a skill that is perishable and must be maintained due to the coordination and endurance needed for the individual methods. Therefore, I use friction fire (most often the hand drill, but also the bow drill and other methods) to start the fires at my home, whether it is an outdoor fire for cooking or smoking hides, or an indoor fire for heating the home. Through avoiding the use of a butane lighter or matches, I maintain a skill and use local materials that were not produced through industry and distributed by long-distance transportation. When the materials have served their purpose, they can be discarded in the forest because they are 100% biodegradable, and came from that setting to begin with. This is similar to many other ancestral technologies in that they do not pollute the landscape through their creation, use, or discarding.

Important "Print Elders" on the topic of fire:

Primitive Technology: A Book of Earth Skills, chapter 2, edited by David Wescott (1999, Gibbs Smith Publisher)
Naked into the Wilderness: Primitive Wilderness & Survival Skills, chapter 2, by John and Geri McPherson (1993, Prairie Wolf)

SHELTER FROM THE ELEMENTS

Of the many contrasting technologies between hunter-gatherers and city builders, one of the most conspicuous is the home. It is not merely the size and materials that comprise the shelter, but even the very social meaning of the shelter is drastically different between these two groups of people. The hunter-gatherer shelters were generally quite small (by modern standards), built entirely of natural materials, and did not afford different levels of prestige between different people because the shelters were largely similar within a particular band (i.e., even those considered to be respected elders or sachems did not have shelters fundamentally different from those of anyone else in the community). Today, homes of people in affluent countries would be considered massive, are almost always built with some materials that are synthetic and harmful to human health, and the larger and more expensive they are, the more status they afford. A home was a place to shelter the family, it is now that and also a place to showcase one's belongings. But beyond these differences, there is a fundamental change that has occurred in the past century: essentially no one in an affluent country can build the homes they live in. While you may dispute this because contractors "build" homes all the time, those contractors use materials such as particle board, vinyl siding, polymer flooring, glass windows, and the like that they did not construct (industry did). They merely purchased these factory goods and assembled them. Assembling is not the same as building, though today we consider home assemblers to be home builders.

As has been mentioned with other indigenous technologies, homes and shelters varied around the world according to the materials available, the prevailing environmental conditions, and the people who constructed them. They also varied in the permanence, with some shelters designed for a short duration (i.e., days), with others meant to last several seasons. From a very basic standpoint, shelters need to create a bubble of habitable environment that the humans within them can withstand without expending too many calories to stay warm or remain cool. This usually means that huts and other small homes need to shield inhabitants from wind, divert precipitation around them, and be able to remain warm (or cool) to prevent hypo- or hyperthermia. Shelters also provide protection from biting insects and intense sunlight, and afford emotionally safe locations where people can find solace from the hazards in their environment or culture. Because most indigenous groups were nomadic, most shelters could be constructed in a relatively short period of time or could be dismantled and transported to a new location. The former method was the most widely used strategy for shelter; therefore, most hunter-gatherers had a relatively small investment in their homes, with most non-mobile homes being constructed in the span of hours or days (with some exceptions, such as bark long houses, which involved a greater investment in time). Consider the investment by most Americans—a thirty-year mortgage taking 17–25% of the household income for younger adults (17–34 years old; according to the Bureau of Labor Statistics, 2013). This means that many Americans are spending 442–650 days (of wage labor) to pay for their home (actually, because many homes have two adults contributing, it is twice these figures in wage-days). On top of this, American homes are increasing in size (according to the Census Bureau), with new homes built in 1983 averaging 160 square meters of floor space. However, over the span of 30 years, there was an increase in home size of 50%, with the average new home having 241 square meters of floor space. This compares with the average indigenous shelter of approximately 19 to 76 square meters (which would be a radius of 8 to 16 feet for more or less circular shelters). While this is not a suggestion for all people to raise their families in a tee-pee (though I know people who have), perhaps we can find a middle of the road approach where homes are significantly smaller and cost much less to build, heat, cool, illuminate, and maintain. To do this, members of affluent countries will need to make several adjustments, including caring much less about what others think of the size of their homes.

Returning to indigenous shelters, there are many variations that can be found on a single continent. Considering just North America, there are a diversity of indigenous homes that were found in use at and for some time after European colonization. In many temperate parts of the continent, bark was peeled from trees in large sheets and placed over a frame made of sapling trees. Shapes varied by groups, ranging from conical frames with a pointed apex to hooped frames with a domed apex. The bark was secured to the frame by various methods (e.g., direct lashing, pinning between inner and outer poles) and formed a kind of natural sheet shingling that kept the inhabitants warm and dry. The Passamaquoddy and Penobscot of Maine were documented to have used a variety of tree barks, though paper birch (*Betula papyrifera*) was the most common covering for their shelter and is completely waterproof. The Ojibwa of the Great Lakes region similarly used several different trees, sometimes using the bark of American elm (*Ulmus americana*). Woven mats of soft bark or various robust, grass-like plants or the branches of evergreen trees often were placed on the floor for comfort and insulation from the ground. Woven mats were also secured to the interior walls by some groups to form a double wall that would hold heat longer during the cold season. This shelter was called a wikuwam (in Passamaquoddy), giving rise to the English wigwam.

There were many types of indigenous shelters found around the world. In the warmer and drier parts of the world (though certainly not limited to those regions), conical or hooped shelters called wickiups were often constructed (the name of this shelter derived from Native American words, such as the Meskwaki word "wiikiyaapi"). These shelters provided shade from the mid-day sun and protected against wind and precipitation. They often differed from the wigwams in that they were not covered by broad sheets of bark, rather they were created by layering grasses, branches, poles, narrow strips of bark, or slabs of dead trees upon the frames. Examples of this shelter come from the Miwok of northern California and the !Kung of the Kalahari region of Africa. The thípi (often spelled tipi in English) of the Great Plains of North America, as exemplified by those of the Apsáalooke and Lakota, was a mobile version of shelter that consisted of bison hides stretched over a framework of lodge poles. This shelter could be disassembled in a short period of time and had smoke flaps near the summit to allow for the use of fire within it. Further to the north, shelters made of blocks of wind-packed snow were used by the Inuit. This famous shelter, the iglu (or igloo in English), varied in its size, with some built for temporary use (e.g., hunting trips) and others constructed for longer periods of habitation (e.g., family dwelling). Wherever indigenous people lived in the world, whether it be the frozen lands of the north or the rain forests of the equator, hunter-gatherers had shelters that protected them from the elements and offered a protective space from which to recuperate, socialize, and prepare for the coming day. In all cases, the shelter reflected the wild humans' interaction with their landscape and was part of their ancestral skill set.

One of the most easily constructed and versatile shelters that can be used for camping and other short-term wild living is the debris hut. This shelter functions not only as the weatherproof covering over a person but also the insulation that keeps them warm. In brief, the debris hut is a relatively small shelter made by propping a ridgepole on something sturdy and leaning against the ridgepole a latticework of sticks, brush, bark, or whatever to support leaves and other debris from the forest floor. The leaves and debris are heaped upon this supporting material to create a deep layer of protection that sheds water and wind and holds heat from the human body. The interior of the shelter, made only slightly broader than the human sleeping within it, is stuffed with dry debris that functions as padding and insulation (much like the filling of a sleeping bag). This shelter has a much lower time commitment, and it is possible to construct one when materials are present in 3–6 hours. This shelter provides an introduction to personal lodging and can be maintained for years if desired. It is deceptively simple—there are some important details that must be incorporated to ensure it will protect from low temperatures and heavy precipitation (this is where finding a competent primitive living skills school will be valuable).

Important "Print Elders" on the topic of shelters:

Wigwam: Building the Traditional Northeastern Domed Shelter by Jeffrey Gottlieb, (2007, self-published)
Primitive Technology: A Book of Earth Skills, section 1, edited by David Wescott (1999, Gibbs Smith Publisher)
Survival Skills of Native California, part 1, by Paul Campbell (1999, Gibbs Smith Publisher)

CONTAINERS AND COOKING VESSELS FROM THE LANDSCAPE

One of the most important skill sets that is virtually lost from modern civilizations is an ability to create containers (of various kinds) from natural materials. These important items are so vital to our living, and yet we rarely even consider them because industry has made bags, sacks, bowls, baskets, cooking pots and pans, plastic containers, bottles, and jugs always available (even as trash on our landscapes). Our drinks come in plastic and glass bottles. Our cut vegetables and butchered meats are wrapped in a thin, translucent plastic wrap that acts as a small container. The fruits we buy (especially the smaller ones) are very often also wrapped in plastic or held within cardboard containers. When we cook, it is generally within a metal container of some kind placed on a modern range top or a plastic container within a microwave. If we cook outdoors, then the food is wrapped in a temporary container of aluminum foil (which often becomes part of the waste stream after a single use). If we harvest from the garden, it can go in a plastic bag, in a plastic bowl, or even a plastic bucket—all made by industry and all ultimately ending up in a landfill with consequences for people who are yet unborn. Despite the ubiquitous use and importance to us, we simply have lost an ability to create effective containers for ourselves. This is especially true when it comes to containers that can hold liquid and be heated (in some fashion) for cooking, sterilizing water, or creating steam for wooden tool shaping.

Because containers of some kind are easy to secure in the modern marketplace, we rarely consider how vital this knowledge is for wild living. Or, for that matter, even a nature-connected living that seeks to make more of the things we use in the home. Many natural containers can be made through non-lethal collection of plant material or the gathering of clay, steatite (also called soapstone), and shells. And when these containers have served their use (which can be a decade or more for some kinds), they can be discarded almost anywhere because they are made of materials that are non-toxic and, for many kinds, completely biodegradable. For example, a bark bowl that I will use for many years can be placed on the forest floor or in my compost pile and will be completely gone in a few seasons. Its breakdown will nourish the growth of new life in the forest, the field, or even the garden. Despite these obvious advantages, many consider ancestral life skills as having no worth in the modern era, often using poor logic like "because the entire world doesn't have access to such natural materials for containers, it won't matter in the end". This is comparable to saying "because some communities don't have access to organically grown food, we shouldn't strive to grow any food in this manner". Clearly, such rationale isn't particularly sound because movements start small and grow larger. Initially, individuals and families benefit by altering their practices, paving the way for communities and larger segments of society. In this case, those who do not use the products of industrial technology create less landfill waste and can keep themselves clean of polymer food contamination (i.e., leaching). Further, those families and communities that readily engage in creating objects from their wild landscapes further their own self-reliance, detaching from industry a little bit more.

One way that the topic of containers can be approached is to examine the materials they will be constructed from (e.g., grasses, branches, bark, clay, wood, stone). We can also study them from the perspective of how they will be used, which I generally think of as having two major categories: containers that can hold liquids, such as water, and those that cannot (i.e., they can hold solid objects, materials that clump together). Most of the containers that can hold water can be cooked in, and they can be further subdivided into those that can be heated directly over a fire or embers and those that must be heated indirectly (through placing heated stones within the liquid they hold). With these three categories in mind—non-watertight, directly heated watertight, indirectly heated watertight—let us briefly examine some useful container designs for those wishing to connect with their ancestral heritage and live more softly in their place.

There are abundant varieties of non-watertight containers. These include baskets that are woven into a tight pattern using flexible branches and shoots. Many hunter-gatherer groups around the world used woody plants with supple growth, as well as the shoots of species of rush (genus *Juncus*) and similar plants that have long, straight, unbranched stems that work well for basketry. Most of these forms of containers were made by using some material as a frame (warp, the passive supports) around which other branches and shoots were woven (weft, that which is actively interlaced). Highly functional, these containers could also be made exquisitely beautiful through the use of different weaving patterns (e.g., twining, twilling) and through contrasting-colored materials. Given that woven containers have so many junctions between the materials, they rarely were made to be water-tight (though some versions were). Likewise, several species of trees have bark that can be peeled during the growing season and can be shaped into different kinds of buckets and bowls. The seams were often stitched together using the roots of conifer species (which are strong and very flexible). Bark buckets are a frequent type of container I use for foraging. The inner bark forms a layer that is impermeable to moisture, helping shoots, leaves, and roots to maintain their moisture and avoid desiccation (similar to a plastic bag, but without the endocrine-disrupting chemicals).

Water-tight containers can be made from a range of materials. Tree bark can be folded in such a way as to avoid any seams that would leak water. As well, bark can be stitched into a bucket or bowl and the seams sealed with some kind of mastic (such as resin from conifer trees mixed with tallow or beeswax, for flexibility, and tempered with wood ash or ground charcoal, for strength—there are other versions of natural adhesives available). Such containers can be used for cooking by heating stones in the fire and placing the heated stones within the water in the bark bucket. The heated stones transfer the heat to the water allowing the user to cook whatever is needed.

Containers that can be directly placed on the heat source are more convenient (similar to modern pots and pans). Clay and steatite pots can be used for this type of cooking or they can be used as a normal bowl for eating. While steatite is merely carved into shape for use, clay requires a more elaborate and nuanced approach for use. Clay items must be mixed with temper (an added material to control cracking during firing), shaped, and fired, the firing process altering the material so that it is rigid and resistant to dampening by water. Wood-fired clay pots can be made relatively thin, making them easier to manipulate than a stone bowl. Clay vessels are a relatively new technology for humans. The oldest earthenware pots are about 20,000 years old (found in China), though they did not appear in North America until about 4500 years ago. However, in that time, pottery was developed into an amazing art form and was vitally important for some American cultures. The Pueblo Cultures and the Diné were groups that formed exquisite pottery that was used for cooking and storage, though earthenware pots were found throughout most of North America (including the arctic). Handmade, wood-fired clay pots represent some of the most outstanding and useful natural containers, though they do require care to prevent breakage.

Containers made from natural materials are another segment of ancestral lifeways that provides empowerment to those who invest the time to learn these skills. There are many kinds that can be made, including several not discussed here, (e.g., carving and sanding wooden bowls and plates). While some forms of containers appear, at first, very complicated or requiring substantial time commitments, like any art form, they can be approached with simpler designs and smaller projects until some expertise is gained in the topic. And for those who are unable to make such products, purchasing or trading for these items ultimately is better for the world because they are non-polluting. The main concern about containers is that the raw materials are collected in a responsible manner. Given that many kinds of containers are made from living plants, these need to be gathered in a sustainable manner and gratitude offered for their gifts. Remember, all humans have ancestors who created functional and beautiful natural containers. It is a memory that can be awakened simply by locating the right mentor.

Important "Print Elders" on the topics of baskets, buckets, and pots:

Baskets from Nature's Bounty by Elizabeth Jensen (1991, Interweave Press)
Handmade Baskets From Nature's Colourful Materials by Susie Vaughan (1994, Search Press)
Primitive Pottery by Hal Riegger (2001, Gentle Breeze Publishing)
How to Make Primitive Pottery by Evard Gibby (1994, Eagle's View Publishing)
Primitive Technology II: Ancestral Skills, section 3 of this work, edited by David Wescott (2001, Gibbs Smith Publisher)
Naked into the Wilderness: Primitive Wilderness & Survival Skills, chapters 7 and 8, by John and Geri McPherson (1993, Prairie Wolf)

BINDING THE WORLD TOGETHER

Another aspect of modern living that has changed dramatically is the issue of cordage. There is nowhere in the world where people did not create cord from plant and animal sources. Today, it is simply purchased in a store, made primarily of synthetic materials, such as polyester, nylon, and polypropylene. While it is possible to find some natural fiber cords in craft and hardware stores (e.g., jute, sisal, raffia palm), these represent a minority of cordage purchases in most affluent countries. And, in any case, people cannot take those raw materials and make cordage themselves but, instead, are reliant on machines to spin them into a functional rope, cord, or thread. It was very different in indigenous cultures. There was a suite of plants that would be used for this purpose, each having its place of growth, timing for collection, and specific preparation method. Fiber plants were simply another item of focus that linked people to their landscapes. And each group had their preferred species due to a combination of characteristics, including abundance, ease of processing, tensile strength, resistance to abrasion, and/or ability to withstand rot. As Paul Campbell noted in his reference on California Natives:

"... the Paiute Indians tied their world together. They tied their wood and willows in bundles to carry them into camp, they tied small game onto their waistbands; they tied the tules to make boats, and cattails to make houses; they tied babies in baskets, and arrowheads to shafts. They used cords in place of buttons and safety pins, to make traps, to catch fish and hang them to dry. In addition to the tough rope of cattails and sagebrush bark, they made a strong string of sinew and human hair. They also used supple young willow withes for tying. But the finest cordage of all was made of Indian hemp, or dogbane."

In the northeastern United States, we see a range of plants used as sources of fiber or cordage. For example, the Penobscot used hemp dogbane (*Apocynum cannabinum*), which they called "nsəsk^{w}", as an important fiber plant. This perennial, herbaceous plant can be used during the growing season and after the plants have senesced in the autumn. At that time, the dried stems can be gathered and stored for long periods of time if kept dry. The fibers were extracted by splitting open the stems and separating the brittle, inner layer from the strong, pliant fibers. Another important fiber plant was the American linden (*Tilia americana*), called "wiigob" by the Ojibwa. It was the inner bark of this forest tree that was used for fiber. Sheets of bark were allowed to soak in water (called retting), which allowed bacterial decomposition to break down the inner bark into the constituent fibers. Sometimes boiling in water with added wood ash was also used to facilitate this process. Other trees were used for fiber, including the inner bark of a tree the Passamaquoddy called "kakskùs", known to English speakers as northern white cedar (*Thuja occidentalis*). Inner bark offers some advantages, including its abundance and very long fibers, alleviating the need for frequent splicing. When the ground was not frozen, the roots of spruces (genus *Picea*) were gathered for binding, basketry, and stitching bark containers. Many groups would split larger roots into smaller strands using a process called split separation, which allowed one to guide the split carefully to get long, equal diameter strands from a thick root. The Passamaquoddy called the split spruce root "wotòp", and used this extensively in their daily living. These are just a small part of the full list of important fiber plants for the northeastern indigenous people. Elsewhere, it was species of milkweed (*Asclepias* spp.), yucca (*Yucca* spp.), and stinging-nettle (*Urtica* spp.), among many other species.

Portions of animals were also used as a raw material for cordage and ropes. Some of the strongest ropes were secured from animal parts. Two parts of animals were generally used: the hide and the sinew. Hides of various animals could be cut into long, narrow lengths and used for various purposes. The Inuit used sealskin ropes for hunting—the rope was affixed to a detachable point for seal and walrus hunts. They also used the ropes for making the harnesses for dog sled teams. Such skin ropes were not confined to northern areas. For example, the Tongva people of southern California also made sealskin ropes. Hide ropes and cords were made from many different animals, with people utilizing those species in their region. The Passamaquoddy of northeastern North America made skin threads (called wolokesqis) for stitching clothing together from caribou (*Rangifer tarandus*), until European colonists caused their local extirpation, and white-tailed deeer (*Odocoileus virginianus*). The Rarámuri of Mexico used rawhide laces to construct baskets used for carrying loads (a practice seen also on other continents).

In addition to the hides, the sinew (tendon) of animals was used for various purposes. Sinew is a remarkable material because it can be stretched along its length with high tensile force and return to its original measurement when the force is removed. Like rawhide, it contracts as it dries, pulling tightly on anything it is tied or affixed to. Sinew has been used for stitching clothing and other objects together, such as by the Maliseet of northern North America (who called the thread of sinew "'tonuwan"). It was used to make strong bow strings by the Nyyhmy (Mono) of California. It was also glued to the back of wooden bows to increase their draw weight and protect the bows from breakage by some western North American indigenous, such as the Olekwo'l (Yurok) of northern California. Such use of sinew was most often seen in drier climates where precipitation and humidity would not affect the strength of the water-soluble hide glue used to laminate the sinew threads to the bow. Where conditions would prevent the glue from functioning well, the sinew could be braided into a thick cable that would be tied at several points along the back of a bow and twisted taught. Sinew cable-backed bows were used by northern cultures, such as the Inuit, allowing relatively poor quality wood (or horn, antler, etc.) to be used as effective hunting tools (the sinew cable functioning like a glued-sinew backing, providing higher draw weight and protecting the shaped wood from breaking).

Two of the most important skills in regard to the manufacture of cordage is (1) an ability to wrap the fibers together to increase the cord's ultimate strength and (2) the ability to add additional fibers to create longer strands of cord. The first necessity was accomplished by reverse wrapping, a method of wrapping bundles of fiber around each other in such a way that opposing twists kept the strands of cord from unravelling. Reverse wrapping can be done with plant fibers, sinew, or even hide. It was used by indigenous people around the world. With certain animal cords, such as hide, or even some inner bark cords, it is relatively straight forward to add more length by joining two strands with a knot. However, this is not feasible with many plant fibers or sinew. In these cases, methods of splicing are needed to seamlessly add material so that the cord can be made longer and longer. Therefore, splicing is the method of satisfying the second required ability. There are several different methods of splicing, all of which allow a person to make a uniform diameter cord of any given length (rather than being limited to the length of the original fibers). Through reverse wrapping and splicing, two complementary skills that were vital for the manufacture of cordage, hunter-gatherers accomplished most of their binding needs.

There were many facets of life that defined different hunter-gatherer groups. Their diets, their hunting weapons, their baskets, their language, their stories, and so on, all distinguished the different regions because they were so highly influenced by their landscapes and the way each group of wild people interacted with those living species found in their region. If one looked around different regions of a given continent, they would notice that indigenous people were using different species of plants and animals for cordage and applying their own techniques to each craft. Again, like so many facets of wild living, fiber arts were one of the ways people uniquely connected to their specific landscape. The plants and animals were part of their lifeway—the people were completely dependent on them, and, as a result, they developed strategies to steward their cooperative connections to these other-than-human persons.

Important "Print Elders" on the topic of cordage:

Primitive Technology: A Book of Earth Skills, section 4, edited by David Wescott (1999, Gibbs Smith Publisher)
Naked into the Wilderness: Primitive Wilderness & Survival Skills, chapter 2, by John and Geri McPherson (1993, Prairie Wolf)

FORAGING FOR THE COMMUNITY

Regarding indigenous people, hunting often gets a disproportionate amount of the space in anthropological works (even the name "hunter-gatherer" demonstrates this, where hunting is afforded a privileged position in the name of these wild people). There are a number of reasons for this, one of which is certainly that many early anthropologists were men and were interested in male activities. But make no mistake, in many parts of the world, it was through foraging that families were fed on a regular basis—as much as 85% of some hunter-gatherer diets was provided by foraged plant foods. While animal foods were of high importance, they were less predictable, and excursions for hunting (and fishing) were not always successful. It was the women (most often) who made forays from the encampments on a nearly daily basis, and who provided a consistent source of calories and nutrition for their families. Though often viewed as having a lower prestige role by members of modern society, and certainly not seen as exciting as the hunt, the foragers of each band were pivotal to the survival of the community. Their deep knowledge of a wide array of plants allowed them to correctly identify the edible species (taxonomy), find them in their appropriate habitats (ecology), and time the collection to when edible portions would be present (phenology). This was true even of people in northern regions, where the short growing season limited the duration of plant collection. While there was certainly worldwide variation in the amount of effort dedicated to foraging, influenced partly by the degree to which the climate, season, and landscape provided for plant food abundance, over much of the world it was the foragers who made sure there was something to eat each day as the families gathered about the fires and shared the stories of the day.

Foraging can be thought of a gateway to wild foods for people interested in rewilding. Most wild plants do not have any rules or regulations around their harvest (so long as you have permission to access the places they grow). While this should not be used as an excuse to gather in an unsustainable manner, it does mean that permits, fees, and tagging are not usually necessary. Equally important, we do not have the cultural baggage around gathering and processing plants that we do with killing and butchering animals, wild or domesticated. Because most people are disconnected from the processing of animals for food, the thought of cutting flesh from a deceased animal is sometimes considered barbaric (though they ask butchers to do this for them when they shop at the supermarket—which begs the question, are butchers barbarians?). However, many purchased plant foods require some amount of processing prior to cooking or eating, including cutting, chopping, peeling, grating, and slicing. As a result, people are still quite comfortable with plant foods and the preparation needed for their consumption. This makes wild plant foods an excellent introduction to wild foods and a wonderful way to bring deep nutrition into the home and begin a path of greater self-reliance.

One of the biggest challenges people face regarding wild plant foods is the tremendous diversity of organisms that can be encountered. Unlike much of the animal world, where people can at least group the observed organisms into major groups (e.g., birds, fish, hooved mammals, cats, dogs), people simply do not have the background education to have a framework of classification for plants. Therefore, a major obstacle that people face is learning plant taxonomy—specifically, how to identify plants. Plant identification relies on the observation of morphological features that most are not used to observing (or even know exist). Further, those who have gained expertise in plant identification have acquired fluency in a descriptive vocabulary that characterizes a plant so that it may be differentiated from other species, including those with close morphological similarity. This is another one of the reasons why anthropological work has focused more on animal foods because botanical training in modern societies is quite poor and researchers can at least generally describe the animals being hunted. For example, when I used terms like waterleaf, flatsedge, and rockcress (all genera containing edible species), do they create images in your head as would animal categories like duck, trout, or deer? Therefore, the most important thing for the neoaboriginal to learn regarding plant harvesting is the process of identification (which can be learned from a variety of resources, including botanists that may not have an interest in wild foods but can, nevertheless, teach plant identification and ecology). Another challenge that people face are the persistent wild food myths that abound in the generations of edible plant books. Some wild food references have little personal experience by the author incorporated into the manuscript, meaning the writer is simply repeating what the previous generation's authors wrote. This leads to some edible wild foods being stated as poisonous, some inedible plants being reported as edible, and some foods lacking the necessary preparation information to make them palatable and edible. There are simply too many of these commonly appearing inaccuracies to give a full account here. For one example, some authors' description of the processing of acorns of the black oak group (*Quercus* section *Lobatae*) are not effective in removing the tannins from the nuts, leaving a food that is bitter, astringent, and with potent antinutrients still in place (not exactly the kind of food you want to serve your family and guests). Given these challenges, it is important for aspiring foragers to find experienced mentors (or their books) who can dispel these myths and allow people to make efficient use of their time gathering. Finding such instructors will then require people to overcome perhaps the biggest challenge of all—finding (read making) time for foraging and other rewilding pursuits.

Modern foragers in affluent countries tend to focus on some of the plentiful and easily collected wild foods, such as spring shoots and leaves, berries and other fleshy fruits, and nuts. While these are important, healthful, and delicious foods to know, it is important to mention that people should not neglect the underground storage organs (USOs). While the aforementioned foods do supply important dietary elements, including micronutrients, phytochemistry, and often (in the case of nuts) lipids, these foods generally have a relatively short window of collection and can be difficult or tedious to store long term. Underground storage organs, which include taproots, rhizomes, tubers, corms, and bulbs, often have long periods over the year that they can be collected, so long as the ground is not frozen. This means that they can be collected before plants appear in the spring and long after they senesce in the autumn (for temperate regions of the world). Knowledge of these subterranean foods allows one to gather carbohydrate- and fiber-rich plant foods, often even when the plant is not actively growing (i.e., the withered remains of the aerial stem and leaves can indicate where the below-ground food store can be found). This fact made USOs vitally important to many hunter-gatherer groups, including those in desert regions where plants would go dormant during dry seasons but their USOs could still be found by skilled foragers. Importantly (especially for modern people), these foods often contain various kinds of resistant starches that are fermented by large-intestine bacteria, promoting the health of the colon. While USOs may have more work involved in their collection (i.e., the digging and unearthing of these foods), they are a valuable part of the ethnobotanical knowledge of one's landscape.

Foraging is much more than simply leaving the home to gather plant foods. Through foraging, humans become reconnected to their landscapes, once again using their senses to scan their environments and find plant allies, learning about their region in the process. We encounter tracks, listen to bird song, and feel the sunlight on our skin while we roam over the land. We become much more in tune with our ecosystems because we are (finally) paying attention to the species that comprise them, their age, and their condition. And we do all this with the younger generation along (if we emulate hunter-gatherer communities), teaching them the ability to feed themselves outside of industrial food systems. The excitement of finding a large colony of valued wild food has been replaced today with the excitement of opening a package that was delivered to the home. But our original enthusiasm for the new was the discovery of food and other needed resources that nourished and supported the community. The focus needed for foraging, and the associated mental state of searching, can help us to return to the present and leave behind, at least for a while, the chronic stress we often endure living in modern societies. Foraging is one of the key skills needed for self-reliance. It provides more nutrient-dense food than any supermarket can, and in the process of acquiring that food, people are immersed in nature, are exposed to the elements, and get feral movement—all valuable aspects of a healthful, nature-connected living. Further, the satisfaction and joy experienced by feeding oneself from wild places (large and small) is both healing and contagious.

Important "Print Elders" on the topic of foraging:

Ancestral Plants volume 1: A Primitive Skills Guide to Important Edible, Medicinal, and Useful Plants of the Northeast by Arthur Haines (2010, Anaskimin)

Ancestral Plants volume 2: A Primitive Skills Guide to Important Edible, Medicinal, and Useful Plants of the Northeast by Arthur Haines (2015, Anaskimin)

The Forager's Harvest: A Guide to Identifying, Harvesting, and Preparing Edible Wild Plants by Sam Thayer (2006, Forager's Harvest)

Nature's Garden: A Guide to Identifying, Harvesting, and Preparing Edible Wild Plants by Sam Thayer (2010, Forager's Harvest)

Foraging California: Finding, Identifying, and Preparing Edible Wild Foods in California by Christopher Nyerges (2014, Morris Book Publishing, LLC)

HUNTING IN PERFECT FORM

Humans are heterotrophs, and, unlike plants (who are autotrophs), they cannot utilize inorganic carbon but must acquire organic carbon from other life forms (through consuming part or all of their bodies). Humans are also predators. And while some who practice modern fad diets correctly point out that our bodies lack features we commonly associate with predators (e.g., fangs, claws), they are overlooking the fact that our intelligence has allowed us to create an array of effective hunting weapons designed for acquiring animal nutrition. These hunting tools, including the aerodynamic throwing stick of the Kumeyaay (Diegueño), the atlatl (or spear thrower) of the Australian Aborigine, the harpoon with a carved, detachable bone point of the Inuit, and the reflexed incense-cedar bow of the California Miwok, are clearly magnificent specializations produced by the human animal for hunting other animals. Given that humans, through intense hunting pressures, have caused the extinction of other animals, there is (perhaps) no greater predator than *Homo sapiens*. While I do not wish to glorify the loss of the earth's biodiversity, humans are clearly apex predators that stand beside a long list of impressive wild animals known for their ability to capture other animals. And like other predators that pursue large prey, humans also hunt high-risk prey species that are capable of injuring, maiming, or killing the hunter (i.e., not all prey species can appropriately be referred to as defenseless). The fact that hunting is a part of the human species is memorialized in our artifacts, our rock paintings, our carvings, and the ubiquitous act of hunting itself found in all indigenous cultures (past and present). To deny that humans are predators is comparable to rejecting that humans are communal organisms.

As was briefly mentioned earlier in this chapter, many members of affluent countries have significant cultural issues surrounding hunting, considering it both unnecessary and cruel, though many of those same people support industrial farming (through their purchases) that place animals in horrendous conditions, feed them diets that lead to illness, and take their lives with little or no empathy. Wild animals represent some of the most conscientious food to acquire because they never spent time in cages, ate biologically appropriate diets, and their living did not cause their ecosystems to become highly degraded. Even still, images of hunters looming over their kills often receive a flood of negative comments concerning over-developed egos, unfair hunting advantage, and no ability to witness the beauty in wild animals. While I agree that all of that is often the case, the fact that modern hunters are emotionally removed from the lives they take is to be expected. Society conditions males (especially) not to demonstrate sadness, fear, anxiety, and similar emotions (as these are signs of weakness). Further, modern society has conditioned people, especially males, to stand out because of their accomplishments. In fact, they must act excessively macho and not show any fear during hunts, even when the animals are capable of maiming or killing the hunter (for the record, while courageous, hunter-gatherers felt comfortably expressing fear to others when discussing dangerous prey). The ever-present images of men reveling over dead animals is the logical outcome of this kind of broken community. However, we can transcend this. Hunting can benefit from several things that would change the way this activity is viewed by the public, including less gloating over kills, hunters who do not use excessive technology to make up for their lack of ecological knowledge, and males that experience sorrow at the loss of life (despite the fact they are simultaneously feeling elation for a successful kill). The fact that a life has been lost, and that animal will never again walk this earth, should produce sorrow. However, that animal can live on through stories told to the younger generations and through the nourishment derived from the animal that becomes part of our being (as has happened for the entire history of *Homo sapiens*). This is a level of intimacy that hunters are not currently allowed to experience, but a truly rewilded human is an empathetic hunter who understands that the loss of life, when the hunt is successful, is a time for both mourning and celebration.

While we do not have space to discuss all the merits of hunting tools used throughout the world and their applications to different environments, I feel it would be useful to briefly mention the bow. The archeological history of this weapon is quite wanting (in my opinion), and it appears to have possibly been independently developed on different continents (despite the fact the oldest artifacts associated with the bow are in the range of 64,000 years old and could have been transported to all the continents from Africa; see Lombard and Phillipson's 2010 article in Antiquity). The bow represents, perhaps, the peak primitive weapon by hunter-gatherers and its appearance in different regions heralded the declining use or outright abandonment of some other hunting tools (e.g., hand-thrown spear, atlatl). The ability to cast a projectile (the arrow) at increased velocity relative to many other weapons is a huge asset—many animals from the size of deer and smaller are very quick and can dodge hand-thrown objects. Further, the act of shooting the arrow requires less movement than with many other weapons, making the bow a stealthier weapon that doesn't alert the animals to the hunter's presence. Finally, it is more accurate at greater distance than many hand-thrown weapons, meaning the hunter has an increased chance of striking the animal in a location that results in a quicker, more humane death. In North American, almost all indigenous groups used bows, though the choices of wood, the style crafted, and the game pursued with those bows were often very different. I strongly encourage anyone interested in the rewilding path to develop the craft of constructing bows and arrows and committing the time to become accurate (for both the hunter's and hunted's sake). Keeping in mind that indigenous hunters understood their landscapes in a way modern people do not, learning of the styles used in your region will likely be beneficial.

I was once highly criticized for hunting with a wooden bow and wooden arrows tipped with stone points. Essentially, the main focus of the argument was that I should use more lethal means of taking animal lives, such as the rifle that modern living has made available. While I appreciated the concern for animals and the suffering they might experience, I was a bit surprised at the superficial aspect of the comment (a perennial problem in a society disconnected from nature). Essentially, the person unhappy with me was claiming that it was more humane to use a rifle because it would result in a more rapid death. In other words, the focus was entirely on the individual animal being hunted. Of course, the creation of that rifle required the leveling of mountains and/or creating massive scars in the ground (to secure iron ore), producing materials for chemical explosives (gunpowder), and polluting the world with a highly toxic metal (acquisition, processing, and dispersal of lead). This stood in contrast to the wooden bow I was using, which required the death of a single tree (from which multiple bows were made) and the non-lethal taking of some shoots from a specific shrub for arrow shafts. The overall ecological harm produced by industry for gun manufacture was never considered in the argument, nor was the emotional detachment of moving a person significantly further from the death of the animal. I would politely argue that the most humane hunting weapons, when all factors are considered, are those made from our landscape and used by people who practice frequently to maintain a high standard of accuracy. Further, the hunter needs to have a high degree of empathy for wildlife so that the only shots they take are likely to result in the rapid death of the animal.

The previous paragraph certainly hints that I am suggesting there is a higher level of ethics when it comes to hunting. And I am. While I do not want to state there is no use for things like stealth cameras, purchased animal scents, thermal cameras, high-powered glass optics, and similar technologies, I also recognize that these are crutches that modern humans use because their knowledge of animal habits and their ability to track, stalk, and observe are often significantly less developed compared with those of hunter-gatherers. Further, the time required to learn the manufacture of a bow and, perhaps also, the knapping of stone points, is simply too long in a society geared for instant gratification and the use of technology made simple for the lowest common denominator. My hope is that people will graduate from such technologies as they learn more about their quarry, ultimately putting themselves closer and closer to the act of killing. Equally so, there is a greater realm of self-reliance through using technologies that one can replicate from their local environment. Firearms often cannot be repaired without tools and spare parts produced by industry, whereas a bow and arrow can be crafted from most landscapes even with tools of natural materials (e.g., stone axes and blades, antler and wood wedges, scouring-rush stems for smoothing). Successful primitive bow hunting requires knowledge of several fields of ancestral living, including plant identification, woodworking, knapping stone for arrow points, adhesives, nature observation, and so on. Even beyond this, crafting hunting tools from one's landscape truly puts the hunter on equal footing with the hunted animal. Both are using their evolutionarily derived adaptations in a very pristine and natural way that connects both the predator and prey with their landscapes. And both are acting as wild animals that are attempting to learn the habits of the other, ultimately promoting greater awareness in both.

Important "Print Elders" on the topic of hunting weapons and stone tools:

Bows and Arrows of the Native Americans: A Complete Step-by-Step Guide to Wooden Bows, Sinew-backed Bows, Composite Bows, Strings, Arrows & Quivers by Jim Hamm (1989, The Lyons Press)
The Art of Making Primitive Bows and Arrows by D.C. Waldorf (1999, Mound Builder Books)
The Traditional Bowyer's Bible, volume 1, by Steve Allely et al. (2000, the Lyons Press—there are four total volumes to this series)
The Atlatl: Primitve Weapon of the Stone Age by Kris Tuomala (2000, Walking on Old Ground)
The Art of Flint Knapping by D.C. Waldorf (1993, Mound Builder Books)
Naked into the Wilderness: Primitive Wilderness & Survival Skills, chapters 3, 4, and 9, by John and Geri McPherson (1993, Prairie Wolf)
The Universal Tool Kit: Out of Africa to Native California by Paul Campbell (2013, Sunbelt Publications)

CLOTHING FROM SKIN

Functional clothing is a necessity for a species of ape that lacks pelage and plumage to protect itself from the elements. Clothing is one of the many reasons why *Homo sapiens* has been so successful at dispersing over the globe and thriving in a wide range of conditions, some of which are extremely harsh. Indigenous peoples created functional garments from animal and plant sources. As with other aspects of hunter-gatherer living, the clothing defined the people because it was made from local materials and designed to function in that place (as you have read several times by this point). It was another example of wild people expressing the intersection of their culture and the land. While the fabrication of beautiful clothing would be celebrated in a traditional culture, clothing was not (as it partly is today) an individual's attempt to demonstrate a certain financial position within a society. The clothing of hunter-gatherers usually came from living beings (i.e., death may have been involved in the sourcing of the materials); however, the fabrication of the clothing did not pollute the landscape nor expose the wearer to synthetic chemicals. Further, it was yet another gift from the earth, not an entitlement to be made overseas by poorly paid workers. Truly, clothing is as important a topic for social justice as it for personal sovereignty. The ability to fabricate the required wares for one's ecoregion is of paramount importance to those who wish to experience a greater degree of autonomy in their lifetime.

Hunter-gatherers make a remarkable diversity of clothing. For example, the Ivilyuqaletem of California made a fiber sandal from the Mojave yucca (*Yucca schidigera*). The Laich-kwil-tach of British Columbia made hats and diapers from the inner bark of western red cedar (*Thuja plicata*), others in the region used the same tree for capes and skirts. The Mamaceqtaw (Menominee) of the western Great Lakes region used the inner bark of American linden (*Tilia americana*) as thread for stitching together fabrics to make clothing. And this list could go on at length. However, this section is more about the use of animal hides for clothing. Further, it is primarily about deer and similar animals that can be used to make a functional leather through a process called brain-tanning. The leather made from the brain-tan method is much unlike commercial leather of today as the finished fabric is supple and soft. Like other leather, it is very durable, blocks the wind, and protects the body from sharp or abrasive plants and stones. It is an ideal fabric for hunting because it does not make loud noises when the fabric touches or slides against other objects and it is a scent-block, which prevents human scent from being carried by wind. Further, it is easy to dye certain colors—one of my favorites is the rich, dark brown color produced by the dried husk of black walnut (*Juglans nigra*). To add to the value of brain-tanned leather (or buckskin), it can be used to make a wide variety of clothes, including shirts, jackets, hats, shorts, pants, leggings, skirts, dresses, shoes, and mittens.

Brain-tanning can be used for a wide variety of animals, including those that are often tanned with the hair on and those from which the hair is removed. For simplicity, I'll here limit the discussion to members of the deer and pronghorn families (e.g., white-tailed deer, mule deer, black-tailed deer, elk, pronghorn, moose). Tanning is a method of creating leather that will remain flexible even after it gets wet. Hides typically become rigid once they dry (like rawhide), in part due to the collagen molecules that act like a glue to bind together the microfibers found in the dermis of the hide. Tanning a hide creates a situation in which the microfibers can slide past one another (rather than being glued to one another) to make a supple fabric. To briefly describe the process, a hide must be scraped clean of all of the muscle and fat (materials that would decompose rapidly and create a foul odor). Through dry scraping or wet scraping, the grain, which holds the hair, is removed. The membrane, a thin layer on the flesh side of the hide, is also removed through scraping. Both of these layers (grain and the membrane) are relatively impermeable to the dressing; therefore, their removal helps the dressing to penetrate for the creation of a soft final product. The dressing was traditionally made from the brains of the animal. The brain is an extremely fatty organ, and the lipids coat the microfibers of the dermis (the interior layer of the hide) and allow them to move past one another. Today, touching brains would be considered gross and uncivilized, so some readers may be relieved to learn that eggs and even certain kinds of soap can be used (though, in my experience, nothing works as well as brains). After the dressing is applied, consisting of brains and often some warm water, the hide must be kept in constant motion while it is drying or it will become rigid. Through stretching, rubbing, manipulating, staking, and cabling, the hide slowly dries and becomes very soft. Finally, the hide is smoked to make the softening process permanent. Smoking makes a permanent chemical change to the hide—without smoke, the hide will become stiff again if it gets wet.

Today, animal hide clothing is often considered a sign of cruelty. And for most of it, it is truly that. Animals used to make clothing are raised in areas (or cages) too small for healthy movement, fed poor diets, and killed by inhumane methods so that people may have fur coats and leather boots. However, the fact that some animal hide clothing is derived from a cruel industry should not cloud our perceptions about all hide clothing. Learning to make brain-tanned buckskin from deer and their relatives allows hunters, friends of hunters, and those who find minimally damaged road kill to fully utilize the animals they have acquired. Buckskin is a marvelous material and those who have learned to make clothing from it are truly grateful for this fabric. Nearly every hunter I know discards the hide, wasting a valuable resource and acting in a manner that does not fully honor the animal. As a result, hides are usually very easy to acquire, especially if a relationship is developed with a game butcher. One of the main obstacles many will face is the discomfort experienced around deceased animals and their hides—this created by a society that is content with other people performing certain tasks necessary for their living. While we do not want to be callous around dead animals (and plants) that support our living, we do need to develop some ease with butchering and processing the fauna that allow us to live in our place. And certainly, if brain-tanning your own hides is simply not something that you will develop a desire for, consider supporting those who brain-tan for a living (i.e., purchase finished brain-tanned buckskin). While this misses an important part of the rewilding philosophy, it is much better for the world to purchase this kind of leather, and it supports those who keep an important skill alive. Either way, brain-tanned buckskin is one of those traditional fabrics that led to greater utilization of animals and allowed people to endure the climates of their region in comfort.

Important "Print Elders" on the topic of clothing:

Deerskins into Buckskins: How to Tan with Brains, Soap or Eggs by Matt Richards (2004, Backcountry Publishing)
Buckskin: The Ancient Art of Braintanning by Steven Edholm & Tamara Wilder (2001, Paleotechnics)
Blue Mountain Buckskin: A Working Manual by Jim Riggs (2003, Backcountry Publishing)

ESSENTIAL SKILLS FOR NORTHEASTERN WILD LIVING

At this point it might be useful to help people understand the full spectrum of technologies and skills required for wild living. A list of such skills will differ for each place on the earth, though individual locations would have some commonalities due to the similar difficulties humans face for living (e.g., acquiring nutrition, creating and maintaining fire, fabricating clothing). While this list (presented below) is not to quench anyone's fantasy of living apart from society, it should provide a realistic understanding of what would be required for this mode of living. It should also help people understand why it may take several generations for people to move to a more nature-connected (i.e., place-based) manner of living. Modern humans (*Homo sapiens domesticofragilis*) initially often have a difficult time replicating these skills; however, for anyone with perseverance, these skills are recorded in our genetic memory and are certainly our birthright.

In order to live sustainably in the wild, one must ultimately be able to do everything that is required of him or her with tools that can be gathered and/or made from the landscape. That means that the tools must also be made from stone, bone, antler, wood, plant fiber and resin, animal parts, or soil particles (such as clay). This "requirement" often adds additional challenges, but should be considered the highest form of practicing a skill; however, those who are first learning these skills need not commit to avoiding modern tools and materials as they learn about a given topic. But, keep in mind, the ability to perform these skills with metal blades, modern adhesives, plastic, synthetic cords, and other highly processed materials misses a key point—much of the challenge of primitive living skills is creating the tools needed for a given project (not just building a specific item). To live indefinitely in the wild, the following set of skills must be both understood and validated through real life performance. It is not acceptable to merely know (intellectually) how these tasks are done. Rather, they must be known through actual practice (experientially). For example, I had built Paiute dead fall traps for several years (without actually using them). I could build beautiful traps and demonstrate the necessary principles. However, when I actually committed to using this trap to secure food, it took me two weeks (and many refinements) before the first animal was captured. My traps, though correctly constructed for a coffee table book, were missing necessary design features for actual functioning in the wild.

The following set of skills is only a partial listing of abilities needed. It does not include aspects of community and spirituality, physical fitness and a host of movement-related skills, art and music, and many other aspects of wild living. It is merely the physical skill set of our ancestors that was needed to secure nutrition, protect people from the elements, heal from injury and disease, and craft necessary items for daily and yearly living. We are extremely fortunate to still live in a time when each of these skills can still be replicated by some person (though few people can replicate all these skills). However, if we do not learn and practice them, the ability to perform them will ultimately disappear from the ethnosphere of *Homo sapiens*, making rewilded living something that can never be realized. It would simply become a distant dream that humans thought of generations ago.

The skills listed below can be used as a checklist of items that domesticated humans will ultimately require for complete rewilding (in the temperate, northeastern region of North America). Some tasks are necessarily repeated under different headings because they are interdisciplinary. While survival experts often present skills in a particular order (the Sacred Order of Wilderness Survival), this order is based on the premise of either being rescued or returning to civilization under one's own power. Fully rewilded humans would be those neoaboriginals who remain immersed in their wild landscapes. Therefore, items are presented below in no particular order (i.e., no hierarchy is implied because all these skills are essential for extended living).

NUTRITION: sustain healthy populations through the generations, providing necessary macro- and micronutrients, along with beneficial phyto- and mycochemistry and bacterial nutrition to produce healthy children (which will ensure all else).
• foraging—knowledge of over 100 species of edible plants, including species that can be gathered during all four seasons
• preparation—understanding of how to prepare plants to deal with toxins and antinutrients (when present) so that nutrition can be maximized
• preservation—ability to preserve a wide array of plant, fungal, and animal foods for lean times
• hunting—finding and effectively acquiring game with a variety of tools (e.g., throwing stick, bow and arrow, atlatl/spear, hand capture)
• fishing—ability to secure fish throughout the year by use of hook and line, trap sets (including weirs), and nets
• collecting—gathering relatively stationary animal foods, such as shellfish
• trapping—knowledge of at least 10 different trap sets (some may reuse a particular type of trigger mechanism), ranging from deadfalls to snares to live capture to drowning sets, and an ability to target a variety of different sizes and different kinds of organisms (e.g., mammal, fish, reptile)

MEDICINE: maintain and restore health through the use of multiple avenues of healing (e.g., plant, fungus, animal, water, mineral, ceremony, trauma medicine), including infection, injury, birth, and chronic disease
• phytotherapy—knowledge of at least 50 species of plants from different ecosystems that can be used for a wide array of remedies
• mycotherapy—knowledge of at least 10 species of fungi that can potentiate the immune system, fight infection and chronic disease, reduce inflammation, etc.
• altered states—ability to produce altered states for divination and self-exploration, though use of entheogens or various practices (e.g., syncopated drumming)

STONE TOOLS: craft different kinds of stone tools from the appropriate rock for each tool, though the use of knapping (percussion and pressure), pecking, sanding, and bipolar percussion, also including the knowledge to change the lithic character of stone through heating
• flakes—for general purpose duties, including cutting, butchering, and scraping (often discarded after one or few uses)

- biface blades—knives for extended use, can be hafted to wood, antler, and bone handles
- hammers—hafted and unhafted, for various pounding purposes
- scrapers—hafted and unhafted, for preparing hides for clothing, cordage, etc.
- axes—hafted and unhafted, from knapped stone and pecked/sanded stone
- drill bits—hafted (usually) drill bits for drilling through various materials

BONE AND ANTLER TOOLS: create various tools for various purposes, using both fresh and aged bone
- smashing—creating tools through smashing bone and collecting shards that can be utilized or further refined
- scoring—grooving bone so that it can be broken into a predictable shape
- abrading—wearing away bone so it can be worked into desired shapes
- drilling—using various methodologies to drill holes and slots in bone (as needed)

BARK SKILLS: understand the use of tree bark in ancestral lifeways and how each species has different applications, also understand of split-separation to divide layers of bark; some important species used in the Northeast include paper birch, American elm, northern white cedar, American linden, and eastern hemlock
- timing—knowing when bark can be peeled
- methods—how bark can be peeled, including those species that can be harvested by special techniques when out of season
- processing—knowledge of necessary processing for different tasks (e.g., retting for cordage, flattening for shelters)
- application—experiential knowledge of which species are used for each task, such as shelter covering, fiber for cordage and clothing, medicine, containers, and water craft

SHELTER: this is essentially a composite of other skill sets, though bringing those together to create effective lodges where people can cook indoors during inclement weather is vital
- temporary—various simple shelters such as debris huts that can be constructed in a day and serve as suitable shelter without fire
- semi-permanent—longer-term shelters that can stand 5–10 years before replacement, generally using bark sheets as the exterior
- lighting—use of fat (best when rendered) and wicks to light the interior space
- mats—constructing mats to provide comfort and insulation from the ground and as an interior wall for cold weather times
- fire—ability to manage fire for heating, cooking, and, to some extent, lighting without filling the interior with smoke

FIBER ARTS: create a variety of different kinds of cordage from various plant and animal fibers, including lashing together shelter poles, cords for traps, bow strings, sewing materials, etc.
- bark cordage—fresh and retted kinds, gathered throughout the year (as possible)
- herbaceous plants—when to gather and how to process to create permanently flexible cordage from both stems and leaves (of different species)
- roots—clear knowledge of the different species and how they can be used, along with an ability to split-separate thicker diameter roots
- rope skills—ability to tie various kinds of knots and lashings suitable for the purpose at hand
- weaving—knowledge of weaving to make various crafts, including knife sheaths, pouches, other containers, ground mats, shelter interior walls, etc.
- coil basketry—creating coil baskets from various plant materials

• net construction—this technology allows for the fabrication of netted bags for carrying and as a means of securing fish

CONTAINERS: construct containers for various purposes, including dry and wet storage, cooking, and carrying
• bark containers—water-tight and non-water-tight kinds, the former allowing cooking through use of heated stones
• branch baskets—use of branches (as well as roots) to weave baskets for carrying foraged goods
• hide containers—pouches and sacks, also an ability to use stomach and intestine for cooking and storing food
• earthenware containers—ceramic vessels for storage and cooking directly on coals
• coal-burned containers—use of embers to burn out hollows in wood
• packs—construction of burden baskets to allow carrying of loads
• woven fish traps—these are essentially basket technologies applied to the capture of fish and decapods (e.g., crayfish, lobsters)

CLOTHING: know how to manufacture clothing to protect body from the elements (e.g., wind, rain, temperature, solar insolation, biting insects, plant armature)
• braintanning—create permanently supple fabric from animal hides (from a variety of species)
• barktanning—create more durable (though less supple) and more weatherproof clothing through use of high-tannin-content plants
• weaving—footwear, body wear, and blankets from plant fibers
• clothing types—ability to make shirts, pants, shorts, leggings, seasonally appropriate footwear, hats, mittens, and jackets
• methods—understanding use of awls and needles, building from intuitive patterns, repair of clothing
• weatherproofing—knowledge of making clothing at least partly weather resistant through use of plant- or animal-based formulas (grease, resins, etc.)
• elemental protection—creating items, such as sunglasses from bone, wood, or hide, to protect from aspects of the elements

WOODWORKING: know how to construct tools and shelters from wood
• green wood—understand working with freshly gathered wood
• dried wood—understand working with aged wood
• bending wood—an ability to use dry heat and/or steam to shape wood (a necessary skill for various hunting tools, skis, toboggans, arrow shafts, etc.)
• hunting weapons—ability to make spears, bows, and similar tools
• shelters—creating poles for sturdy shelters

MASTICS: know what materials to use as adhesives, waterproof coatings, hafting, and protecting
• hide glue—creation and use
• pine pitch—locating, tempering, and use
• birch tar—creation and use

FIRE AND LIGHT: fire is the primary tool that allows creation of complex tools, it is a pivotal skill
• fire creation from at least 3 different methods (e.g., hand drill, bow drill, pump drill, strap drill)
• ability to maintain fire in less than optimal settings
• ability to carry fire for an entire day of travel

- use of fire for food preparation, including cooking, sterilization, and detoxification
- use of fire to create dry heat or steam for tool construction
- use of fire for heating shelters
- use of fire (embers) for burning hollows into wood to make utensils, containers, etc.
- illumination for shelters, navigation, and torch fishing

WATER: procure clean water from the landscape and manufacture the ability to carry and store it
- finding water on the landscape, even during periods of drought
- sterilizing water when necessary
- use of watertight containers to carry water from place to place

NATURE OBSERVATION: understand deeply the biotic and abiotic elements in the landscape that are crucial for finding the necessary resources for survival
- plant, fungus, and animal identification
- locating and identifying necessary lithic and clay resources
- weather forecasting
- deep knowledge of tracking, including track and sign identification, interpretation, and following, along with ecological tracking
- heightened awareness and bolstering of the senses

MOVEMENT AND STEALTH: move and navigate across the landscape (even great distances) and sometimes do so unseen and unheard for hunting purposes
- familiarity with macro- and micro-features on the land to allow navigation by landscape
- navigation by sun, moon, and stars
- ability to move day or night, and in the presence of snow (requiring a understanding of the construction of snowshoes and skis)
- knowledge of concealment (stationary) and stealth (moving)

PERSONAL HYGIENE: keep good hygiene practices to avoid infection, dental caries, and external parasites
- oral hygiene—creating tools for cleaning teeth, locating suitable clay, and knowledge of plants for making tooth powders with anti-adhesion properties
- washing—plants that foam for soap, clays, and other suitable items for washing the body
- nails—keeping nails trimmed to avoid splinters and accumulating debris
- hair—washes for cleaning hair and protecting from problem dandruff
- sunscreen—ability to make protective sunscreen from animal lipids
- insect repellent—plants that can keep away biting insects and ticks , smudging practices to keep shelters clear of problematic insects

NEOABORIGINAL STRATEGY FOR ENGAGING IN PRIMITIVE TECHNOLOGIES

Ancestral lifeways are the original form of affluence experienced by *Homo sapiens*. They represent a suite of strategies for living on wild landscapes around the world and are infinitely adaptable (i.e., some skills practiced in eastern Africa can be applied to eastern North America). They are as relevant today as they were 15,000 years ago, they simply must be interlaced with those necessary modern technologies in use in the home or community. These skills allow for true autonomy. Every aspect of ancestral skills brought into a person's life allows for an increment of detachment from industrial living. This is not meant to be a push for anyone to abruptly leave society and live off-the-grid in the wild—this is a sure way to put yourself at risk of injury or harm. Wild living must be learned, no different from learning how to live in society. Most people were raised for 18 years (or longer) by their parents, relatives, elder friends, and educators, during which time they learned about the safety and day-to-day details for modern living. Nature-connected living also requires a long period of experiential learning. However, each craft you learn for your family requires less money to be spent on industrial goods. A lifeway that requires less money also requires less time spent earning wages, providing more time for enjoying life, socializing with friends, rearing children, observing the natural world, and connecting with place.

I've added further reading suggestions at the end of each section in this chapter for several reasons. First, most people who have an interest in some aspect of ancestral lifeways, be it foraging, wildcrafting medicine, bow hunting, wood-fired pottery, or knapping stone, do not have access to mentors. Our society is not populated with elders who still teach the Old Way. While there do exist people who keep these skills alive, they are in the minority, scattered within our respective countries, and distant from most people. Therefore, books become our elders or as I refer to them, our print elders. We are now a society that learns from books (in stark difference to how humans formerly learned: we watched and attempted to replicate). Print elders are poor versions of mentors, but they are much better than nothing and can give people direction when they are needing assistance. Second, this chapter was not a how-to chapter on primitive living. That requires many volumes to contain the information needed for wild living within a single ecoregion. Therefore, the print elders I refer to can provide actual instruction to get someone started on their path to learning primitive living skills. Ultimately, a deep knowledge of any topic will require human-to-human instruction and ample opportunity to put that learned knowledge to work as real experience.

The real difficulties for most people interested in any or all aspects of ancestral lifeways are going to be (a) finding a highly skilled practitioner to learn from and (b) finding a band that practices a broad array of primitive living skills so that the union of ancestral technologies and community can be observed. While many instructors out there are skilled relative to the general population, they are quite amateur when compared with hunter-gatherers. My recommendation is to find mentors who actually live what they teach, rather than merely teach a particular skill but are otherwise immersed in modern living. People who truly live what they teach have learned so much more than is known by a hobbyist and have gained more awareness of a topic and have developed efficiencies that can't be known by merely dabbling in a subject. Of course, these ancestral skills were not practiced by a single person in a vacuum, rather they were part of a communal species' lifeway that bound the people together and connected them to their location. Ultimately, it is through the practice of such place-based technologies with other like-minded people that we find our original community.

While there will always be people who cannot see past the comfort and convenience that modern living provides those in affluent countries, ancestral lifeways are the only approaches of human living that are demonstrated as sustainable, leaving the world in a relatively similar condition for each successive generation. Even if we ultimately do not incorporate these methods into our lifeways, we will need to incorporate the concepts of place-based technologies into our manners of producing goods. Until that time, individuals, families, and communities can benefit immensely from the practice of primitive technologies. Miles Olson summarized my own thoughts well when he wrote[11]:

[11] Miles Olson. 2012. Unlearn, Rewild. New Society Publishers, British Columbia, Canada.

"Truly sustainable technologies are renewable and place based, meaning the necessary components can be harvested from one's bioregion, giving those with practical knowledge a deep level of autonomy or freedom."

Following are ten ways to incorporate ancestral lifeways into modern living for health and self-reliance.

1. **Consider the ways in which you are dependent on and support industry**. The current manifestation of industry, despite some of the useful and beautiful products made, is a highly damaging manner of manufacturing the things we need (when taken collectively) that is responsible for tremendous ecological harm. Without recognizing this, the true value of ancestral lifeways will never be fully appreciated.

2. **Disengage from industry** as much as possible, and help the next generations to reach even greater levels of autonomy. Finding quality primitive skills schools and gatherings allows you to put into practice sustainable living skills, which is one of the best strategies you can employ for living lightly on this planet. If your situation does not allow for pursuing these technologies, foster them in your children and grandchildren so that they may disengage from those modern industries that are destructive.

3. **Learn to steward fire**. Take this skill as far as you can, starting with maintaining fire and progressing to initiating fire. While you may begin with modern methods (e.g., lighter, matches), strive to gain a mastery of this essential skill and work toward creating fire from your place. While friction fire methods may be beyond of your physical ability (at the moment), you can still support your community by learning about the ways fire can be used as a tool for sustainable living. Controlled use of fire is a unique trait that binds all of humanity together. Engage in this ancestral practice.

4. **Constructing shelter** is something all humans knew how to accomplish in their place with the materials on hand. Regain this skill through camping without modern tents and tarps. Spending time in a functional shelter built with your own efforts is a very rewarding experience and provides you with real skills for a variety of situations, including civil emergencies. Every day you spend in a traditional structure helps you reconnect with the earth—even if the shelter is in your backyard.

5. **Build containers** of all kinds. Learn to weave, twine, fold, coil, and carve plant materials. Study the methods of fabricating earthenware pots from wild-gathered clays. Use these containers in place of the polymer bags, cups, bowls, and plates that are so frequent in our world today (including on the landscapes, in the oceans, and buried in our landfills). Ultimately, learn to cook within the watertight containers you build, generating even more sovereignty for your family. Even if you do not use this set of skills on a daily basis, these are talents that are there for you when you need them.

6. **Forage for wild plants**. Learning to identify, locate, conscientiously harvest, and process undomesticated plant foods brings to the family and community the most nutrient dense leaves, shoots, fruits, and roots available. These are foods rich in beneficial phytochemicals that thwart chronic disease. One of the easiest ways to control a population is through access to nourishment. True freedom cannot be experienced without the ability to acquire healthful foods.

7. Become a knowledgeable, effective, and respectful predator through **participating in hunting**. Learn the animal's habits so that you may connect with the organism that will sustain your life. If you cannot or will not hunt, consider helping to process the animal or participate in other ways to secure animal nutrition, like fishing or gathering shellfish. Omnivory is not an excuse to be cruel to animals, it is a responsibility to take life in an ethical manner and utilize as much as the animal as possible.

8. **Knapping stone** to create blades, points, scrapers, axes, and other stone tools is one of the early paths in the human journey of tool-making. Indigenous people learned the location of quality, knappable stone and often made long trips to secure this valuable rock. Knapping stone allows us to create tools that we currently require highly processed metal for. This aspect of ancestral lifeways is very important for successful primitive hunting.

9. **Construct clothing from natural materials**. Buckskin is one of the most durable and versatile fabrics, being used for many kinds of clothing. Other kinds of hides can be used to make blankets and durable soles for shoes. Hides and plant fibers give us a greater ability to live within our place with less dependence on industry.

10. **Express gratitude** for our ancestral lifeways and the people who keep these skills alive and pass them on to the next generation. We are extremely fortunate to still have access to many of the technologies that allowed our ancestors to thrive, and they will help us to regain health and develop a greater level of independence. True human sovereignty is difficult to achieve without a rekindling of ancestral lifeways in our communities.

13. Rewilding: tying it all together

The rewilding of modern *Homo sapiens* is a crucial step in our development as a species. For the last 10,000–12,000 years, we have experimented with a path of greater and greater divorcement from nature. This separation has manifested in a desire to control every aspect of our lives and the very planet we inhabit. The control mentality is now so firmly entrenched in our societal mindset that we can think of no other means of interacting with nature and resolving the problems that our species faces. While this path has brought a material knowledge that has allowed us to manufacture remarkable structures, machines, and computational devices, it is also a path that has created an unfathomable level of chronic disease, discontent, and ecocide. Many in a position to benefit from this industrial path would claim it has been a wonderful road and will go to great lengths (are going to great lengths) to prevent a transformation in the way we view nature. However, such a change is vitally necessary. We need a new path that recognizes our fundamental nature as autonomous, wild animals that celebrate our intimate connection to Gaia. Fortunately, such a path is clearly available to us, but to start down this route, it will require us to examine our lifeway with radical honesty. Once we truly understand the nature of our hesitations, we can progress in a way that merges the strengths of two, starkly different lifeways. We can have a near zero incidence of cancer (hunter-gatherer) with life-saving trauma medicine (domesticated human). We can experience fulfilling community and avoid chronic depression (hunter-gatherer) and support those people half-way around the globe who are struggling with a natural disaster (domesticated human). We can demonstrate respect for our ecosystems through an eco-conscientious living (hunter-gatherer) and have a greater scientific understanding of the cosmos (domesticated human). We can have all of this and much more if we are willing to commit to the rewilding path. But first, we must rewild our minds and our hearts so that our bodies will take the first steps.

THE ELEPHANTS IN THE ROOM

Many are familiar with the saying "the elephant in the room", a phrase that represents a very obvious and hugely important issue that no one is talking about or is talking around without really addressing it. While some of these topics have been broached already in this book, there are others that need to be mentioned and, more importantly, dealt with if humans are ever to rewild in large numbers. Dealing with major issues is something that modern humans are very poor at. This is because we are divided on most of them and cannot come to consensus. There are many reasons for the division, though one of the most critical to recognize is selfishness. With any proposed change, there will be those who see themselves as negatively affected. They will fight to prevent change, even if the change benefits almost everyone (and everything) involved, especially when considered in the long run. This is even true of people who are employed in the manufacture of items injurious to people's health, work in fields that discharge massive volumes of pollution, or function within governments that are knowingly repressive of their populations. Such persons will expend tremendous energy and sometimes even commit unlawful acts to keep the current situation in place, allowing them to continue to derive benefit—even though others are harmed. Such selfishness, which is epidemic in most countries of the world, is truly a sickness that prevents consensual decision making. If we all acted for the benefit of people who are yet to be born, allowing our decisions to be guided by a philosophy of health and sustainability, we would live in a very different world than we do today. But, this is how societies operate. Whether we choose to admit it or not, each society acts in its best interest in the short run, and then to the greater benefit of the wealthy, political, or religious elites within each society. It is rare for choices to benefit everyone equally, and even when such seeming conclusions are reached (such as protecting the quality of air), allowances are made for some to continue with their former practices. The recognition of this selfishness is a necessary step in deconstructing why some large issues, no matter how serious, are never dealt with in a timely and constructive manner (e.g., climate change). There will always be those who act on their own behalf, rather than that of the earth. With this is mind, let us examine three critical issues that stand in the way of large-scale rewilding.

The first elephant in the room we must discuss is human population. As of July 2016, it was estimated to be 7.3 billion humans by United States Census Bureau. I want to be very clear with this statement—this is too many people for the world to support in a way that both humans and the world are healthy. We are not only creating a more stressful place for humans, but the very climate itself is changing as a result of our industry. Considering that natural disasters (most of which related to climate or epidemics) are becoming more frequent, with the number tripling between 1980 and 2000, it should be clear that this many people living this particular lifeway is deleterious to our very well-being. Intense storms and droughts also exacerbate conflicts among humans, who fight wars over resources and flee their countries (for various reasons) in large numbers, creating stress and humanitarian issues in the locations they arrive. Many people are convinced that we can feed everyone alive, thinking that somehow this will remedy all the problems. High-quality food that supports human health is not possible for this many people, and even if it were, it is only one part of the problem—people are rarely examining what is happening to the globe as we feed all the people. With more mouths to feed, we are simply converting more wild land into agricultural fields, spraying more chemicals to protect domesticated plants from pathogens, depleting more water sources for irrigation, and ultimately producing more deserts with the loss of topsoil and the increasing salinity of the soils. And by feeding more people, those people have more children (and the problem worsens). One way or another, the world population of humans is going to decrease. We simply have to choose whether it will be voluntary or involuntary.

There are voluntary solutions to the issue. While none of these are a perfect answer, they do make inroads into the world population problem. The most obvious part of the strategy to reduce human numbers over time is to have fewer children per couple. By willingly choosing to have no children, a single child, or even two children, regional population will decline once the death and birth rates even out. Such a practice applied to large areas of the globe would, given time, help substantially. We are simply living in a time when the choice to have a large family is not an eco-conscientious choice to make (said another way, previous generations' choices have taken away this privilege from those families alive today). While this solution is not seen as a viable one for many people due to various lifestyle choices and beliefs (e.g., some religions consider their members to have an obligation to populate the world with children of their particular denomination, some agricultural families require child labor to produce surplus food), everyone who decides to follow this approach is making one of the most significant contributions they can to world health. This is especially true of people living in financially affluent countries, whose children will grow into adults that use a disproportionate amount of natural resources (much of which were living beings). Furthering this approach is to wait until later in life to have children. From a mathematical perspective, having children approximately every 20 years means that in 60 years there will have been three generations of humans born. However, parents who increase the generation time by waiting until thirty to have children will produce only two generations each 60-year interval. For most people, waiting later in life means they can provide more opportunity for their child or children and have begun to incorporate better lifestyle choices, which also benefits the health of the child. While I have encountered some geneticists who decried this strategy, they failed to understand that diet and lifestyle choices can maintain healthy genetic expression even into later years (I was 44 years old when my daughter was born, a young person who today is healthy and advanced with respect to cognitive development). Together, these two methods (along with others, such as adoption) provide us with an ability to beneficially alter the path humans are currently following, which is one of greater and greater overpopulation.

The second elephant in the room is both more difficult for people to perceive and much harder an issue to solve. It centers on governmental legitimacy. It may not seem relevant at first, but I'll make the case (shortly) that this is a major obstacle to rewilding as individuals approach the end point of this path. First, we need to open this topic by asking a simple question: what establishes the validity of a government? While some would posit that a legitimate government protects its citizens and creates laws to protect them from human rights violations, the fact is there are many governments in the world that do not value the civil liberties of its own people. Further, many other countries allow these violations to occur and even engage in peaceful trade with them. Certainly, some governments are highly repressive and invade other sovereign countries. What gives them legitimacy? Following are a number of other items that people might believe give validity to regimes, but as Christopher Cantwell points out, most of these are fallacious reasons:

"The length of time an institution has existed cannot be the measure of its legitimacy, because to say so would make it impossible for them to get established in the first place. The mere presence of a military cannot establish legitimacy, because it is the legitimacy alone which separates a military from a terrorist cell. The writing of a constitution does not establish legitimacy, otherwise I would publish one on this website right now and become my own republic. Having legislative, executive, and judicial branches does not establish legitimacy, otherwise I would simply declare myself president, and appoint my closest friends and relatives to the other branches. A majority vote does not establish legitimacy, otherwise I would simply hold an election within my own household to expel the United States from my homeland (house). The opinions of well paid [sic] lawyers cannot establish legitimacy, because Russian and US lawyers come to completely different conclusions based on the same information. The UN cannot establish legitimacy, because the UN is created by institutions that already gained their legitimacy without its assistance."

What we must understand is that governments gain legitimacy because of their ability to use force (i.e., violence), through which they are capable of compelling their citizens to abide by various laws and customs and keep other nations from invading them. On the surface, this might seem like a win-win situation, but not all governments use this threat of force for the benefit of their people (in fact, no government is completely innocent of human rights violations). To demonstrate this, we can raise the question of North Korea. This country was documented by the United Nations Commission of Inquiring to be a highly repressive regime with unparalleled abuses of civil liberties. The government uses enslavement, torture, sexual violence, forced abortions, and murder to coerce and control its population. Given all these mistreatments, it would seem logical that other countries would feel compelled to invade and remove the controlling government and replace it with one that is more benign. But this does not happen because North Korea has a nuclear arsenal and a very powerful ally (China). As a result, other countries are held at bay because they fear the retaliatory response. North Korea's highly repressive government continues (i.e., is legitimate) because of its ability to subjugate its own population and violently strike back if attacked.

Some people reading the last paragraph might dispute the use of the word "legitimate" in describing a cruel government (such as North Korea or others). However, if we look at the etymology of the word, it comes from the Latin *legitimatus*, which means "make lawful". Each country has its own take on the idea of what makes something lawful. The reality of this is that a country can enact any laws it chooses (or break those laws), so long as it has the necessary ruling strength to enforce them. For example, the United States Executive Branch implemented a domestic spying program in 2002. Despite the fact that its citizens were protected from warrantless surveillance by the Fourth Amendment of the United States Constitution, the government was able to perform the unlawful secret observations and escape consequences because … it can. The United States government has one of the strongest police and military forces in the world. It, like other governments, can impose its will on its citizens, even when it is enforcing illegal activities or unhealthful practices. This practice will continue until a country cannot enforce the laws it has established, and then there may be various outcomes, including the intentional overlooking of law breaking, lawlessness, and revolution.

What does governmental legitimacy have to do with rewilding? Ultimately, quite a lot. Initially, as people further their personal autonomy and become more capable of doing for themselves, it is quite easy for them to remain integrated within a ruling society. However, at some point, if people follow this path to one of several logical outcomes, they may live a relatively wild life that is largely detached from not just industry, but also governmental bureaucracy and law. I am not stating rewilded communities will be malicious groups looking to harm others, only that they may operate outside of various state laws, especially in regard to food sovereignty, vaccination schedules, and education programs. And even though such communities may experience greater overall health than the general population of the country, it is likely that the government will impose its will and force various conditions on such a community. Further, a rewilded community will experience financial burdens of local, state, and federal taxes (among other monetary penalties). While I agree that a portion of tax money does benefit people, some is used in ways people may not agree with or ultimately benefit from (e.g., invading sovereign nations, supporting GMO agriculture, furthering an education system that does not present an accurate view of the country's history, public works projects that degrade natural areas). Yet, rewilding communities will be forced to generate income to satisfy their tax burdens, especially true if they have been successful in securing large areas of land on which to live. These are people that may be utilizing reciprocal gift economies that do not generate financial wealth (i.e., they do not contribute to state and federal income tax like most members of society). This will require innovative solutions, such as establishing non-profit land trusts and organizations to escape property and sales taxes, respectively. And we could go on with other topics, such as hunting regulations, which would prevent neoaboriginals from feeding themselves with wild foods, even if they were harvesting in a demonstrably sustainable fashion. The point of this paragraph is that governments of affluent nations have a very difficult time allowing a segment of its citizenry to live in a self-governing manner, especially if that number were to grow to thousands of people in each of the different ecoregions of the country.

The third elephant in the room is the parenting that occurs in affluent countries, including the education system parents choose for their children. While this obstacle to rewilding is under our control more than the others and, in theory, the easiest to overcome, it is also the most invisible to domesticated humans. Essentially, the root of the problem lies in the fact that children are not treated as sovereign humans, meaning that their parents and caregivers are allowed (by their governments) to act in a dominating manner that is indicative of the social hierarchy found within their respective countries. In most affluent nations (e.g., United States), children have little or no control over their lives and are raised in a manner that enculturates them into a pecking order, with children near the bottom, sitting only above other-than-human persons.

While you may dispute that statement, the fact that parents can strike children for "misbehaving", an act that if performed on another adult would have them arrested for assault, is highly indicative of the children's lack of the rights and privileges afforded to grown-ups. Children are generally commanded to do things, may not be comforted when they cry (e.g., Ferber Method of sleep training), and often have to show a greater level of respect to their elders than do elders to their peers. All of this indicates they rank below adults in society and conditions them to follow authority (often without question), even when authority is moving a nation of people in a clearly detrimental direction.

Adding to this child sovereignty problem (which has ramifications for the adults later in life) is the current model of public education. While offering students a large body of information, it does not teach people how to live in their place. Equally important, it is designed to create a skilled worker within the industrial system, one who may have creativity in the work place but does not consider if that industry is even worth supporting. Nor does the skilled worker question the legitimacy of its government, or many other items she or he is taught, such as the sanitized version of history presented in schools (one that generally lacks the discussion of genocide and ecocide committed by Europeans and their colonists). In the end, public education often creates another automaton that must be woken up from The Matrix, a human who must undo decades of conditioning within an inherently damaging lifeway. Because of this, an entire book (forthcoming) will be dedicated to this topic so that children do not have to spend much of their adult lives overcoming physical, emotional, social, and spiritual deficits produced by human domestication.

Currently, human overpopulation means there is simply not enough space in the world for all people to benefit from healthy lifestyles that require open, undisturbed spaces where people can live, work, and play outdoors. Governments of the world can prevent people from fully rewilding if they so choose, and can even take necessary resources from these communities at some point (through various mechanisms, such as eminent domain). Further, the parenting and education children receive makes them willing to accept the direction of their country's leadership and not understand why rewilding is a fundamentally important strategy for the health of humans and the world. These are three huge obstacles that stand in the way of any nature-connected living that can be experienced on a larger scale. While some might state these are reasons that rewilding is an approach is doomed from the outset, it is clear that the current, industrial approach is also not successful in generating human health, contentedness, and serenity. It, too, is doomed to failure because of these elephants in the room and many other reasons that have been discussed in this book. Confronting these three issues are some of the most important topics that humans need to contend with.

WHAT BIRTHING PAINS MAY LEAD TO

Humanity has been on a steady path of transformation, marked over the previous millennia by increasing divorcement from nature. This change has fostered other transformations across many aspects of living, leading to a population that is content in its quest for excessive comfort and longevity. We have changed from a people who could endure the hardships of the landscape to ones who require climate control. We are now fearful of death and pursue the egocentric erection of monuments to ensure our name lives on in case the afterlife is not as we have been told. And while we seek those physical and emotional comforts, we are overlooking critically important facets of our lifeway that are detracting from the overall quality of life experienced by humans and other-than-human persons. We are making it harder and harder for each generation to reach their full genetic potential (as evidenced by the increasing rates of childhood disorders and adult chronic disease). But, perhaps, this is all a necessary step in the evolution of *Homo sapiens*, a wake-up call that will become so disastrous that finally all can perceive it. Given the loss of awareness in domesticated humans, the need for awakening must be obvious.

We humans have a way of focusing on all the good that comes of our technological worship, even though that technology causes us to be more and more maladapted to the world we inhabit. It can be accurately described as a cage without walls because once we have forgotten how to do for ourselves, or no longer have a body that can, we are dependent on the very industry that erodes our health and takes our autonomy (in many cases without a person's realization). This nature-divorced path has run long enough for us to understand what has occurred to this point and where this will likely lead. As Charles Eisenstein writes in "The Ascent of Humanity"[12]:

"The progression of social and ecological disintegration was written into the future long long ago, at the very dawn of the Separation which took a series of quantum leaps with stone and fire technology, and again with agriculture, and again with modern science and technology. While the catastrophic effects of Separation are flagrantly apparent to many people today, it was not so obvious in the past, when vast amounts of social, natural, cultural, and spiritual capital were yet to be depleted, that disaster was in the works. Who could have guessed, when the first granary was built in prehistoric Mesopotamia and the first forest cut down in Sumer, where it would all lead?"

And here we are, with a clear view of the path of nature divorcement—both forward and backwards. We are entering a traumatic period in human history, with human disease, ecosystem deterioration, civil strife, and tensions between religions, races, and nations collectively degrading the quality of life for many and contributing to a palpably tense global mood. As we vie for physical space, important resources, and religious territory, we are feeling the pains that come prior to the creation of a new lifeway. Much like the birthing pains experienced by a mother prior to the arrival of her child into the world, humanity is experiencing discomfort from the metaphorical contractions of 7.3 billion people who are approaching the transformation of their species. Most do not consider that the pain of human childbirth serves an important purpose—it contributes to the intensity of the birthing event that helps ensure the mother deeply values the life she has carried and brought into the world. Likewise, it may be that humans will not value a return to a nature-connected lifeway in the same way as one that is hard fought from the clutches of a technological catastrophe. Perhaps what we are passing through now is a necessary step, something that must mimic the trial of birth.

The appearance of a new and beautiful life follows a stressful transition period (birthing), a change that is stressful for both the mother and her child. Likewise, the current situation can be seen as traumatic to the earth (mother) and her children (humans). But such a period can be a catalyst for the creation of a new and beautiful life. Unfortunately, many people have lost the capacity to visualize the prospect of a wonderful future (which is made possible by changing our behaviors now). They are too wrapped in grief to be able to allow themselves to consider that this period is not only the spark for a new fire, but possibly even necessary to promote transformation. Such people often display one or more of the **11 Signs of Grief**. These were passed to me by Mike Douglas of the Maine Primitive Skills School, who has given me permission to share them with you in order that they can be used to identify grief wrought by our current situation in our family, friends, and community.

---

[12] Charles Eisenstein. 2013. The Ascent of Humanity. Evolver Editions, Berkeley, CA.

Mind to the mound: The preoccupation with thoughts of what is causing pain, a dwelling on a past that can't be changed or a future that has not yet occurred, all of which degrade the quality of the present time.

Eyes clogged with the dust of death: The visual perception of the world that all things are wrong, with no ability to see the good, any solutions, or the possibility of a bright future.

Ears clogged with the dust of death: Hearing only the ill things in the world, with each story being interpreted as presented in sarcasm, selfishness, with hidden plans, or as another conspiracy theory.

Throat choked with the dust of death: With only the capacity to speak about how wrong things are, with little expression of warmth, funny stories, or happy endings. This person is the curmudgeon in the group, always talking about how poorly things are and how much worse they are going to be.

Yellow spots in stomach: The general feeling of dis-ease, a recognition that something is missing, the yearning for purpose that can't be fulfilled, and no amount of material gain or pharmaceutical use will calm the sensation of wrongness (because these are not the cures).

Clouds on path: The inability to fulfill a personal vision or supply the world with one's unique gift to the world because there are always perceived obstacles that prevent these coming to fruition. In essence, the prisoner builds their own prison with bars of doubt, anguish, and languor.

Black disk covering the sun: This is demonstrated by a person who is lost in apathy, and simply has given up trying to make a difference. The sensation of disconnection from that which is right and worth fighting for. The idea that this issue is "not my problem", and the person simply stays in the home, lights down low, shades drawn, and doesn't involve themselves anymore.

Your fire is out: No concern for personal health or well-being. More than just disconnecting from the world (black disk covering the sun), but now disconnecting from oneself. Epitomized by constant health issues that are preventable, a house that is cluttered, with many dishes to be done, poor hygiene, and no focus on diet.

Blood on your chair: Someone who is always preoccupying themselves with distractions from the present state, and always having a place to be or something to do rather than making time to be part of the solution. Rather than work toward an improved self or a better world, there is always an excuse to focus on something other than the things that need to be changed.

Reaching for the poisonous plants: The chronic and abusive use of alcohol, drugs, and addictive substances. This is a desire to escape the pain experienced by this manifestation of the world, and any attempt at escapism (such as deep involvement in hobbies) is part of this sign of grief.

No thankfulness: No desire to honor or express appreciation for people, never any reason for gratitude, and no general appreciation for anything. This sign of grief is also demonstrated in the entitlement of some people in affluent countries who believe they deserve better than others because of the fortune of where they were born.

As can be seen by aware individuals, many alive today have several of these indicators of grief as a result of industrial living, a lifeway that influences tremendously our interactions with other people and the environment. Dealing with these signs requires a multi-faceted and individualized approach; however, in essentially all cases, individuals dealing with anguish will almost always benefit by addressing the root cause issue: separation from nature (literal and figurative). In my experience, the best way to treat grief caused by separation from nature is to become part of a community of people who are themselves dedicated to healing the separation. These are people who understand (at least to some degree) and likely have experienced the wall of grief. Even a loose community of people who meet occasionally can help one another immensely to ease the birthing pains felt by all as humanity transforms its relationship to the earth. The common problem is that many people openly share their grief with those who are also overwhelmed with grief, with those who are not receptive, or those who have never even considered how nature divorcement affects the human soul. Sharing one's grief requires a safe setting in order that the grief be healed to any degree (otherwise, it can be amplified). Often, it is those who are attempting to build a place-based community who most understand that nature divorcement is a powerful stimulus and potentiator of grief. Being among such people, talking through our sources of sorrow, and working to regain connection with the land can be strong medicine to comfort the dis-ease during this period.

THE SEVEN FIRES PROPHECY

Prophecies are stories that carry a message with implications for a future time, and sometimes serve to provide motivation for a culture to follow a certain path (i.e., make a particular set of choices) in order to avoid some kind of catastrophe. In this way, prophecies carry a message, one that can be vital to the survival of the people. Whether or not prophecies are real messages delivered to one or more people or merely stories that provide inspiration is almost irrelevant (at least to me), as what is most important is the content of the prophecy itself. The Seven Fires Prophecy is perhaps one of the most important stories for everyone in the United States (and elsewhere) to listen to. It was first shared with me by Caleb Musgrave, a member of the Anishinaabe People, who has given me permission to present this story here. It is a pertinent and powerful story that is very much in-line with the vision of rewilding presented in this book. However, I am unqualified to present the full story, so what will appear here is a brief narration and discussion of the prophecy's teaching. The reader is directed to "The Mishomis Book" by Edward Benton-Banai to experience this story told from the First Nations' perspective.

The Seven Fires Prophecy is a telling of seven individual prophecies (called fires) given in as many time periods. The entire story speaks of the migration of the Anishinaabe People and a foretelling of a time that will come when an important decision will be need to be made that affects all of humanity. The First Fire tells of a necessary movement of the people away from the Atlantic Coast to an inland location. Along the way, there will be stopping points—seven in all—that will be recognized by the sacred miigis shell (known as a cowry shell, which is a large, marine snail). The beginning and end of the migration would be marked by a turtle-shaped island. The people would know when they had reached the end of their journey when the locate the land where food grows on the water, a reference to wild rice (genus *Zizania*). The first fire also speaks to the importance of Midewiwin (Grand Medicine Society) and that its traditional ways will be a strength for the people.

The Second Fire speaks of a time when the Midewiwin would diminish in strength. Further, the evidence of the sacred miigis shell would be lost. The Anishinaabe divided into two groups (a southern and northern group). The southern group further fragmented into three distinct bands. Within one of those bands, called the Potawatomi, a boy was born who pointed the people back to the traditional ways and the path of the miigis shells. The Third Fire speaks of the Anishinaabe finding their path to their new home where food grows upon the water. The Fourth Fire was delivered by two prophets. The first spoke of knowing the future of the Anishinaabe by the face of the light-skinned race. The prophet told that if they come wearing the face of brotherhood then there will come a time of beneficial change for many generations. The light-skinned race would bring a bring a new knowledge not held by the native people, and that that knowledge could be joined with that of the all the First Nations People to make the mightiest nation of all. This face of brotherhood would be recognized if the new people came carrying no weapons. The second prophet warned the Anishinaabe that the light-skinned race may come wearing the face of death, which would look very much like the face of brotherhood. The prophet told the people that if the new race comes in suffering and greed for the riches of the lands, then the rivers will run with poison and the fish will be unfit to eat.

The Fifth Fire speaks of a time where all the native people would be involved in a great struggle. If the Anishinaabe and the other Native Americans accept the promise of the new way and abandon their traditional teachings, then the struggle would last for many generations. Essentially, it tells that the acceptance of the way of the light-skinned race will cause the near annihilation of the native people. The Sixth Fire tells of the evidence that the false promise of the Fifth Fire has become true. During the time of the Sixth Fire, native people will not teach their children the traditional ways, and grandchildren will turn against their elders. When this happens, the elders will lose their reason for living. During this time, a new sickness will also come to the people, and grief will spread.

The Seventh Fire was told by an unusual prophet that was said to have a strange light in his eyes. He described the emergence of a new people. These people will return to the traditional path and seek elders. However, many of the elders will have fallen asleep and will have nothing to offer, and other elders will remain silent because they have not been approached. During this fire, the new people will have a difficult task and will need to learn how to speak with the elders who are still awake. The new people will need to be fearless in their quest. In this time, the light-skinned race will have to choose among two paths. One of these paths is materialism. If that path is chosen, then the destruction brought by the light-skinned people will come back upon them and there will be much misery and death to all the World's inhabitants. The other path is that of spirituality—one that is infused with a deep respect for nature. If that path is chosen, then the Seventh Fire will light the Eighth and final fire, an eternal fire of peace, love, and comradery.

The Seven Fires Prophecy speaks of a choice between two different worlds—one where people rush headlong into greater reliance on technology that furthers materialistic gain and one where technology is guided by a nature-based philosophy. This latter choice does not abandon technology, but instead unites the strengths of material knowledge (held by the light-skinned race) with that of traditional ecological knowledge and wisdom (held by indigenous people). In essence, it joins the Europeans and their descendants on other continents with the Native People of the world so that they may all walk on the same path. It provides humanity with the strengths of both lifeways, and makes possible a world where our children can experience landscapes that are equally pristine (or more pristine) ecologically than those of the generation before them. This means that the rivers will once again have fish that are safe to consume. This also means that pregnant mothers do not have to avoid foods that support the central nervous system development of the children they carry because of toxins found in the flesh of the fish. And people don't have to fell the last forests to grow yet more grain because some of their meals will come from the very rivers their grandparents needed to avoid. This world is entirely possible, and it is not only a vision I have but one that the Anishinaabe have as well.

When the Seven Fires Prophecy was first shared with me, I was fascinated by the obvious teaching it held. At that time, I was exploring and consolidating my own views on how possibly to move forward within a society where most people were focused on the unhealthy quest for comfort and status without much thought for the physical and emotional harms wrought by these pursuits. In fact, most of the country is focused on sports teams, political races, and disputes over which brand is the best smartphone on the market while the very land they need for life is being desecrated. I am not an advocate of the doomsday scenario, where most of the human population will be eradicated by some calamity because relying on mass devastation as a solution is a symptom of grief (would any healthy human actually want this for the world?). Nor do I subscribe to the phoenix scenario, where from the ashes of civilization a nature-based society will arise who will unexplainably learn how to live in cooperation with wild ecology without elders to show them how. Elders are produced by people living for many generations in one place, where they learn how to engage in cooperative connections through observation of their world (and the shared observations of their ancestors passed down to them). I was seeking a way forward that would preserve life and allow for a transformation. The Seven Fires Prophecy spoke of elders who would be asleep and have nothing to share (i.e., they had become olders). It also told of a new people who would once again seek the traditional ways. I would contend that these new people are the neoaboriginals described in this book (or at least are one manifestation of them).

THE GIFTS OF THE HUNTER-GATHERERS

This section could alternatively be titled "Why We Need to Preserve Indigenous Culture". Many inhabitants of modern civilization consider indigenous people who still live as hunter-gatherers, or at least possess a significant proportion of their traditional lifeway, to be merely relics of the past. City builders are convinced that humanity's path forward does not need to take into account the evolutionary history of our species. Despite the fact that all modern humans have hunter-gatherer ancestry, this is assumed to be superfluous information, and that we have transcended our natural selves. *Homo sapiens*, living in the industrial age, is now cared for by electronic, fossil-fuel, and polymer technologies and is free to pursue, without restraint, any number of different diets and lifestyles that the present day world allows. Such a belief, especially common among citizens of affluent countries, can be maintained only through a concerted effort of ignoring obvious information about our health and well-being (much of which has been described in this book). Modern people display observable biases against cultures that lack industrial technology. Further, civilization must convince its inhabitants that they are living in the best period humanity has ever experienced in order that those people overlook the genocide, ecocide, wage slavery, physical and emotional health insults, lack of equality, and loss of sovereignty that any unbiased individual would observe. The focus is generally on the comforts and conveniences we currently enjoy, the expanded understanding of the cosmos we have garnered, and the increases in longevity that humans experience. But these are (clearly) not the whole story.

Following are seven reasons that summarize why we need to preserve all the remaining hunter-gatherers as an endangered species, some of which has been discussed previously in this book (but is placed here in one location for convenience). These are seven seemingly selfish reasons, but they do not just benefit us, they benefit all of humanity. I do not here discuss reasons of social justice that would also suggest leaving the remaining hunter-gatherers alone. The information contained in their lifeway and the very manner they view creation is incredibly valuable to people living in the industrial world. Once we confront our biases, it can be seen that their lifeway has some real benefits that can be emulated today in a wide variety of settings.

1. We are very proud of our medical system. It has made amazing advancements in life saving technology for all age classes of humans. However, there is one thing it deals with poorly: chronic disease. According to the US Center for Disease Control and Prevention, about ½ of adults experience chronic disease and ¼ of adults have two or more chronic diseases. Chronic disease is a euphemism for "preventable disease" because it takes a long period of time of insulting the health of the body with poor diet, lack of movement, and/or exposure to environmental toxins to manifest the disease. We are frequently led to believe that the reason we experience such a high rate of chronic disease is because we live so much longer than our ancestors. This is patently false. Research into hunter-gatherer cultures showed that adults lived relatively long lives, with the mode of the age of death (i.e., the most frequent age of death) at 72, with individuals living into the 80s and 90s—and experiencing an extremely low incidence of chronic disease (in fact, some populations were free of various diseases altogether). While we modern people have incredible diagnostic tools and the most advanced trauma care (ever), we are also some of the sickest people in the world. Given that hunter-gatherers living their traditional lifeways experienced a near zero frequency of cancer, heart disease, and diabetes, their lifeway holds the key to real prevention measures.

2. Today there is a dizzying array of different diets, most of which make extraordinary claims about promoting health and offering protection from chronic disease. Amazingly, most of the popular diets do not examine how health, physical form, and cognitive development are promoted (or compromised) in the next generations. Prior to agriculture, *Homo sapiens* consumed a tremendously different diet than that experienced in most affluent countries, one that was omnivorous and documented as more nutrient dense, more diverse, included plants with greater levels of beneficial phytochemistry and fiber, and had a different essential fatty acid ratio compared with modern diets. This diet was protective of chronic disease and cancer, as evidenced by numerous physicians and surgeons living on what was the frontier in the late 1800s and early 1900s among indigenous populations. These medical professionals observed essentially no cardiovascular disease, diabetes, or neoplasties. More importantly, this diet supported bone, dental, and structural health. Modern people demonstrate less dense bones and narrower faces with a high frequency of crowded, crooked, and/or impacted teeth. Observations of hunter-gatherers from all six continents show different facial structure and room for all teeth (including the wisdom teeth). While vegetarian and vegan diets are touted as the most healthful diets on the planet, research shows they have elevated rates of cancer and heart disease compared with omnivorous hunter-gatherer diets (and there is evidence of some suppression of cognitive development relative to omnivorous diets). Hunter-gatherer diets are the only dietary patterns with proof of nearly complete disease prevention.

3. Modern therapeutic approaches are heavily reliant on drugs with a documented litany of side-effects, one of which includes death. While drugs save many lives, they also kill many lives and cost affluent nations that rely on them billions of dollars each year (the US spent 374 billion dollars on pharmaceuticals in 2014). The American society is absolutely prejudiced against natural medicine despite its widespread use in the world, its extremely low incidence of lethality, and tens of peer-reviewed scientific journals (published in countries outside of the US) that demonstrate efficacy for this healing modality. Even when headlines demonstrate that certain infectious diseases, such as malaria, are treated with the highest efficacy using herbs, the bias is unwavering. Hunter-gatherers developed an extensive medical pharmacopoeia using both awareness and trial and error. Many of their medicines have been confirmed as effective in the laboratory setting. In an age where antibiotic resistance is a growing threat, herbal remedies for bacterial and viral infections show promise because they consist of suites of antimicrobial compounds that work in a synergistic fashion (i.e., they are not a single, laboratory produced compound that is easier for microbial populations to thwart). The vast majority of our modern drugs are based (originally) on natural remedies located, primarily, in plant tissues (but also sourced from fungi and animal venoms) used by native people.

4. Anthropologists have documented a broad array of commonalities among hunter-gatherer populations, even among groups living in widely disparate regions. These observations provide important clues to how humans lived and the kind of social environment they have experienced for all but a relatively short period of time. Hunter-gatherers lived in egalitarian communities that practiced extensive harvest sharing and had a high degree of gender equality. They used consensual decision making, and each member experienced a high level of autonomy. Political states with social hierarchy, competition among members, privileged classes based on ethnicity, religion, wealth, or heredity, and limited ability to direct social outcomes is a new experience for *Homo sapiens*, first beginning around 5400 years ago. Understanding the historical communal environment can provide important clues for helping allay the social strife observed in many affluent countries. Keeping in mind that depression and suicide were virtually non-existent in hunter-gatherer cultures, it may be important for social planners to rethink our political and social design to incorporate features that humans may be evolved to experience for feelings of happiness, contentedness, and freedom.

5. Relatively recent work has demonstrated that hunter-gatherers practiced often strikingly different child care patterns than those observed in affluent countries. Again, despite the groups examined, there were a number of commonalities observed among groups. For example, hunter-gatherer parents and alloparents demonstrated a high degree of responsiveness to crying children. Contrasting this is the commonly used Ferber Method, where children are required to cry it out. Research shows this latter method of child care maintains high levels of stress hormones that increase the incidence of Attention Deficit Hyperactivity Disorder and similar mood disorders. Another example, hunter-gatherers rarely use physical punishment, a common method of disciplining children in the US (a method employed by over 70% of parents). Physical punishment has been shown to suppress cognitive development in children, which lowers IQ scores, and can be shown to role model bullying (given that it is a larger person using physical violence or the threat of violence to direct behavior in a smaller, physically weaker individual). The anthropological work done to date clearly demonstrates that hunter-gatherers used different child-rearing methods and produced children without depression, mood disorders, identity crises, or abrupt changes in temperament. Modern science is building a larger and larger tome of evidence that our methods of parenting may be interfering with proper cognitive and emotional development of the next generation.

6. Linguists have documented over 7000 different languages on the planet, some of which are now without fluent speakers, and a large proportion are critically threatened by extinction. It is estimated that 90% of these languages will be lost by 2050. Languages are not simply another similar way to express ideas. Each language harbors a unique world view that is important for expressing different ideas and vantage points. Therefore, the loss of linguistic diversity represents a further homogenization of ways to think about the world and the cosmos humans are part of. We are in a time where diversity of thought is vitally important to aid in solving the problems we face. Industrialized countries have but one primary way of solving problems—use of technology, which can be shown in example after example to create additional problems that require additional technological fixes (which in turn create their own set of problems). What is needed is a concerted effort to protect against language loss (as depicted in George Orwell's *1984*), which can supply novel ways of approaching contemporary difficulties due to the unique world view embedded in each language.

7. Hunter-gatherers have a unique way of interacting with the world and understanding its phenomena. Modern science considers this native way of viewing the universe as antiquated, ineffective, and often outright incorrect. However, an unbiased examination of native knowledge will show it to be highly complementary to contemporary science. Modern science works through reductionist approaches, studying the individual pieces in an attempt to understand the whole. Further, it seeks to be an unbiased observer in an effort to avoid influencing the experiment (even though science has documented that this is not fully possible and that the presence of an observer affects the experiment). These approaches have their strengths and limitations for understanding complex systems. Native knowledge approaches this from a completely different angle, considering humans to be part of the system, and therefore possessing greater respect for landscapes and feeling a heightened responsibility for the state of the world. Further, it does not dissect its parts in an attempt to understand the whole, rather it celebrates the complexity and unknowable mysteries. Native knowledge also sees the world as holy and imbued with spirit, rather than profane and merely representing a collection of physical and chemical reactions. As such, it fosters a completely different relationship between humans and the natural world, one in which dominion and exploitation are not the logical outcomes.

None of this writing is meant to portray hunter-gatherer lives as perfect and idyllic. They weren't. They experienced some hardships that we do not today. For example, they had a higher infant mortality than we do for a number of reasons. Today, we are able to protect neonates (and mothers) from some of the serious complications that can occur during birth. This is a reason to embrace this particular aspect of modern medicine. However, the absence of cancer in indigenous cultures with long-lived inhabitants is a reason to consider the advantages of that system and how features of it can be emulated today. This is not an all-in or all-out approach but a call for common sense to embrace the strengths of both systems. We need living hunter-gatherers who are still experiencing their traditional lifeways. In other words, we need to stop acculturating them against their will—which is the usual pattern because we assume all aspects of our lifeways are better. However, study after study shows that when hunter-gatherers become civilized, they experience chronic disease (including cancer), depression, fractured community, disrupted sharing networks, and a loss of contentedness and feelings of connection. Hunter-gatherers need to be considered as a critically endangered species, one that holds important clues to solving some of humanity's current dilemmas.

Of course, hunter-gatherers are sovereign people who must make their own choices on how to proceed. I'm not here attempting to present that I know what is best for them—I am simply discussing important aspects of their lifeway that modern humans should seriously consider. This consideration should occur in a way that requests, acknowledges, and properly compensates hunter-gatherers for this valuable information (i.e., we should not appropriate it). Whether or not they move forward with modern technology is no one else's decision to make but theirs. However, at the very least, we can avoid interfering with them because we believe they require spiritual salvation. We can cease to push the industrial world on them because they lack electricity. We can recognize them for what they are—wild humans who are as much a part of the landscape as the other animals that live in that place. And just like those animals, wild humans require familiar land on which to live. Therefore, when we establish wildlife refuges in regions where hunter-gatherers live, we need also to include their ecological needs in the park design. We need to preserve all of the wildness of that region, including the wildness embodied in *Homo sapiens*.

CONSERVATION THROUGH USE

The current paradigm of conservation is to protect the organisms of concern from any and all insults they may experience. This amounts to hiding those species or assemblages of species (i.e., natural communities) from the public in refuges and behind no trespassing signs. In this model of conservation, only academics are worthy of interacting with the species of concern; the public is not invited to be part of the collaboration. While this may be the appropriate method for some species that are limited to very few remaining populations in the world and/or locations that receive profuse human traffic, it is a strategy that is now applied to most life when people discuss conservation. While with the best of intentions, this method has a serious shortcoming—it alienates people from the very resources (read: life) that they are trying to protect. With this separation comes a loss of awareness as to why the organism was important in the first place. Once the cooperative connection is completely severed, there is no understanding of the need to protect the organism in the first place, and then the population acts, votes, and lives in a manner that is inconsistent with conservation. The method ultimately fails in most cases, and local and global extinctions continue at the accelerated pace we are witnessing today.

The hands-off approach to conservation used by many biologists and land planners today is very different from the form of conservation used in the past. Indigenous conservation was based on a model of human use. Through use, people were constantly reminded how valuable a particular plant or animal was to their living. As such, those populations were utilized in a sustainable way that would allow the continued thriving of both the human and the species of interest. While indigenous people were not perfect (as extinctions did occur as a result of human hunting pressures, though there is some exaggeration of this idea), their record of resource stewardship stands strongly above our industrial model (refer back to the section "sustainability" in chapter 2 for an expanded discussion of this). Wild people, through living in their place for long periods of time, developed a large body of information called traditional ecological knowledge and wisdom, information that guided their taking of life. As the Director General of United Nations Educational, Scientific and Cultural Organization (Mayor, 1994) defined traditional knowledge:

"The indigenous people of the world possess an immense knowledge of their environments, based on centuries of living close to nature. Living in and from the richness and variety of complex ecosystems, they have an understanding of the properties of plants and animals, the functioning of ecosystems and the techniques for using and managing them that is particular and often detailed. In rural communities in developing countries, locally occurring species are relied on for many—sometimes all—foods, medicines, fuel, building materials and other products. Equally, people's knowledge and perceptions of the environment, and their relationships with it, are often important elements of cultural identity."

This knowledge and wisdom protected two important aspects of a place: biodiversity and bioproportionality. Biodiversity can be described as a measurement of the number of kinds of life present in a location (which can range in size from a small parcel of land to a continent to the entire globe). In other words, it measures the total variability of living organisms within an area. The more kinds of life that are present, the more biodiverse a region is (note: the concept of biodiversity is actually more complex than this and includes additional topics, such as landscape heterogeneity, but this brief definition will suffice for this discussion). Bioproportionality is the idea that there is more to conservation than just protecting the number of species living in a place. It examines the abundance of life in a place and seeks to protect species above a minimally viable population. This abundance of life can be measured and comparisons made between a pristine location with one influenced by an industry. Bioproportionality is a very important concept because a strict focus on biodiversity as a measure of ecosystem health allows populations to be suppressed due to overuse or habitat destruction, but so long as there are still many kinds of species present, the measure of biodiversity can still be considered high (and industry can continue as normal). Bioproportionality states that these organisms should occur in an abundance, which would be specific to each life form's natural history traits. While modern conservation focuses very strongly on biodiversity (a tact that allows habitats to be degraded and still be considered diverse), indigenous methods protected both biodiversity and bioproportionality. We know this to be the case because the European colonists who first explored and exploited the natural riches of each new continent described an abundance of life that is no longer present on those continents. For example, we know that prior to widespread settlement by European colonists, the northeastern United States had more acreage of forest covering the region and that those forests were composed of larger and older trees than what exists today. As Mathews' states in the 2016 article in the journal Biological Conservation:

"To insist that biological resources be distributed more equitably than they currently are amongst the world's species does indeed mean re-designing human civilization so that it becomes a system of affordances for the rest of life, thereby re-integrating the interests of other species with our own, as eco-modernists advocate. But it also means conceding that as the biosphere was shaped for earth-life and by earth-life just as surely as it was shaped for ourselves and by ourselves, it belongs to the rest of earth-life as much as it belongs to us. Since we have already annexed most of the terrestrial surface of the planet and are in the process of ecocidally depleting and degrading the oceans, we have not only to create new spaces for earth-life within the interstices of all the environments currently co-opted to human use; we also need to cede any remaining ecological estates to the species to which they belong, together with Indigenous peoples who have culturally co-evolved with them."

People must be able to interact with the life we want to conserve. While this does not mean people must be allowed to harvest rare orchids, it does mean that the forests or peatlands that sustain those rare orchids must be open to some sustainable human use—a truly sustainable use that does not degrade the natural community and allows for the continued existence of life in abundance. This use may have to be non-commercial (i.e., personal use), because corporate industry does not understand sustainability, and in some locations it may need to be non-consumptive use. In any case, through use, humans will value those habitats that support rare orchids (or whatever species we are seeking to conserve). However, it requires those who interact with natural communities to gain a greater understanding of the local ecology before they cooperate with that place. Humans must also be trained (or learn through mentorship with elders) to recognize the life they share the planet with and not just those species that are of interest commercially. In doing so, they will come to recognize that a landscape is composed of more than just the species of interest to them. People with natural history talent have a greater awareness and the potential to utilize more organisms from their area. From a seemingly selfish perspective, the more life we can recognize, the more organisms we are able to use for food, medicine, or utility. While this seems very self-serving, it is through wide and varied use that we come to understand the full value of natural places and ultimately rewild ourselves. Being barred from using natural areas forces people into a deeper dependency on modern technology. Much like when the !Kung hunter-gatherers were initially prohibited from hunting in the newly formed game preserve within their ancestral homeland, they were forced away from their relationship with the earth and into wage slavery. The conscientious use of wild beings in a fashion that is not motivated by profit establishes cooperative connections between humans and them, and these ties lead to understanding, collaboration, and empathy in emotionally healthy humans.

Let us not forget that some species of plants benefit from (i.e., require) frequent interaction to remain present at a given site. Let us use the example of common evening-primrose (*Oenothera biennis*). This is an early successional plant species that colonizes disturbed areas where the vegetation and leaf litter has been scraped or removed, exposing mineral soil where the seeds can germinate. Common evening-primrose is eventually lost (as growing plants) to a site as it becomes more densely vegetated, the leaf litter becomes deeper and covers the soil, and as taller species, like shrubs and trees, shade the site. Digging in the ground for the taproots of the first-year plants provides foragers with a high-quality root vegetable. It also disturbs the soil, exposing the mineral soil underneath the vegetation and duff, allowing the seeds to germinate and perpetuate the population. Essentially, the conscientious foraging, which leaves some plants to fruit and re-seed the site, disrupts the progression to a forest (for example), allowing the plant to continue living on the site. In this case, lethal collection of the plant (i.e., digging the taproots) actually keeps the species growing at the location (so long as the collection pressures are not so intense as to gather all the plants). This idea, that plant populations can actually benefit from harvesting that kills some individuals, is an example of how the commonly used method of preservation (i.e., a hands-off approach) is not a suitable way to protect all species from loss.

To conclude this section, I will present an important question that must be asked concerning our usual focus on protecting species: are we focusing on the wrong thing when we try to educate about and conserve life? Perhaps the individual animal (for example) is not what is most important but the connections it has to the rest of the world. We tend to focus on the animal (or plant or fungus) because it is the most apparent thing that can be seen, but that entity is just the connection point, the hub of interaction, and not the interaction itself. Much like in chemistry, we know that the end byproduct of chemical reaction is important, but chemists focus on the reactions (they understand that the process is of fundamental importance). Our identification, biology, and conservation measures focus on the result of connections (the noun), but don't seem to highlight the idea that it is the act of connecting (the verb) that must be maintained. For example, if we provide space for an insect pollinator but do not protect its interactions with preferred species of flowers (through eradicating all of the flowering plants it utilizes), the insect of interest will be eventually lost to that area. Perhaps we are seeing the obvious (the physical life form) and missing the process. Without connections, the lifeform (which is the point of connection) will ultimately end. In this way, the cooperative connections that exist between life on this planet must be maintained in order to conserve all life. We simply need to remember that humans must be considered in this discussion of ecology. They too must have cooperative connections or they cease to value the life they are disconnected from.

SUBMERGING INTO THE WILD MINDSET

Many wild animals live longer in a captive setting. While there are some exceptions (such as elephants), most animals provided with shelter, a constant supply of food and nutritional supplements, and protection from the wild interactions that might wound, maim, or kill them experience increases in longevity. And despite the greater life expectancy and longer lifespan, most people understand that wild animals held in a zoo setting do not live the lives they were biologically intended to. For example, a lion living in a relatively small enclosed area that is fed beef and poultry on a regular schedule is not experiencing what it means to be a lion. In other words, while it is still a lion, some of its "lion-ness" has been taken away from it by its captors. Almost everyone would agree that in spite of the easier life, a healthy lion would prefer to be in the wild, even though this involves living with risk and uncertainty. Wild lions experience many adversities, including hunger due to failed hunts, injuries from hooves and horns during chases, and sometimes fierce battles against other lions. Through these hardships—perhaps only because of the hardships—the animal fully lives the life of a lion only when in the wild.

But, for some reason, humans are seen differently. The greater life expectancy and increased longevity experienced in the modern world is used as rationale for why this version of living is better than that experienced by any previous people (especially wild humans). No matter what freedoms are taken away from us and how much we are forced to work for others, we live longer and that makes everything acceptable. We spend much more time laboring than indigenous people, often performing jobs that are deprived of fulfillment, ultimately experiencing a form of captivity that is without fences. Worse, our education makes it impossible for us to be wild because we have both forgotten how to live outside of our human zoos and have been convinced that being wild is a step backward. The chronic disease and frequent depression indicates very clearly we are not living as humans were biologically intended to. Could it be that we are unwilling to see that we are no longer fully human, that some of our "human-ness" has been taken away from us? Perhaps we traded a significant part of our sovereignty for a longer life, the same longer life that many zoo animals experience.

And so here we find ourselves, much like the domesticated crops in agricultural fields. During dry periods, the farmers must use precious water and energy to irrigate the crops to prevent them from drooping, wilting, and ultimately desiccating, even though the wild plants that grow in those same fields as weeds are still green and vigorous. (I've always wondered but never asked: do the farmers see that the wild species are more than just tolerating the dryness, but actually becoming more vital and resilient as a result of it?) Modern humans are much the same, requiring more resources to remain within an ever narrower range of living conditions so that they can experience a greater degree of comfort than the wild species they originated from. Is this really humanity's calling, to use industrial technology to create more and more luxury, so that we can be coddled throughout our lives (like the cultivated plants in the field)? Do we not see this ultimately creates weakness in *Homo sapiens*, or are we just unwilling to explore that question? Ultimately, individuals will need to decide what they want to be adapted to. The current path has allowed some wonderful human endeavors, such as arts and sciences. However, it is also one of relative inactivity, social media in lieu of actual community, climate-controlled environments, and pronounced nature deficit. Is this truly what you want for yourself (and your children)? Do you want to be adapted to your landscape or to the inside of a home?

Those who decide to embark on rewilding their lives will be embracing a holistic hormesis, one that touches their physical bodies, their emotions, their spirituality, and the very lens (the ego) that they view the world through. It is one that can be lonely at times, especially for those living in areas with limited contact with like-minded individuals. However, their time walking this path will benefit them with greater awareness, health, self-sufficiency, and sense of wholeness—even if they never reach the endpoint. For example, incorporating more wild foods into the diet that are prepared by traditional methods will bolster total nutrition in the diet, something of great benefit to the individual, even though the diet will still depend on cultivated foods to a large extent. Likewise, a lifetime of sitting in classrooms and wearing heeled shoes means that some changes have occurred to the body that cannot be totally undone. The shortened connective tissues of the lower leg mean that most modern humans cannot ever sit effortlessly in a flat-footed squat for extended periods of time like many hunter-gatherers—but our work on this position still benefits us and role models this to the next generation so that they do not lose physical ability as a result of domesticated living. Rewilding offers a peace that comes with both a heighted connection to nature and a greater ability to live within that setting that must be experienced to truly understand its value—it is similar to trying to describe dreaming to someone who has never dreamed. Further, and very importantly, this path ultimately leads to softer footsteps upon the earth.

As part of this movement, those who aspire to rewild will once again need to value place over space. To help illustrate this concept, we can use the forced relocation of the Ani-Yu^{n}wiya (Cherokee) from their ancestral homelands in the southeastern United States (Georgia) to areas west of the Mississippi River (Oklahoma). Following the discovery of gold in their ancestral lands, the indigenous people were moved against their will over 900 km (straight-line distance, they actually travelled over 1600 kilometers on their journey) to a landscape that would have been unfamiliar to them. This move to a new place along the Trail of Tears would have severely impacted their ability to live in a traditional manner because the natural communities and local ecology differed dramatically from where they had lived for generations. If you are still having a hard time understanding the value of place, let us use an analogy of a family that fishes by vessel in the Atlantic Ocean off the coast of Maine. This family fishes for lobster and shrimp, among other species, utilizing special kinds of traps that allow easy entrance but difficult egress. They have fished in the same location as their grandparents and great-grandparents (i.e., they have elders that can share ecological knowledge of their place). Then, along comes a government with its military strength that forces this family inland 900 km, to the Ohio River just inside the state of Ohio. Despite having fished for generations, the relocated family would have much less proficiency in the new space. Their elders would be of diminished value, and their ability to maintain their traditional lifeway would be highly compromised. This occurred because the government saw space as the important attribute, rather than place. The fictitious family was bound to place with their livelihood, a connection that was severed by the forced relocation. Rewilders will need to once again establish deep connection to place and develop true elders there. Without this depth of knowledge, reconnection to nature can proceed only so far.

Rewilding will require us to examine the very way we express ideas about creation. Many have never considered how the very language they use affects their worldview. Consider that the English language is not an indigenous language but rather a verbal system that began around the fifth century A.D. and was subsequently modified by later invasions. It is a language of agriculturalists and imperialists (i.e., it is a language of people who farm and conquer other races). It does not have embedded within it a systematic manner of referencing the landscape as does Peskotomuhkati-latuwewakon (Passamaquoddy Language) and other Eastern Abenaki dialects, which incorporate the land into many of their verbs of motion. In this way, one is constantly reminded of the place of focus. Using several samples from Peskotomuhkati-latuwewakon, one can observe the constant reference to place in the following verbs of walking: kisahqewse (s/he walks uphill); motapewse (s/he walks downhill); milawuhse (s/he walks out into water, into field, onto the ice); kcitawse (s/he walks far into it, like a forest or opening); and ksokawse (s/he walks across something, like a trail or stretch of forest). While these concepts can be presented in English, they are not a fundamental part of the system of expression. Such indigenous (i.e., hunter-gatherer) languages have been molded by a close association to their local landscape and incorporate important features of the environment into the language. In this case, they are also verb-based languages, and many aspects of the environment that English considers to be nouns are viewed as dynamic processes, like the wind and the rain, both of which are verbs in Peskotomuhkati-latuwewakon—wocawson (it blows) and komiwon (it rains). Thinking of the world in this manner makes it more difficult to extract portions of the environment for ownership or sale. We don't have to rely exclusively on indigenous language to understand how language changes the way we interact with our world. Consider the fact that gender-neutral languages are shown to have a greater equality in pay between men and women who perform the same job than languages that have evident gender distinctions (e.g., English, German, French). The case I'm making here is that the very language we speak can impact our belief in human dominion over the environment, equality between the sexes, and other important issues. Examining our language biases is one important step in the total process of rewilding.

It is sometimes presented that we have two worlds today—the modern technological world and the primitive natural world. Unfortunately viewing the earth in this manner has some repercussions. It can be frequently seen that some people who have dedicated significant time to rewilding practice a softer version of living with the world only when they are in nature. Once they arrive back in civilization (i.e., their home) after a camping trip of some length, they often return to the dominant mode of living, one highly influenced by consumerism and often without regard to what goes down the drain. The reality is this: **there is only one world, with two extremely different methods of interacting with her**. Thinking of our world in this way helps people realize that a return to civilization should not be used as justification for a return to an unhealthy manner of interaction. The above statement is clearly a false dichotomy because there are many ways of interacting with the world, the modern technological world and the primitive natural world are simply the endpoints on the spectrum. But this statement makes clear we are responsible for how we treat the planet regardless of the setting we are in. The fact is, it would be best if we incorporated as much of our ancestral lifeways and other eco-centered practices as possible into our daily living.

The rewilding path is one that most alive today, regardless of their enthusiasm and dedication, will not see the endpoint (not for the individual or community, and certainly not for society). But how do we gauge our progress? How will we know when we are approaching the endpoint? It is actually straightforward to measure our progress: when we and our immediate community are directly responsible for taking all the lives we require for our continued living. Humans must kill to live; this is a truth of our existence that we cannot escape. However, we do not need to kill excessively for unnecessary material gain and we do not need the death that occurs as a byproduct of industry (as a result of pollution, deforestation, water extraction, wetland draining, long-distance transportation, etc.). The less life that is taken on our behalf, both directly and indirectly, by people and machines in distant states and nations, the closer we will approach the end goal of rewilding. While some would declare that a plant-based diet accomplishes this goal, it can be clearly seen that growing plants in agricultural fields carved from natural communities, places that once supported wildlife, and shipping these foods across and between continents by polluting transportation manufactured through a process that levels mountains and fouls rivers, is not a real solution. It relies heavily on others to do the killing for us (and there is much unintentional death). It is a choice that simply maintains the current form of industry, which is a version of living that reinforces disconnection from nature. Once we recognize and accept that every human must kill to live, we can move forward with embracing the fact that it is best for humans to take lives for themselves directly from their local landscapes (or as close to them as possible). The entire essence of the rewilding movement, which is possible to describe in a variety of ways, can be simplified down to this fact. Engaging in the direct taking of life moves us closer to the least impactful living possible, epitomized by wild humans (the hunter-gatherers). We may never reach the goal of 100% accountability for our killing, but our progress on this path, the neoaboriginal path, will ultimately benefit all of life.

MALOM-OTE NSAPI-PUNOMON NÌT WIKHIKON

It is perhaps most fitting to conclude this book with a summary of what happens to hunter-gatherers when they are forced to adopt the prevailing agricultural and industrial lifeway. They gain access to caloric consistency, life-saving drugs, trauma medicine (including that which can be used to save mothers and neonates from birthing complications), electricity, fabricated goods, and wage income. However, they concurrently adopt a diet that provides less nutrition, lose part of their traditional medicine, begin to treat birth as a medical condition (even when there are no issues that require intervention), develop higher rates of obesity as a result of more work becoming automated and endocrine disruption, lose part of their traditional skills, and experience interrupted sharing networks. As a consequence of these results, they also begin to experience chronic disease, depression, cancer, and higher rates of addiction. Perhaps most important, some members of the community also experience poverty (a phenomenon unknown to hunter-gatherers with intact lifeways). None of this is to assert that hunter-gatherers should not gain access to industrial technology, but perhaps these outcomes, consistently seen in acculturated hunter-gatherer groups around the world, suggest that an industry separated from nature is not the best path forward for anyone involved.

Many would state that human rewilding is not a solution that can be adopted by large segments of society. Essentially, that it is a failed approach (from the start) to deal with our present dilemma. However, our current industrial paradigm is certainly a failed approach, and we are witnessing the multitude of problems that are becoming more apparent as we continue down this road. Only through a loss of awareness or intentional refusal to study the current state of the world can one believe this tactic will result in securing long-term health, happiness, and environmental sanctity. The fact is, the industrial lifeway is likely to result in substantial discord, meaning that a refusal to change our path will simply result in one being forced onto us. One way or another (i.e., by choice or by circumstance), humanity will need to rewild to some extent as civil strife, pollution, war, disease, population pressures, starvation, climate change, and other human-caused or human-exacerbated issues combine to interrupt the comforts and conveniences that people in financially affluent nations have come to expect. While many may interpret this message as gloom and doom, I intend it as one of hope—we still have the opportunity to change our worldview and manner of interacting with creation. If we rewild by choice, we incorporate practices that are documented to produce vitality and contentedness. If we rewild by circumstance, we develop a greater ability to adapt and survive. Either way, rewilding benefits humans. However, this will never happen until we address the domestication of our species.

Human wildness has been tamed through the process of domestication. Wildness is not a state of chaos. It is not disrespect for other beings. It is not selfishness that ignores beneficial customs. Nor is it a failure to cooperate with others. Wildness has been framed in these ways by civilization because it requires that people accept the loss of their sovereignty. It must glorify the present and disparage all aspects of the past in order that most people willingly spend the majority of their adult life working to support excessive resource exploitation (and never even question it). Tamed humans follow the appointed leaders even when those leaders commit to choices that will clearly produce unfavorable outcomes for the majority involved and those yet to be born. This new path is simply a restoration of human wildness. It is a path that can regain lost aspects of consciousness, strength, and connection. It can produce sovereign individuals who engage in the ecological connections found in their place. Rewilded humans can focus on healthful practices, instead of attempting to transcend their biology. Rather than merely trying to immerse in nature, *Homo sapiens* can again become part of the whole of nature—inseparable from the ecological fabric of place. Despite the dominant culture, the potential hardships, and difficulty in learning with so few elders, we must rewild to heal the separation that has occurred between humans and nature. It is the very rebirth of an eco-centered human spirit that is at stake. And as explained in the Seven Fires Prophecy, we must be fearless in our pursuit of wildness.

Nìt-te psìw. (the end)

Index

About the author

Greetings! My name is Arthur Haines and I've been helping people explore human ecology for over 20 years. I've done this with the mission of developing deep awareness of and connection to nature, promoting individual health, and fostering self-reliance. Wild food is a passion of mine, and through this, I offer a glimpse of our past and a new picture of our future. Numerous independent studies attest to the health benefits of wild plants that were consumed by indigenous people around the world. These foods are documented as both the most nutrient-dense plants available and having the greatest concentrations of beneficial phytochemicals, which offer protection against premature aging and insults to health. Wild plants offer a magnificent gateway to real food and wild living. Through this knowledge, and many other facets of our shared ancestral lifeways, we can awaken a rewilding of our body, mind, and heart.

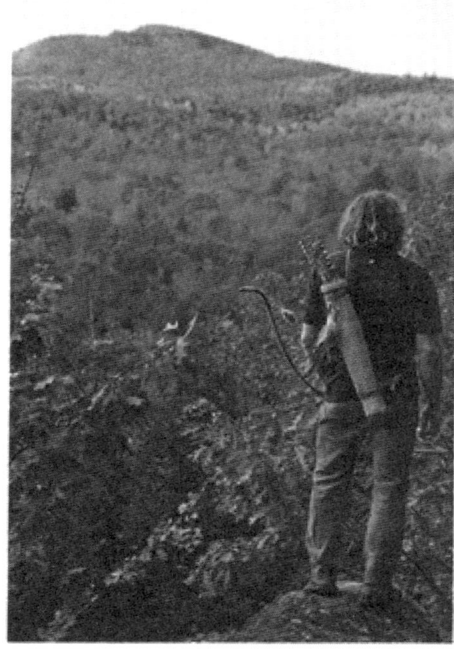

I believe we are at an important crossroads in our existence, one where domestication of the human species has led to an inability for most to nourish, heal, and care for themselves. This process has created profound blindness to the consequences of modern industry and the illnesses associated with nature disconnection. It is critically important to recognize that this point in history, where conversion of the remaining wild lands to intensively managed landscapes and urban areas, is where each person's unique inherited potential is becoming more difficult to achieve. That is, there is a diminishing opportunity to live up to our full genetic capability.

Despite this awareness, I remain positive and hopeful for my family, my students, and my extended community. It is the very skills I practice (i.e., the skills I live)—foraging, wildcrafting medicine, tracking, and many other aspects of wild living—that provide me with grounding and peacefulness in these times. These ancestral technologies provide a reliable means to attain health, become self-reliant, and disenthrall people from the wage slavery that suppresses their true selves. I propose that any solutions that are offered must come from the understanding that we are infused with seven million years of hominid history that has shaped our physical bodies, patterned our ways of thinking, and created nutritional, social, and spiritual needs that must be satisfied. Likewise, I consider nutrition to be of prime importance (i.e., a starting place) because the health of the physical body so strongly affects many other aspects of our living. This belief is reflected in my daily life through the gathering and consumption of wild foods (and sharing this bounty with guests).

My goal as a teacher and mentor is to share my experience and offer real solutions to individuals and families at all stages of life. Examining modern scientific research through the lens of historical evidence provides a unique perspective with which to filter the numerous and often conflicting studies that serve to confuse people and paralyze them with inaction. I endeavor to share knowledge garnered from this perspective, one that merges the material knowledge of present-day people with the ecological knowledge of ancestral people. I sincerely hope our paths cross, perhaps here in Maine at the ancestrally aligned community (Wilder Waters Community), and I offer best wishes to everyone seeking an alternative to the current paradigm of living.

Also from the author

Ancestral Plants: A Primitive Skills Guide to Important Edible, Medicinal, and Useful Plants of the Northeast is a two-volume set that details the human use of nearly 200 species of wild plants found in northeastern North America and beyond. This set differs from most foraging guides in that it is a more holistic resource for food, medicine, fibers, dyes, tools, adhesives, fire making, basketry, and more. Each volume begins with a different set of introductory chapters that discusses important aspects of useful plants, including identification terminology, instructions for making medicine, nutritional analyses of wild plants, and collecting protocols. Every plant species included in this set is given a thorough discussion that includes the distinguishing characteristics, ecology, when to collect various parts, and the food and/or medicine and/or utilitarian use that the plant offers to humans. A calendar of collection dates is also included in each volume to help aspiring foragers learn who is available on their landscape at different times of the growing season. These books are an excellent contribution to learning the ecology of one's place.

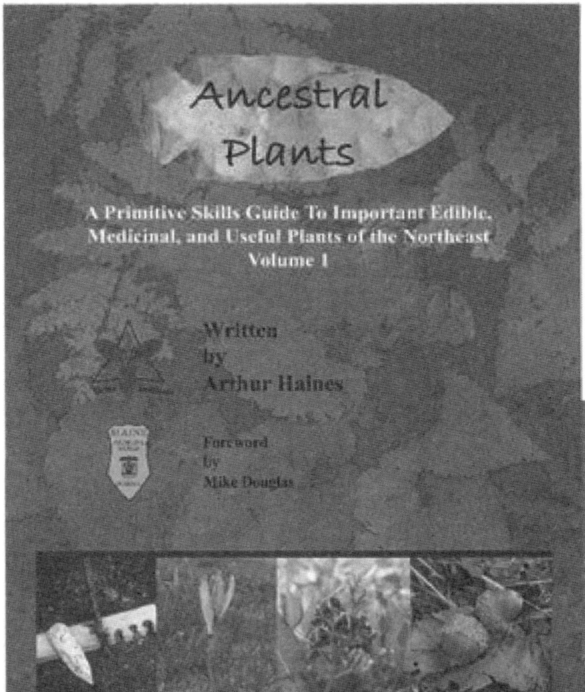

Volume 1 is 218 pages long and covers 94 species of plants. It includes a foreword by Michael Douglas (Maine Primitive Skills School) and can be ordered at http://www.arthurhaines.com/books/.

Volume 2 is 253 pages long and covers 104 species of plants. It includes a foreword by Daniel Vitalis (Surthrival, ReWild Yourself Podcast) and can be ordered at http://www.arthurhaines.com/books/.